Presbyopia

A SURGICAL TEXTBOOK

Presbyopia

A SURGICAL TEXTBOOK

Edited by

Amar Agarwal, MS, FRCS, FRCOphth

Dr. Agarwal's Group of Eye Hospitals
Chennai, India
Bangalore, India
Dubai, United Arab Emirates

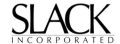

SLACK
INCORPORATED

an innovative information, education, and management company

6900 Grove Road • Thorofare, NJ 08086

Cover image used with permission from Refractec®, Inc, Irvine, Calif

The procedures and practices described in this book should be implemented in a manner consistent with the professional standards set for the circumstances that apply in each specific situation. Every effort has been made to confirm the accuracy of the information presented and to correctly relate generally accepted practices. The author, editor, and publisher cannot accept responsibility for errors or exclusions or for the outcome of the application of the material presented herein. There is no expressed or implied warranty of this book or information imparted by it.

Care has been taken to ensure that drug selection, dosages, and treatments are in accordance with currently accepted/recommended practice. Due to continuing research, changes in government policy and regulations, and various effects of drug reactions and interactions, it is recommended that the reader review all materials and literature provided for each drug use, especially those that are new or not frequently used.

Presbyopia : a surgical textbook / edited by Amar Agarwal.
    p. ; cm.
Includes bibliographical references and index.
  ISBN 1-55642-577-5 (hard cover : alk. paper)
  1. Presbyopia. 2. Presbyopia--Surgery.
  [DNLM: 1. Presbyopia--surgery. 2. Cornea--surgery. 3. Lens Implantation, Intraocular. 4. Sclera--surgery.
WW 300 P9265 2002] I. Agarwal, Amar.
  RE938.5 .P739 2002

2002003774

Printed in the United States of America.

Published by: SLACK Incorporated
                6900 Grove Road
                Thorofare, NJ 08086 USA
                Telephone: 856-848-1000
                Fax: 856-853-5991
                www.slackbooks.com

Contact SLACK Incorporated for more information about other books in this field or about the availability of our books from distributors outside the United States.

For permission to reprint material in another publication, contact SLACK Incorporated. Authorization to photocopy items for internal, personal, or academic use is granted by SLACK Incorporated provided that the appropriate fee is paid directly to Copyright Clearance Center. Prior to photocopying items, please contact the Copyright Clearance Center at 222 Rosewood Drive, Danvers, MA 01923 USA; phone: 978-750-8400; website: www.copyright.com; email: info@copyright.com.

Last digit is print number: 10 9 8 7 6 5 4 3 2 1

DEDICATION

To the doctors, staff, and patients of
Dr. Agarwal's Group of Eye Hospitals.

Contents

Section I. Presbyopia, Accommodation, Anatomy, Physiology, and Optics

Section II. Scleral Modifications to Correct Presbyopia

Section III. Corneal Modifications to Correct Presbyopia

Section IV. Lenticular Modifications to Correct Presbyopia

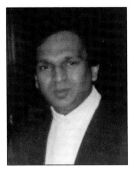

Amar Agarwal, MS, FRCS, FRCOphth is credited as the first surgeon in the world to perform no-anesthesia cataract surgery, phakonit (cataract removal through a 0.9-mm incision), and Favit, a new technique to remove dropped nuclei. He is a very dynamic speaker and has a double FRCS. His parents, Drs. Jaiveer and Tahira Agarwal; sister, Dr. Sunita Agarwal; wife, Dr. Athiya Agarwal; and brother-in-law, Pankaj Sondhi, help him in his goal of perfecting ophthalmological techniques. He practices at Dr. Agarwal's Eye Hospital in Chennai, India. Dr. Agarwal's Eye Hospital is the only one in the world shaped like an eye and has been included in "Ripley's Believe It or Not" series. The hospital's website is www.dragarwal.com.

CONTRIBUTING AUTHORS

Athiya Agarwal, MD, FRSH, DO
Dr. Agarwal's Group of Eye Hospitals
Chennai, India
Bangalore, India

Jaiveer Agarwal, FORCE, DO, FICS
Dr. Agarwal's Group of Eye Hospitals
Chennai, India
Bangalore, India

Sunita Agarwal, MS, FSVH, DO
Dr. Agarwal's Group of Eye Hospitals
Chennai, India
Bangalore, India

Tahira Agarwal, FORCE, DOMS, FICS
Dr. Agarwal's Group of Eye Hospitals
Chennai, India
Bangalore, India

David J. Apple, MD
Storm Eye Institute
Medical University of South Carolina
Charleston, SC

Guillermo Avalos, MD
Guadalajara, Jalisco
Mexico

Georges F. Baikoff, MD
Clinique Monticelli
Marseille, France

Brian S. Boxer Wachler, MD
Jules Stein Eye Institute
Los Angeles, Calif

Luis Alberto Carvalho, PhD
Institutó de Fisica de São Carlos
São Carlos, Brazil

Jarbas Caiado Castro, PhD
University of São Paulo
São Paulo, Brazil

Wallace Chamon, MD
Institutó de Fisica de São Carlos
São Carlos, Brazil

J. Stuart Cumming, MD
Anaheim Eye Medical Group Inc
Anaheim, Calif

Arthur Cummings, MB, ChB, MMed(Ophth), FCS(SA), FRCS(Ed)
Wellington Ophthalmic Laser Clinic
Dublin, Ireland

Kenneth Daniels, OD, FAAO
Pennsylvania College of Optometry
Philadelphia, Pa
Hopewell-Lambertville Eye Associates
Hopewell, NJ

Jonathan M. Davidorf, MD
Davidorf Eye Group
West Hills, Calif

Daniel S. Durrie, MD
Hunkeler Eye Center
Overland Park, Kan

Nora Emmons, RN
Zdenek Eye Institute
Reseda, Calif

Christopher J. Engelman, MD
Stanford University School of Medicine
Stanford, Calif

Gregg Feinerman, MD
Zdenek Eye Institute
Reseda, Calif

I. Howard Fine, MD
Oregon Eye Institute
Eugene, Ore

Hideharu Fukasaku, MD
Fukasaku Eye Center
Yokohama, Japan

Richard S. Hoffman, MD
Oregon Eye Institute
Eugene, Ore

Andrea M. Izak, MD
Storm Eye Institute
Medical University of South Carolina
Charleston, SC

William Jory, FRCS(C), FRCOphth
The London Centre for Refractive Surgery
London, England

Vivek Kadambi, MD
Bangalore Hospital
Bangalore, India

J.T. Lin, PhD
SurgiLight Inc
Orlando, Fla

Richard L. Lindstrom, MD
University of Minnesota
Minnesota Eye Consultants, PA
Minneapolis, Minn

Edward E. Manche, MD
Stanford University School of Medicine
Stanford, Calif

Odemir Martinez Bruno, PhD
University of São Paulo
São Paulo, Brazil

Richard L. Nepomuceno, MD
Jules Stein Eye Institute
Los Angeles, Calif

Mark Packer, MD
Oregon Eye Institute
Eugene, Ore

Venkatesan Palanivel, MS
Dr. Agarwal's Group of Eye Hospitals
Chennai, India
Bangalore, India

Ioannis Pallikaris, MD
University of Crete
Crete, Greece

Gregory J. Pamel, MD
Manhattan Eye, Ear and Throat Hospital
New York, NY

Suresh K. Pandey, MD
Storm Eye Institute
Medical University of South Carolina
Charleston, SC

Nishanth Patel, DipNB, DO
Dr. Agarwal's Group of Eye Hospitals
Chennai, India
Bangalore, India

Louis E. Probst, MD
TLC, The Laser Eye Centers
Windsor, Ontario, Canada

Ronald A. Schachar, MD, PhD
Presby Corp
Dallas, Tex

Paulo Schor, PhD, MD
Escola Paulista de Medicina
São Paulo, Brazil

Ariadna Silva, MD
Guadalajara, Jalisco
Mexico

Cristina Simón-Castellví, MD
Simón Eye Clinic
Barcelona, Spain

Guillermo Simón-Castellví, MD
Simón Eye Clinic
Barcelona, Spain

José Mª Simón-Castellví, MD
Simón Eye Clinic
Barcelona, Spain

Sara I. Simón-Castellví, MD
Simón Eye Clinic
Barcelona, Spain

José Mª Simón-Tor, MD
Simón Eye Clinic
Barcelona, Spain
Société Francophone d' Histoire de l'Ophtalmologie

Barrie D. Soloway, MD, FACS
The New York Eye and Ear Infirmary
New York, NY

Jaya Thakur, MD
Storm Eye Institute
Medical University of South Carolina
Charleston, SC

Luiz Antonio Vieira de Carvalho, PhD
State University of Maringá
Maringá, Brazil

Leonardo P. Werner, MD
Manhuaçu, Brazil

Liliana Werner, MD, PhD
Storm Eye Institute
Medical University of South Carolina
Charleston, SC

M. Edward Wilson, MD
Storm Eye Institute
Medical University of South Carolina
Charleston, SC

Anna Lisa T. Yu, MD
Jules Stein Eye Institute
Los Angeles, Calif

Gene W. Zdenek, MD
Zdenek Eye Institute
Reseda, Calif

FOREWORD

The surgical correction of presbyopia is an art that is currently in its earliest stages of development. This field is currently the domain of the ophthalmic surgeon innovator, much like intraocular lenses and refractive surgery for myopia in the 1950s to 1970s. Yet, success in the surgical correction of presbyopia will potentially impact a greater number of individuals than either of these two monumental innovations.

In the United States alone there are more than 100 million individuals with presbyopia. Worldwide, this number is over 2 billion. Every patient who undergoes cataract surgery with a monofocal intraocular lens is rendered presbyopic. Every individual who reaches the age of 45 also suffers some symptoms of presbyopia. The impact of a true restoration of accommodation on the quality of life of these individuals would be enormous. Clearly, this is an area that demands significant investment of intellectual and financial resources.

Fortunately, this investment of resources has begun in earnest. In their book *Presbyopia: A Surgical Textbook*, Dr. Agarwal and a strong faculty of basic and clinical science investigators bring us up-to-date on the current state of the art and science in this exciting field. The quality and scope of the book is superior, and the material is timely and useful to every ophthalmologist.

My personal goal at age 54 is to return to the vision I enjoyed at age 35: 20/12 at distance in each eye, J1+ at near in each eye, full stereopsis, normal motility, and a full field. It is the goal of the innovators in this book to bring me, and others with similar goals, that vision. I applaud their efforts and look forward to personally enjoying the fruits of their labors.

Richard L. Lindstrom, MD
Clinical Professor of Ophthalmology
University of Minnesota
Managing Partner
Minnesota Eye Consultants, P.A.
Minneapolis, Minn

PREFACE

Presbyopia, a bane for eyes in old age,
Like a bird that can fly but captured in a cage,
Along came the LASIK laser that can laze,
Lo and behold magically disappears the haze.

Have we really reached the final frontiers of presbyopic correction? Are the final answers yet to be found considering that the evolution of medicine as it relates to the homo sapien will continue to evolve to higher and higher levels? From the time that spectacles first came into being and Benjamin Franklin discovered the advantage of bifocal spectacles, aging and subsequent presbyopia have been studied in order to find solutions.

This book addresses another methodology for correcting reading difficulties encountered by those who are 40+ years of age. Of course we have bifocals and contact lenses with bifocal correction, but they are not the only technical advantages available today. Those of us who are approaching age 40 will need reading glasses and most would like some sure-fire technique to do away with the added power.

Taking the reader through various segments of the eye that can have an impact on presbyopic correction, this book addresses the surgical management of decreasing the tenacity of the zonular support by placing implants and scleral supports. This viewpoint takes into consideration that the zonules are overtly stretched, and if we are able to relax them then we should be able to correct presbyopia. There is also the advantage of corneal refraction, which plays a major role in today's changing scenario, especially with added effort from the LASIK laser, which seems to have minimized problems for the refractive surgeon. Many a surgeon and scientist have come up with their own theories and nomograms in treating the added power to read for near. Thus, in some format—either through concentric rings or eccentrically placed myopic corneas—the person with presbyopia seems to be able to improve near vision.

On the other hand, many cataract surgeons still vouch for the friendly and tested technique of monocular focus binocular vision. This means giving one eye a small myopic shift while keeping the other eye emmetropic. The intraocular lens power management effectively treats the problem of the patient having good vision for distance and near without the need for glasses and with the full advantage of fusion of images in the brain. We all know the human brain is far more powerful than the portion of it that is routinely used. In these circumstances binocular vision is obtained through techniques in which no-injection, no-stitch cataract surgery is utilized.

Many a quest still need to be conquered and many a battle in this arena won with the same diligence that we have been conquering other medical frontiers. It is imperative for us to understand the basic science of the formation of presbyopia. Some chapters give a leading thought process in this area, thus setting the stage for understanding the rest of the book. This book also offers food for thought to prompt ophthalmologists to focus their own energies on the treatment of presbyopia. *Presbyopia: A Surgical Textbook* includes chapters written by the best surgeons all over the world who provide their insights into the liberating field of spectacle-free living.

Amar Agarwal, MS, FRCS, FRCOphth

SECTION

I

Presbyopia, Accommodation, Anatomy, Physiology, and Optics

.

Chapter 1

The History of Presbyopia

José Mª Simón-Tor, MD; Guillermo Simón-Castellví, MD; Sara I. Simón-Castellví, MD; José Mª Simón-Castellví, MD; and Cristina Simón-Castellví, MD

Presbyopia (eye strain) is an eye condition in which, despite having practically normal distance vision (with or without optical correction), due to age-related factors the affected person is unable to see with clarity at short distances (ie, normal reading and writing distance [between 30 and 35 cm] or that distance which is common to certain tasks [sewing, etc]) (Figure 1).

Sturm (1697)[1] definitively established the name *presbyopia* for this physiological defect (from the Greek *présbys*, meaning "elderly"; and *óps*, *ópos*, meaning "eye"), which is the symptomatic and lexical opposite of myopia.

The French also call it *presbytie* (1793) and the person suffering from it a *presbyte*. The Spanish terms *presbicia* and *présbita* are derived from these words. In both languages these terms were used before presbyopia and continue to be the most widely used.

Although presbyopia is undoubtedly as old as humanity itself, the first known reference to eye strain is probably by Aristotle (384-322 BC),[2] who referred to the person suffering from it as *presbytes*, from which the relatively modern term presbyopia is derived.

Other ancient references to presbyopia can be found from the following Latin authors:

+ Cicero (Marcus Tulius Cicero, 106-43 BC)[3]
+ Cornelio Nepote (C. Cornelio Nepos, 24 BC)[3]
+ Suetonius (Caius Suetonius Tranquillus, 70 BC)[3]

Johannes Kepler (1611),[4] in addition to physicians of the period, assumed the existence of three classes of sight: short (good close vision), long (good distance vision), and natural (good distance and close vision), considering near-sightedness or the current term *myopia* and long-sightedness or today's presbyopia as two opposite conditions (Figure 2).

The first correct description of presbyopia was made by the Spaniard Benito Daça de Valdés[5] in 1623 (Figure 3). In Chapter V of Book I of his work *Uso de los Antojos (Para Todo Género de Vistas)** (*Use of Glasses [for all Classes of Sight]*), he described "strained or poor sight, which is that of the elderly," in clear, precise fashion. In Chapter IV he refers to the two defects or conditions that can be corrected with spectacles: the "lack of natural sight, which is that which affects the young" (myopia) and "the strained sight of the elderly" (presbyopia). Interestingly, at the end of

Chapter XI, Daça de Valdés mentions cases that correspond to what is now known as *hypermetropia*, although they are not described or separated into a different category of sight defects that are correctable with spectacles (Figure 4).

The history of presbyopia is closely linked to this history of ocular accommodation and glasses. Therefore, the historical highlights of these are described as follows.

THE HISTORY OF ACCOMMODATION

Accommodation is understood as the eye's ability to focus when the distance to the object being observed varies. The phenomena of accommodation is characterized by a triple pseudosynergy of movements (usually simultaneous but in special circumstances can act independently), which are:

1. Accommodative tension or accommodation itself
2. Ocular convergence
3. Pupillar contraction (accommodative miosis) or the Scheiner phenomenon[6]

For the purposes of this chapter, reference will only be made to accommodation itself.

Donders (1864)[7] believed that presbyopia was not a defect of refraction but of accommodation. Consequently, it was not to be classified with myopia and hypermetropia, but rather with accommodation alterations.

According to Villard,[81] accommodation does not seem to have interested ancient physicians in excess. The first to propose (in writing) the existence of an accommodative mechanism was the Italian monk Francesco Maurólico (Maurolycus or Maurolyci) (*Photismi de Lumine et Umbra*, Venice, 1575). Later, the German Johannes Kepler (*Dioptrice*, 1611)[4] and the Frenchman René Descartes or Cartesius (*Dioptrice*, 1637)[9] wrote on this optical mechanism.

Nevertheless, while Maurólico and Descartes** believed that ocular accommodation depended on modifications in the shape or curvature of the crystalline lens, Kepler explained it by a displacement of the crystalline lens, which would approach or distance itself

---

*Antojos: primitive name for what are now called *anteojos* in Spanish, or glasses.

**As the existence of the ciliary muscle was unknown, Descartes attributed modification of the crystalline lens to the action of its contractile fibers. For a long period, the lens was erroneously considered a muscular organ, the *musculus crystallinus* of Leuwenhoeck and Pemberton.

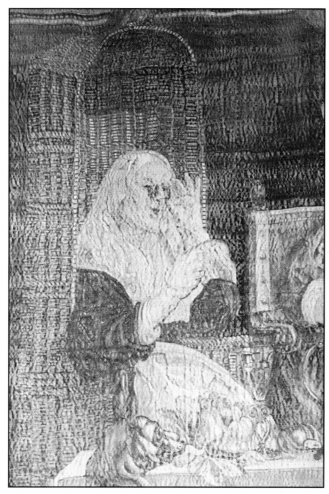

Figure 1. Old woman with presbyopic eye glasses (tapestry, Brussels, 17th century; Catedral de Tarragona, Spain).

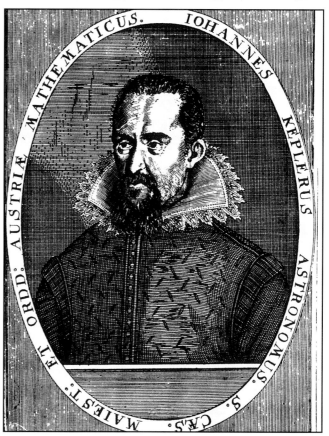

Figure 2. Johannes Kepler (Weilderstadt, Württemberg, 1571; Regensburg, Bavaria, 1630).

from the retina according to the necessary focus. Maurólico was the first to compare the crystalline lens with a convex lens. He believed it to be flatter in cases of presbyopia and more convex in myopia.

The existence and necessity for ocular accommodation was definitively shown by the classic experiment of the Jesuit Christoph Scheiner:[6] if two vertical pins placed one before the other are observed from the proper distance through two close-set orifices separated by a space shorter than the pupillar diameter, when one is looked at the other will be seen double.

Sturm (*Dissertatio de Presbyopia et Myopia*, 1697)[1] explained accommodation through his belief in possible modifications in the shape of the bulbus oculi due to the action of the abducens muscles.

William Porterfield (*A Treatise on the Eye*, 1759)[10] showed the existence of the accommodative phenomena with an experiment that was a simplification of Scheiner's. The Porterfield experiment showed that if two pins placed at different distances are observed directly (without the orificial screen), it is impossible to see them clearly, as when vision focuses on one, the other appears blurry.

THE 18TH CENTURY

In the 18th century, the Englishman Henry Pemberton[11] used the word accommodation for the first time to describe the eye's action and effect of adapting to varying distances, although he did not reach a proper or indisputable explanation of the accommodation mechanism. In keeping with its possible theoretical mechanisms, as of the 17th century other hypotheses were developed.

Pansier proposed the following six hypotheses:

1. The muscular or bulbus oculi change theory (theory of Sturm, Le Moine, Buffon, and Boerhaave),[1,12-14] which explained accommodation by the lengthening and shortening of the anteroposterior axis of the eye consecutive to compressions made on the bulbus oculi due to the total or partial contraction of the extraocular musculature. This explanation was derived from the primitive Kepler theory,[4] in which the retina would be able to distance itself and come closer to the lens reflexively.

2. The Scheiner, Plempius, and Porterfield[6,10,15] theory or that of crystalline lens displacement (withdrawal and propulsion) was powered, according to the common belief, by the ciliary body. The displacement theory also had some advocates in the next century. Ruete[16,17] still believed in it in 1846, without a shred of proof.

3. The Haller and Le Roy,[18-20] or iris movement, theory (the narrowing of the pupil would diminish the circles of diffusion for nearby objects).

4. The Home and Ramsden,[21] or change in cornea curvature, theory. This was conclusively and definitively refuted in the 1800s, first by Young,[22] with his well-known experience, and later by Cramer (1853)[23] and Helmholtz (1855)[24] through ophthalmometric measurements.

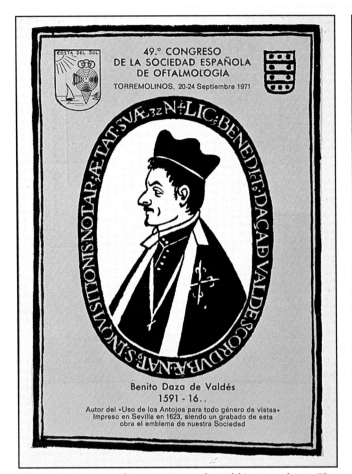

Figure 3. Portrait of Benito Daça de Valdés (woodcut). The author of *Uso de los Antojos* is seen in profile, with a cap, an inquisitorial cross around his neck, and a Santo Domingo cross on his cloak. In the upper righthand corner, the silver coat-of-arms of the House of Valdés, with three "azure fesses" and 10 "besantes" (coins) of "gules" (red).

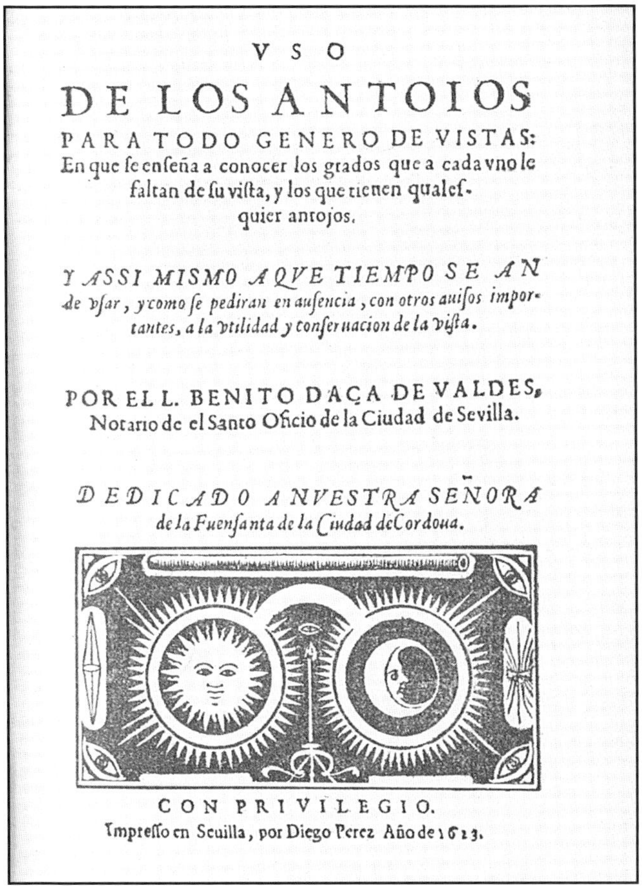

5. The Jurin theory[25] addressed a change in the crystalline lens shape (and curvature) due to the displacement of the Morgagni humour (liquid supposed to exist between the capsule and mass of the crystalline lens).

6. The Descartes, Pemberton, and Camper,[9,26,27] or the change in the crystalline lens curvature, theory. It was not demonstrated that this purely theoretical hypothesis was the one that came closest to reality until the 19th century.

19TH AND 20TH CENTURIES

Thanks to the experiments of Thomas Young (1801) and later expounded on by Helmholtz (1867),[28,29] the hypothesis that the power of accommodation depended on a change in the crystalline lens shape was no longer far-fetched.

Langenbeck (1849)[30] was the first to indicate, following a simple visual examination of the images reflected by the faces of the crystalline lens, that in accommodation for nearby objects the anterior face of the crystalline becomes more convex.

A proper microscopic examination of the reflected or catoptric

Figure 4. Front page of Daça de Valdés' book *Uso de los Antojos*, which apppeared in Seville, Spain in 1623. It is the first book on ophthalmic optics.

Purkinje-Sanson images (Figure 5), whose two posterior or retrocorneal images are formed, as shown by Meyer (1846),[31] on the faces of the crystalline lens, allowed Antoine Cramer (1851)[32] to deduce that during accommodation the anterior face of the crystalline lens becomes more convex and approaches the cornea.

Helmholtz (1853),[33] using the Purkinje-Sanson image procedure as well, confirmed Cramer's conclusions (Figure 6), showing that the posterior face of the crystalline lens was also modified, although it only became slightly more convex without approaching the cornea.***

Knapp (1860)[34] proved that the changes undergone by the crystalline lens in ocular accommodation sufficiently explained the range of accommodation.

Finally, Helmholtz observed that in aphakia in both the elderly and young, there is no real power of accommodation, thus definitively proving that this power depends exclusively on a change in the shape of the crystalline lens.

William Clay Wallace[35] showed that the modifier of the crystalline lens for accommodative focusing was the internal muscle of the eye. Cramer[32] believed that this muscle could be the iris itself. Helmholtz[24] correctly concluded (having been demonstrated in numerous experiments since then) that the active accommodation organ was the ciliary muscle,**** which transmitted its action to the crystalline lens through the zonule of Zinn.

***In 1851, Cramer used an instrument with a microscope he had created, which he called an *ophthalmoscope*, showing that accommodation came about from a change in the shape of the crystalline lens. Nonetheless, he asserted that the posterior face of the crystalline lens was not displaced or modified.

****This muscle, first described by Ernst Brücke[36] as the *choroid tensor muscle*, was later called the *ciliary muscle* by William Bowman,[37] which has proven to be the definitive name.

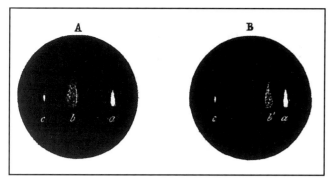

Figure 5. Purkinje-Sanson images. A: Relaxed or distance accommodation. B: Near accommodation. a: Corneal image (the brightest). b: Anterior lens image (moves nearer the cornea image and becomes smaller during accommodation since there is increased convexity of the anterior surface of the lens). c: Posterior lens image (inverted).

The idea that the ciliary processes or bodies could be active accommodation agents had already been supposed, although based on the wrong mechanisms, by Fick (1853) and Czermak (1854).[38]

In 1856, Heinrich Müller[39] and Rouget[40] independently discovered the existence of circular (in addition to longitudinal) fibers in the ciliary muscle that constitute a smooth muscular ring parallel to the edge of the crystalline lens (the Müller-Rouget muscle). This arrangement facilitates its action on the zonule.

THE YOUNG-HELMHOLTZ THEORY (1853)

In accommodation for nearby objects, the contraction of the ciliary muscle would provoke a relaxation of the zonular fibers and, consequently, a bulging of the crystalline lens because of its own elasticity (crystalline lens elasticity theory) (Figure 7).

THE TSCHERNING THEORY (1894)

According to the main author of this theory (Figure 8),[41] accommodation occurs due to the temporal formation of an anterior lenticonus. This phenomenon is possible because the superficial layer of the crystalline lens (the Tscherning accommodative layer) would have the ability to change its shape because of its consistency, like that of a thick rubbery solution.

Accommodative contraction of the pupil would eliminate the peripheral parts of the crystalline which, due to their flattening by zonule traction, would make the image too blurry.

The Tscherning theory differs from the Young-Helmholtz theory in these two basic events or phenomena: when the ciliary muscle contracts, the zonule—instead of relaxing—would tighten and the anterior face of the crystalline lens would suffer, not from a uniform increase in its curvature but from a central lenticonical increase (along with a flattening of its periphery).

The strongest opposition to this theory was given by Hess (1896)[42] when he agreed with Coccius (1867)[43] that in an eye subjected to intensive miotic action, it is easy to provoke a phakodonesis (tremor of the crystalline lens), which can only be explained by a strain of the zonule of Zinn.

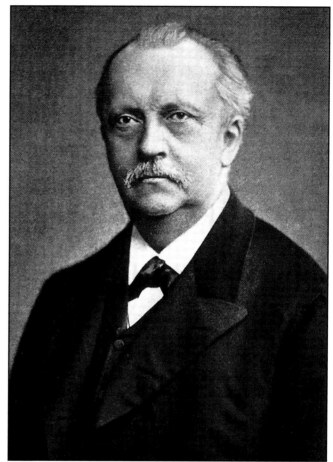

Figure 6. Hermann Ludwig Ferdinand von Helmholtz (1821-1894). German physicist, physiologist, and inventor of the ophthalmoscope. His theory of accommodation is the base of a large part of the modern idea of accommodation.

THE FINCHAM PLASTICITY THEORY (1924)

According to this theory,[44] the crystalline lens is a plastic organ lacking its own shape, as it is not elastic. Its shape would be imposed by the elasticity of the capsule (Figure 9) so that the bulging or deformation would be at a maximum in the thinnest parts of the capsule, mainly in the central anterior zone.

THE GULLSTRAND INTERNAL ACCOMMODATION THEORY (1911)

This theory[45] proposes that almost one-third of the total accommodation would be due to intracapsular mechanisms, by which the crystalline fibers would be incurved mainly in their central section and would slide toward each other, thus increasing the refractive index of the central or optic zone of the lens during accommodation. This internal accommodation would reinforce the external accommodation or that produced by the increased curvature of the crystalline lens' anterior face (Figure 10).

OPTIQUE PHYSIOLOGIQUE

PAR

H. HELMHOLTZ

Professeur de Physiologie à Heidelberg

TRADUITE

PAR

ÉMILE JAVAL ET N. TH. KLEIN

I

PARIS

VICTOR MASSON ET FILS

PLACE DE L'ÉCOLE-DE-MÉDECINE

MDCCCLXVII

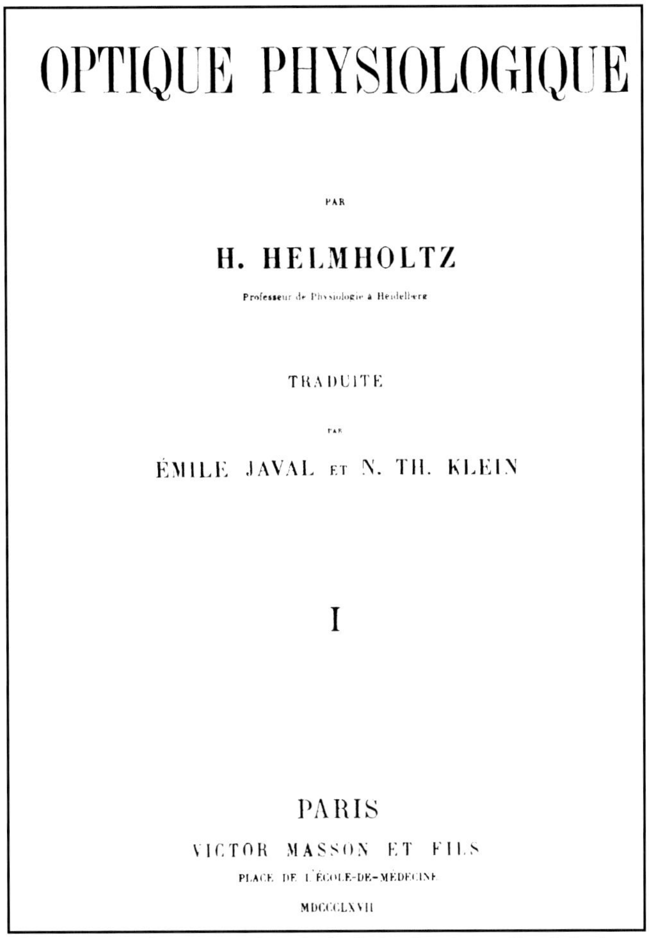

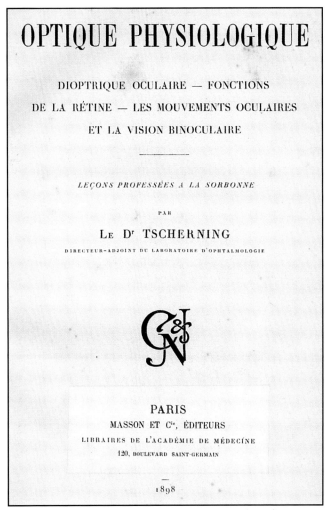

Figure 7. Title page of Helmholtz's *Optique Physiologique* (1867), French edition of *Handbuch der physiologischen Optik* translated by Émile Javal and Klein.

OPTIQUE PHYSIOLOGIQUE

DIOPTRIQUE OCULAIRE — FONCTIONS
DE LA RÉTINE — LES MOUVEMENTS OCULAIRES
ET LA VISION BINOCULAIRE

LEÇONS PROFESSÉES À LA SORBONNE

PAR

LE Dr TSCHERNING

DIRECTEUR-ADJOINT DU LABORATOIRE D'OPHTALMOLOGIE

PARIS

MASSON ET Cie, ÉDITEURS

LIBRAIRES DE L'ACADÉMIE DE MÉDECINE

120, BOULEVARD SAINT-GERMAIN

1898

Figure 8. Title page of Tscherning's *Optique Physiologique*.

Other Theories

There have been several other theories, but the following are the most worthy of mention:

- The Schön theory (1885):[46] zonular fiber duality theory
- The Pflugk theory (1906):[47] vitreous force theory
- The Henderson theory (1926):[48] anatomophysiological duality theory
- The Hudelo theory (1930):[49] muscular ciliary antagonism theory
- The Ronchi theory (1948):[50] hydrodynamic theory

Due to its supposed worth in the surgical treatment of presbyopia, there has been an upsurge in advocacy for the Schachar theory[51] for many years. Its analysis constitutes subject matter outside the scope of this chapter, as it should be dealt with from the physiopathological fundamentals of surgical correction.

Influence of Age on Accommodation

The changes undergone by accommodation and refraction of the eye due to the influence of age are represented in the classical Donders curve (Figure 11), corrected later by Duane (1912).[52] Even so, both curves have become purely historical mementos, as they do not show with sufficient precision the beginning of presbyopia in the emmetropic eye. Therefore, as David Michaels[53] correctly indicates, this initiation is actually presented at least 20 years before the time Donders stated and 10 years before that concluded by Duane.*****

Because presbyopia is an accommodative failure manifested in old age, the following statement by Duke-Elder[54] can be considered true: "In presbyopia the configuration of the structures of the eye, with the increase in size both of the lens and the ciliary body, lessens the effect of any pull by the zonule, while with the loss of elasticity in both the lens substance and the capsule, the balance between the two is upset and the lens retains its natural (unaccommodated) form."

Presbyopia and Hypermetropia (Hyperopia)

For centuries, although it seems impossible, hypermetropia and presbyopia were mistakenly believed to form part of the same anomalous ocular condition, which Christian Ruete (1845)[16] named *hyperpresbyopia*.

*****Donders claimed that diminished ocular refraction (presbyopia) did not decidedly manifest until 60 to 70 years of age.

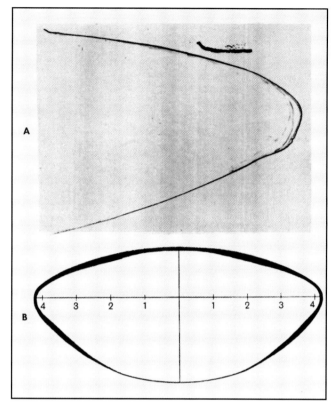

Figure 9. Diagram of regional differences of the human lens capsule (thickness magnified).

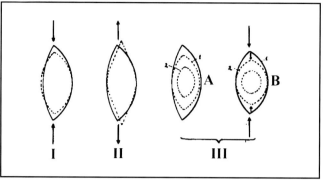

Figure 10. Accommodation according to Helmholtz (I), Tscherning (II), and Gullstrand (III). Dotted line: lens in accommodated state according to Márquez.

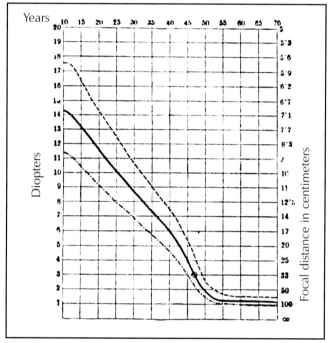

Figure 11. Classical curves of Donders and Duane showing the decrease in monocular accommodation amplitude related with age.

Karl Stellwag Von Carion[55] was the first to study the *punctum remotum* and the behavior of reading distance (*punctum proximum*) to hypothesize the existence of two different (though more or less subordinated, according to him) processes, *hyperpresbyopia* (the future *hypermetropia*, which he described quite accurately) and the so-called presbyopia.

Nevertheless, it was the Dutch physiologist Franciscus Cornelius Donders[56] and his disciple Mac Gillavry who, in 1858, definitively established that hypermetropia and presbyopia were two completely different ocular conditions. Thanks to his prestige, in 1859 Donders was able to discredit the word hyperpresbyopia and have hypermetropia accepted to describe the condition opposite myopia and different from presbyopia. Helmholtz (1859) proposed the word *hyperopia*, a synonym of hypermetropia that fell into disuse over time.

The presbyopia-hypermetropia confusion continued during part of the second half of the 19th century. Thus, Arthur Chevalier[57] (Figure 12) wrote in *Hygiène de la Vue* in 1862: "It is generally believed that presbyopia is exclusive to the elderly. Nevertheless, although it usually appears in elderly persons who, when young, had long sight (*vue longue*), it is also quite frequent in young people... When presbyopia is accentuated, it will be necessary to use lenses of a certain graduation to see nearby objects, and of another to see those that are distant."****** Chevalier also stated that high presbyopia is called hyperpresbyopia. Undoubtedly, in most cases, this is the result of the concomitant existence of the now well-known and correctly termed hypermetropia.

PRESBYOPIA TREATMENT: GLASSES

As described by the aforementioned authors (Figure 13), in ancient times elderly people with eye strain had to have a slave read for them. As can be imagined, before the invention of glasses, a great many useless eye drops were used in hopes of improving sight. Daça de Valdés,[5] in Chapter XI of Book I (*Why the Elderly Have Long But Not Near Sight* [translation]), states that deteriorated sight must be aided and reinforced with convex spectacles.

In Book II, Chapter X (*For Those With Deteriorated Sight to Be Able to Order Spectacles, in Absence* [translation]), he shows the reader how to calculate, based on age and gender, the degree of convexity needed in spectacles to correct what is now called presbyopia. It is interesting that the makeshift table for correction accord-

---

******The use of two different lenses (depending on the usual distances for viewing near and distant objects) was already suggested by Descartes in *Dioptrique*.

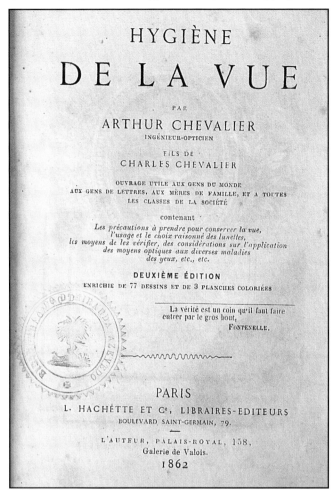

Figure 12. Title page of *Hygiène de la Vue*, by Arthur Chevalier.

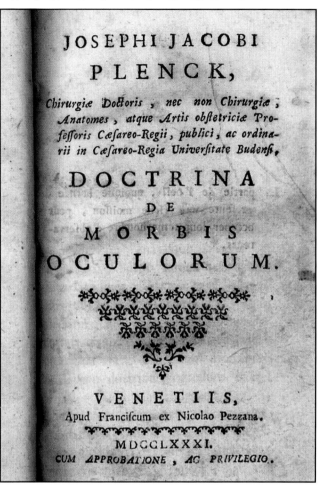

Figure 13. Josephi Jacobi Plenck, in *Doctrina de Morbis Oculorum* (1781), stated he only saw two refraction defects; although among nine varieties of presbyopia, he included one that he called *presbyopia senilis*. A previous edition of this book was published in Vienna, Austria by Rudolphum Graeffer, 1777.

ing to age begins with the age of 30 up to 40 years (2 degrees of convexity) and finishes with the age of 80 years and up (lenses of 5 or 6 degrees), which is an indication that within deteriorated vision other defects were included (mainly the then-unknown hypermetropia). He recommends spectacles with higher degrees for women (Figure 14).

CORRECTIVE LENSES

The primitive monofocal lenses were followed several centuries later by bifocal lenses (with double foci or correction), which combine the corrective lenses for near and long sight in a single block.

To avoid the discomfort of having to change glasses, Benjamin Franklin commissioned a pair of bifocals (1784),[58] which he brought into fashion, especially in aristocratic circles, during his stay in Paris as ambassador of the United States to the French Court.

The *Franklin lenses*, or primitive bifocals, consisted of two pieces of simple glass or semilenses properly joined at the edge by the arch of the frame. The upper part was for long sight and the lower corrected for near. They were separated by a centrally traced straight, horizontal line.

The need to improve their aesthetic appearance, in addition to solving their many and significant problems, soon led to the creation of new types of bifocal lenses, now substituted by trifocal or polyfocal (progressive) lenses.

THE ORIGIN OF GLASSES

It is not known who invented glasses. According to several historical documents, it seems certain that glasses first came into use in the region of Venice (Italy) at the end of the 13th century (around 1285).

The Venetian capitulations or regulations (*I Capitolari Veneziani*) from 1300 is the oldest document in which reference is made to the *roidi da ogli*, or lenses for the eyes. Therein, the first mention is also made of an augmentative lens for reading (*lapides ad legendum*).

In February 1305, the well-known Italian preacher Father Giordano da Rivalto gave a sermon in the Santa Maria Novella Church of Florence, in which he said, "Not even 20 years have passed since the invention of the art of making spectacles, which make one see well and which is one of the best and most necessary arts in the world, and it was invented a short time ago: a new art that had never existed. I knew the man who invented it, and I spoke with him."

In a fragment of the well-known *Chronicle of the Convent of San Catherine of Pisa (Pisan Chronicle)* from 1313, it is written that

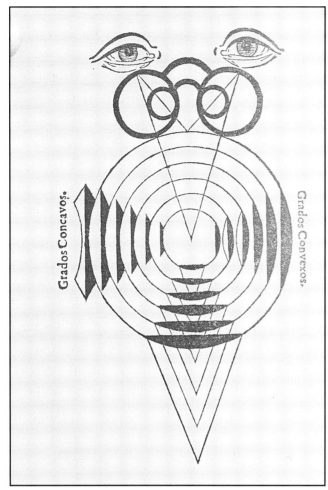

Figure 14. Depiction of the degrees of the concave and convex lenses according to Daça de Valdés. The difference in diameter between the largest (2 "varas" [approximately 1 yard] diameter) and smallest (small sphere of the size of the bulbus oculi) sphere is divided into 30 parts. Daça's degree would be approximately equivalent to 1.19 D.

"Father Alexander de Spina (Alessandro della Spina), a good and modest man, could do anything once he had seen it done. The spectacles (*ocularia*) made first by others who did not want to tell their secret, were made by him, and all were notified spontaneously and enthusiastically."

Thus, Father Alessandro della Spina, who died in 1313, receives the credit for having disseminated throughout Tuscany the procedure for manufacturing glasses, which he probably learned in Venice while in the Dominican convent of this city, today the Hospital Civil. Nonetheless, it should be noted that he was not the inventor.

For the sake of the history of ophthalmology, it is necessary to do away once and for all with fables and tales that are devoid of truthful foundation or based on an erroneous interpretation of passages of texts from past periods on the antiquity of ophthalmic lenses or glasses.

Some untrue tales include:
+ In Confucius' time (500 BC), true spectacles were already in use in China. This falsehood is so evident that the Chinese have never claimed to be the inventors of spectacles.

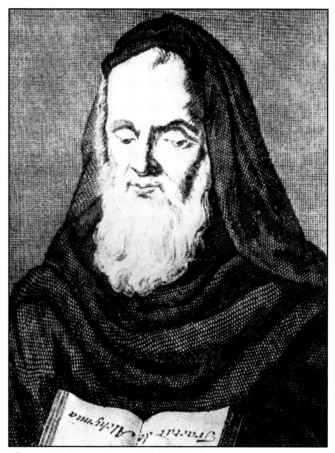

Figure 15. Roger Bacon (1214-1294).

+ The Roman emperor Nero (Claudius Caesar Nero, 54 to 68 AD) used an emerald to correct a supposed optical defect and be able to watch gladiator contests. Pliny (C. Plinius Secundus), called the Elder (23 to 70 AD), the renowned Roman naturalist who governed Spain, writes in his *Natural History* (Book XXXVII, Chapter V): "But their (emeralds) bodies, which are elongated in the same way as mirrors, present the images and shapes of things as if suspended. The Roman emperor Nero watched gladiator contests in an emerald." The only conclusion that can be drawn from this passage is that Nero watched indirectly through an emerald plate that served as a mirror, probably in order to avoid the glare from the sunlight reflected by the sand.

+ The English monk and philosopher Roger Bacon (1214-1294) invented spectacles (Figure 15). With regard to this theory, it must be borne in mind that:

Perspective (published in Frankfurt, 1614) was created and put in circulation 400 years after the death of Bacon, mainly by Molyneux, who based his work, as he admitted, on fragments of Bacon's writings translated from Latin and quoted by other authors, as he still had not been able to read the original Latin version of *Perspective,* later incorporated as Part 5 of Bacon's *Opus Majus*.

Molyneux's Thesis gained momentum when the publisher of the late first edition (1733) of Bacon's *Opus Majus*, Samuel Jebb, presented this work, stating that Bacon "described the

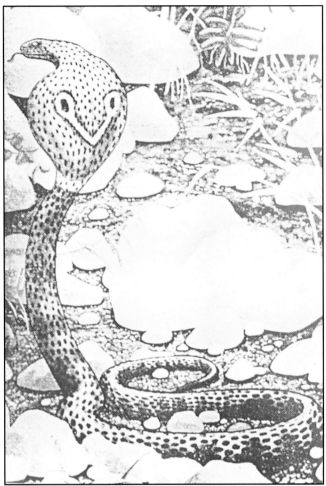

Figure 16. Indian snake (cobra de capello) or spectacled cobra (courtesy of A. Chigi's *Vita degli Animali*).

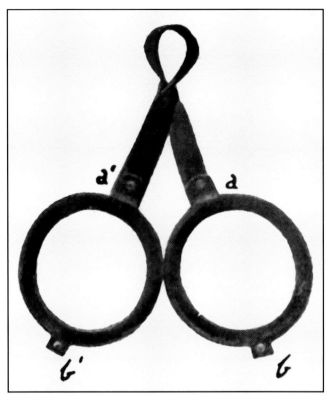

Figure 17. Spring eye glasses, 15th century (courtesy of Simón de Guilleuma).

use of spectacles and the correct manner of manufacturing them." This theory was masterfully refuted as early as 1738 by Robert Smith, who concluded that there was nothing to indicate that Bacon had invented spectacles, a claim later seconded by Montucla.

According to Rosen, although Bacon was not the true inventor of glasses, he was the first to acknowledge in writing the possibility of aiding presbyopes through an augmentation provided by a piece of glass. Further, it can be supposed that due to the period in which some of his texts were issued (1260-1268, during his lifetime), Bacon's work stimulated the creative imagination of the real inventor of glasses. Nevertheless, it is to be understood that this has always been and still is a mere supposition.

✦ Marco Polo, in his renowned book *The Travels of Marco Polo*, implied or referred to the existence of corrective glasses in China before the birth of Christ. After consulting several translations and editions, it is clear that in all of them Marco Polo refers to things that were new or strange to him, but in none does he mention spectacles, which would have undoubtedly caught his attention. The clumsy hypothesis that he could have inspired the joining of two monocles by the handles, thereby inventing glasses upon his return to Venice (in 1295, incidentally the period in which spectacles

were supposedly invented) is also inappropriate. Further, this is attributed to his story about having seen the feared spectacled cobra (*Naja tripudians* or *cobra de capello*, as it was called by the Portuguese) in India, which was trained by snake charmers and given that name in the 19th century because of the design on the cobra's neck, similar to a pair of spectacles that can be dilated by the snake at will when in the vertical position. This design becomes larger and more visible with movement (Figure 16).

The truth is that Marco Polo does not mention real snakes in his book. However, when seeing it for the first time, he does confuse a crocodile with a corpulent two-legged snake.

✦ It is also false that the first spectacles were brought from the Orient by Florentine merchants and the Florentine gentleman Salvino degli Armati, deceased in 1317, invented spectacles. This tale was definitively refuted over 80 years ago.

The first spectacles had metal rivets that came loose after a short period of use. They were followed by spring-loaded spectacles.

The first to mention the existence of spectacles with torsion springs (without metal brads) was Simón de Guilleuma,[59] who in 1922 discovered them in a late 15th century or early 16th century anonymous altarpiece (Museo de Bellas Artes, Barcelona) that depicts Saint Zacharias registering his son Saint John (Figures 17 and 18).

Until well into the 15th century, in which concave lenses for myopia appeared, spectacles (convex lenses) were only used for near sight, as is depicted by certain historical paintings.

Early evolution of spectacles can be depicted from the 14th century paper watermarks (Figures 19 and 20) and marking irons for horseshoes.

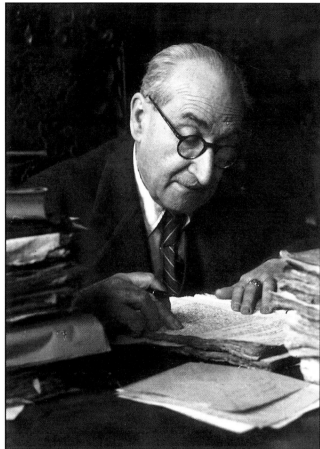

Figure 18. José María Simón de Guilleuma (Barcelona, 1886-1965), an ophthalmologist who was considered the greatest Spanish historian (and collector) of eye glasses. Unfortunately, his major work was only published in the Catalonian language. The photo shows Simón de Guilleuma working at the Archivo de la Corona de Aragón, Barcelona, in 1959.

Angulema or Besançon Miniature

At present, the oldest iconographic document of spectacles in the world is the *miniatura angumesina*, which can be found in the old psalter manuscript used by the Angulema diocese and was first admitted into the library of the Besançon (France) Capuchin Convent in 1776. Later, it was admitted to the municipal library of the same city, leading to its secondary name, *miniatura besontina* (Figure 21).

This psalter is made up of three parts from different periods. The second, copied toward the middle of the 14th century, begins with a mass for the dead, whose initial "D" is illuminated in the miniature. It depicts four clerics standing before a catafalque and singing from the book while laying on a lectern—the oldest of them is wearing spectacles with a fastening brad or rivet. This detail is quite visible. If the face wearing spectacles is observed closely, the main drawback of these (riveted) spectacles becomes apparent: they rest only on the nose, requiring large rims or frames to facilitate setting upon the cheeks and obliging the wearer to tilt his head back to lessen the tendency of the frames to slide down the dorsum of the nose.

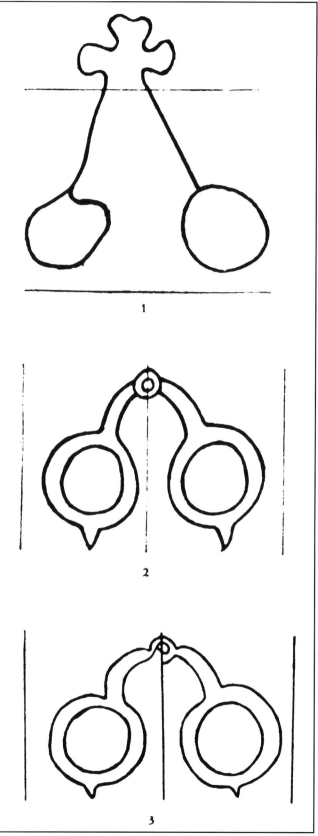

Figure 19. Early paper watermarks illustrating eye glasses (courtesy of Simón de Guilleuma).

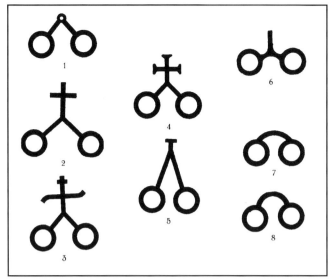

Figure 20. Early horseshoe marking irons depicting sequential types of eye glasses (courtesy of Simón de Guilleuma).

Treviso's Fresco

The first or oldest iconography (1352) of spectacles (riveted) in mural artwork (the second painting with spectacles to exist in the world) is a fresco painted by Tomaso (or Tomasso) da Modena (1325-1379). It depicts Father Hughes de Provenze, the first cardinal of the Dominicans. It can be found in the Chapterhouse of the Episcopal Seminar of Treviso (Venice Province, Italy), a prior monastery of Dominican monks (Figure 22).

The Use of Spectacles

In 1623, Benito Daça de Valdés,[8] who claimed not to know who the inventor of spectacles was, published the book entitled *Uso de los Antojos (Para Todo Género de Vistas) (Use of Glasses [for All Classes of Sight])* in Seville. It is the oldest known work that exclusively deals with the use of eyeglasses. A 17th century French manuscript translation of this work exists. It is in the National Library in Paris (Figure 23).

Despite the clear interest to keep up the Venetian monopoly on their manufacture, spectacles with convex lenses for reading (ie, for the correction of presbyopia) spread quickly through monks and monasteries and among the cultured, rich minority of Europe, first in Germany, where the glass manufacturing industry was quite advanced. We believe the theory of Murube del Castillo[60,61] to be correct: that the appearance of spectacles for presbyopia, as they prolonged the active professional life of many intellectuals and artisans, probably contributed to the scientific, artistic, and social explosion of the Renaissance.

REFERENCES

1. Sturm H. *Dissertatio de Presbyopia et Myopia.* Altdorfii; 1697.
2. Aristotle. *Problems.* Cambridge, Mass: Harvard University Press; 1957.
3. Pansier P. Histoire de l'ophtalmologie. In: *Encyclopédie Français d'Ophtalmologie.* Paris, France; 1903.
4. Kepler J. *Dioptrice, seu demonstratio eorum, quae visui et visibilibus propter conspicilla non ita pridem inventa accidunt.* Augsburg: Frank; 1611.
5. Daça de Valdés B. *Uso de los antojos.* Seville, Spain: Imp Diego Pérez; 1623.

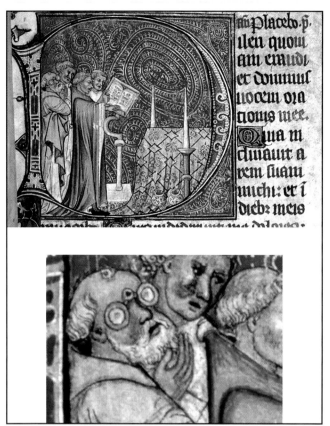

Figure 21. Earliest iconographic document depicting eye glasses (1340): Psalm book miniature (Psaulterium ad usum Engolismensis Dioecesis, Bibliothèque Municipale of Besançon, France).

6. Scheiner C. *Oculus, sive fundamentum opticum, in quo radius visualis eruitur, sive visionis in oculo sedes cernitur et anguli visorii ingenium reperitur.* Innsbruck, Austria: Danielem Agricolam; 1619.
7. Donders FC. *On the Anomalies of Accommodation and Refraction of the Eye.* London: New Sydenham Society; 1864.
8. Villard H. Histoire de l'ophtalmologie. In: de Bailliart et al, eds. *Traité d'Ophtalmologie.* Paris: Masson; 1939.
9. Descartes R. *Dioptrice.* Amsterdam, Netherlands: D. Elzevirium; 1637.
10. Porterfield W. *A Treatise on the Eye, The Manner and Phenomenon of Vision.* London: A Miller; 1759.
11. Pemberton H. *Dissertatio de facultate oculi qua ad diversas distantias se accomodat.* Batav, Netherlands; Lugdun: 1719.
12. Le Moine. *Quaestio an obliqui musculi retinam a crystallino removeant.* Paris, France; 1743.
13. Boerhaave H. *De morbis oculorum praelectiones publicae ex codicibus auditorum editae.* Gottingae, Germany: A. Vandenhoeck; 1708.
14. Boerhaave H. *Praekectiones academ.* Taurino, Italy; 1755.
15. Plempius. *Ophthalmographia.* III. Amsterdam, Netherlands; 1632.
16. Ruete CGT. *Lehrbuch der Ophthalmologie für Aerzte und Studirende.* Göttingen; 1845.
17. Ruete CGT. *Leerboek der Ophthalmologie* (trans: Donders). Utrecht/Amsterdam: Van der Post; 1846.
18. Haller AV. *Elementa Physiologiae Corporis Humani.* Lausanne, Switzerland: Marci-Michael Bousquet; 1763.
19. Le Roy. *Memoires de l'Acad. des Sciences.* Paris, France; 1755.
20. Le Roy. *Mémoire sur le mécanisme par lequel l'oeil s'accommode aux différentes distances des objets.* Paris, France; 1771.
21. Home E, Ramsden J. *Philos Transact RS.* 1796;82(2).
22. Young T. On the mechanism of the eye. *Philos Transact.* 1801;I(23).
23. Cramer A. *Het Accommodatievermogen der Oogen, Physiologist Toegelicht.* Haarlem, Netherlands: De Erven Loosjes; 1853.
24. Helmholtz H. Ueber die accommodatio des auges. *Graefe's Archiv für Ophthalmologie.* 1855;I(2):1.

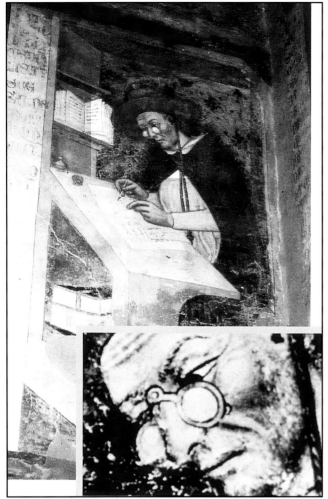

Figure 22. Riveted eye glasses in an Italian fresco (1352) (Cardinal Hugo of Provence by Tomaso da Modena, Seminary of S. Nicolò, Treviso, Venecia).

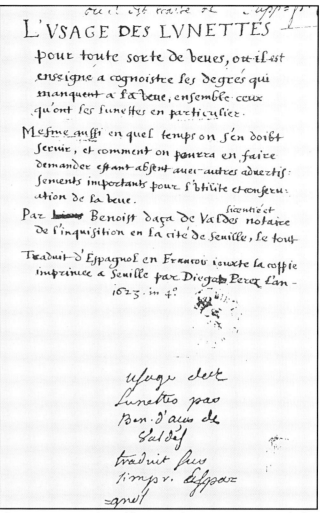

Figure 23. Daça de Valdés' French manuscript, *Uso de los Antojos* (1627, Bibliothèque Nationale, Paris).

25. Jurin J. *Essay on Distinct and Indistinct Vision*. Cambridge, UK: Smith's Optics; 1738.

26. Pemberton H. *Dissertatio de Facultate Oculi qua ad Diversas Distantias se Acomodat*. Batav, Netherlands: Lugdun; 1719.

27. Camper P. Disert. Physiol de quibusdam oculi partibus. *Lugduni Batavorum*. 1746;23.

28. Helmholtz H. *Optique Physiologique*. Paris, France: Victor Masson; 1867.

29. Helmholtz H. *Handbuch der physiologischen Optik*. Leipzig, Germany: Leop Voss; 1867.

30. Langenback M. *Klinische Beiträge aus dem Gebiete der Chirurgie und Ophthalmologie*. Göttingen; 1849.

31. Meyer H. *In Henle und Pfeuffers Zeitschrift für Rationelle Medicin*. 1846;V:262.

32. Cramer A. Mededeelingen uit het der ophthalmologie. Tijdschrift ned maatsch. *Tot Bevordering der Geneeskunst*. 1851;99:119.

33. Helmholtz H. Uber eine bisher unbekannte Veranderung am menschlichen Auge bei veranderter Akkommodation. *Monatsberichte d Akad zu Berlin*. Feb, 1853.

34. Knapp JH. Ueber die lage und krümmung der menschlichen krystalinse und den einflus ihrer veränderungen bei accommodation auf die dioptrik des auges. *Archiv für Ophthalm*. 1860;VI(2):1; VII(2):136.

35. Wallace WC. *The Structure of the Eye With Reference to Natural Theology*. New York: Wiley and Long; 1836.

36. Brücke E. Uber den musculus cramptonianus und den spannmuskel der chorioidea. *Müller's Arch*. 1846;370.

37. Bowman W. *Lectures Delivered on the London Royal Ophtalmic Hospital*. London: Moorfields; 1847.

38. Czermak JO. Akkommodationslinie. *Wiener Sitzungsber Akad Wissensch*. 1854;XII(322).

39. Müller H. Über einen ringförmigen muskel am ciliarkörper. *Arch für Ophthalmologie*. 1857;III:1; IV:2.

40. Rouget C. Recherches anatomiques et phisiologiques sur les appareils érectiles. Appareil de l'adaptation de l'oeil. *C R Soc de Biol*. 1856;113.

41. Tscherning. Étude sur le méchanisme de l'accommodation. *Arch De Phys*. 1894.

42. Hess C. Bemmerkungen zur akkommodationslehre. *Arch für Ophthalmologie*. 1896;XLVI:243.

43. Coccius A. *Über den Mechanismus der Akkomodation des menschlichen Auges*. Leipzig, Germany: Bergmann; 1867.

44. Fincham EF. The changes in the form of the crystalline lens in accommodation. *Trans Opt Soc*. 1924;26:239.

45. Gullstrand A. *Einführung in die Methoden der Dioptrik des Auges des Menschen*. Leipzig, Germany: Bergmann; 1911.

46. Schön W. Zur Ätiologie des glaucoms. *Arch für Ophthalmologie*. 1885;XXXI(4):1.

47. Pflugk AV. *Über die Akkommodation des Auges der Taube nebst Bemerkungen über die Akkommodation des Affen und des Menschen*. Wiesbaden, Germany: Bergmann; 1906.

48. Henderson T. The anatomy and physiology of accommodation in mammalia. *Trans Ophth Soc UK*. 1926;46:280.

49. Hudelo. Surl'accommodation. *Archivesd'Ophtalmologie*. 1930;fév:70.

50. Ronchi V. *Occhi e Ochiali*. Bologna, Italy: Zanichelli; 1948.
51. Schachar RA. Zonular function: a new hypothesis with clinical implications. *Ann Ophthalmol*. 1944;26:36.
52. Duane A. Normal values of the accommodation at all ages. *Trans Ophthalmol Am Med Assoc*. 1912;383.
53. Michaels DD. *Visual Optics and Refraction*. St Louis, Mo: Mosby; 1975.
54. Duke-Elder S. *System of Ophthalmology*. Vol V. London: Henry Kimpton; 1970.
55. Stellwag Von Carion K. *Die Ophthalmologie von naturwissenschaftlichen Standpuncte aus*. Erlangen; 1855.
56. Donders FC. Winke, betr. den Gebrauch un die Wahl der Brillen. *Arch für Ophth*. 1858;VI(1):62. 63.
57. Chevalier A. *Hygiène de la Vue*. 2nd ed. Paris, France: L Hachette; 1862.
58. Smyth AH. *The Writings of Benjamin Franklin*. New York: Macmillan; 1905.
59. Simón de Guilleuma JM². *Notes per a la Historia de les Ulleres*. Barcelona: Imp Badia; 1922.
60. Murube del Castillo J. Sobre el origen de los anteojos. *Studium Ophthal*. 1983;3(3):95.
61. Murube del Castillo J. Evolución y denominación de los anteojos en relación con el sistema de sujeción de su montura. *Studium Ophthal*. 1984;4(3):98.

BIBLIOGRAPHY

Albertotti G. *Lettere Intorno alla Invenzione degli Occhiali all'Onorevolissimo Senatore Isidoro del Lungo*. Rome: Ann D'ottalm E clin Ocul; 1922.

Bidault R. Deux miniatures du Moyen-âge intéressant l'Ophthalmologie. *Aesculape*. 1937;117.

Brücke E. Über den musculus cramptonianus und den spannmuskel der chorioidea. *Müller's Arch*. 1846;370.

Brücke E. *Anatomische Beschreibung des Menschlichen Augapfels*. Berlin: G Reimer; 1847.

Buffon GL. Histoire naturelle. Paris, III, 331, 1749.

Catalogue. *Géneral des manuscrits des Bibliothèques publiques de France*. Paris: Départements. Tome 32, Besançon; 1897.

Cortejoso L. La invención de las gafas. *Jano Medicina y Humanidades*. 1984;616:101.

Cotallo De Caceres JL, Hernandez-Benito E, Munoa JL, Leoz De La Fuente G. *Historia de la Oftalmología Española*. Madrid: LXIX Ponencia Soc Esp Oftalmol: 1993.

Chevalier C. *Manuel des Myopes et des Presbytes*. Paris; 1841.

Del Lotto E. *Dallo smeraldo di Nerone agli occhiali del Cadore*. Belluno: Tip Silvio Benetta; 1956.

Den Tonkelaar I, Henkes HE, Van Leersum GK. Antoine Cramer's explanation of accommodation. *Documenta Ophthalmologica*. 1990;74:87.

Donders FC. Beitrage zur kenntniss des refractions und accommodationsanomalien. *Arch Für Ophth*. 1861;VIII(2):185.

Donders FC. Reflexieproef van purkinje en sanson en accommodatie van het oog naar max. *Nederlandsch Lancet*. 1849-1850;132.

Donders FC. Cramers ontdekking van den grond des accommodatievermogens van het oog. *Nederlandsch Lancet*. 1851-1852;529.

Duane A. Anomalies of accommodation clinically considered. *Trans Am Ophthal Soc*. 1915;14:386.

Fincham EF. The mechanism of accomodation. *Brit J Ophth*. 1937;Supp 8:1.

Gil Del Rio E. *Fisiología de la Visión. Apéndice de Fisiología Aplicada del Ojo de Lyle*. Barcelona: Ed Toray; 1961.

Gilson M. Histoire des lunettes (lunettes et lorgnettes insolites). *Hist Sci Méd*. 1992;26(2):141.

Gilson M. Histoire des lunettes. *Bull Soc Belge Ophthalmol*. 1997;264:7.

Helmholtz H. *Beschreibung eines Augenspiegels zur Untersuchung der Netzhaut im lebenden Auge*. Berlin; 1851.

Hernandez-Benito E. Oftalmología española del siglo XVII. In: *Historia de la Oftalmología Española*. Madrid: LXIX Ponencia Soc Esp Oftalmol; 1993.

Janin J. *Mémoires et Observations sur l'Oeil*. Paris, France: PF Didot; 1772.

Le Grand Y. *Optique Physiologique*. 3rd ed. Paris: Masson; 1964.

Levene JR. *Clinical Refraction and Visual Science*. London: Butterworth; 1977.

Mac Gillavry. *Onderzoekingen over de Hoegrootheit der Accommodatie*. Utrecht; 1858.

Mackenzie W. *A Practical Treatise on the Diseases of the Eye*. London: Longman; 1854.

Marquez M. *Sobre la Invención de los Anteojos y Comentarios Acerca del Libro de Daza de Valdés' Uso de los Antojos*. Madrid: Imp Cosano; 1923.

Marquez M. *Lecciones de Oftalmología Clínica General*. Madrid: Tipog Blass; 1928.

Marquez M. *Lecciones de Oftalmología Clínica y Defectos de Refracción del Ojo*. 2nd ed. Madrid: Tipog Blass; 1934.

Murube Del Castillo J. ¿La lente o el lente? *Studium Ophthal (Barcelona)*. 1987;6(4):67.

Pansier P. *Histoire des Lunettes*. Paris: A Maloine; 1901.

Pansier P. Histoire de l'ophtalmologie. *En Encyclopédie Française d'Ophtalmologie*. 1903;I:1.

Simon-Tor JM². Esbozo de una historia de los lentes o anteojos. Conf magistral. V reunión grupo historia humanidades oftalmol. *Decisions Mediques*. 2000;(Suppl).

Stellwag Von Carion K. Die akkommodationsfehler des menslichen auges. *Wiener Sitzungsber. d. Akad. d. Wissensch*. 1855;XVI:187.

Stellwag Von Carion K. *Lehrbuch der Praktischen Augenheilkunde*. Vienna, Austria: W. Braumüller; 1861.

Wallace WC. *A Treatise on the Eye: Containing Discoveries of the Causes of Near and Far Sightedness*. New York: S Colman; 1839.

Wallace WC. *The Accommodation of the Eye to Distances*. New York; 1850.

Peacock G, ed. *Miscellaneous Works of the Late Thomas Young*. London: J. Murray; 1855.

Chapter 2

The Human Crystalline Lens, Ciliary Body, and Zonules

Their Relevance to Presbyopia

Suresh K. Pandey, MD; Jaya Thakur, MD; Liliana Werner, MD, PhD;
M. Edward Wilson, MD; Leonardo P. Werner, MD; Andrea M. Izak, MD; and David J. Apple, MD

PRESBYOPIA: SIGNIFICANCE AND ECONOMIC BURDEN

Presbyopia, literally meaning *old eye*, is the most common ocular affliction in the world. This is a condition of insufficient accommodative amplitude for clear near vision. Human accommodative amplitude progressively declines beginning in the second decade of life, or perhaps earlier, and is completely gone between the age of 50 to 55 years.[1-7] Presbyopia occurs as the near point of the eye recedes toward the far point so that small objects must be held farther from the eye to be clearly visualized. No individual appears exempt from this condition. However, high myopes who remove their spectacles may have their far point close enough to the eye to function satisfactorily.[8] While presbyopia is certainly not a blinding complication and it is correctable by various optical means such as bifocal or reading spectacles, its cost lies in the manufacture of the devices and in the lost productivity of the population, potentially totaling on the order of tens of billions of dollars annually in the United States alone.[9-15]

PRESBYOPIA VERSUS AGING OF THE CRYSTALLINE LENS

The human crystalline lens, together with ciliary zonules and ciliary muscles, are the important structures of accommodation in humans. The loss of the physiological function of accommodation that leads to presbyopia occurs as the human crystalline lens undergoes profound optical and physical changes with increasing age. These changes occur mostly after the age of 40 years. However, several experiments have suggested age-related changes in the human crystalline lens begin from birth and continue as aging progresses. The reasons for the occurrence of these anatomical and physiological changes are not clear, and it is also uncertain whether the changes may be a cause or a consequence of presbyopia. In brief, the changes associated with aging of the human crystalline lens include increased mass, increased thickness and hardness, increased posterior and anterior surface curvatures, and possible changes in refractive index distribution. Some of the other changes include loss of the ability to undergo accommodation, changes in spherical aberration, increase in shortest attainable focal length, and decreased ability of the capsule to mold the lens. It is important to consider these morphophysiological factors associated with the aging of the human crystalline lens, ciliary body, and zonular apparatus to achieve the long-term success of several surgical modalities aimed at restoring accommodation.

In this chapter we will focus on the anatomy and histology of the human crystalline lens, ciliary body, and zonules. A basic understanding of this anatomy is helpful in order to understand the morphological changes associated with aging of the crystalline lens, ciliary body, and zonules, which may be associated with presbyopia.

GROWTH OF THE HUMAN CRYSTALLINE LENS

The pediatric ocular structures, including the crystalline lens, are significantly smaller than in the adult, especially in the first 1 to 3 years of life.[16-18] The mean axial length of a newborn's eye is 17 mm, compared to 23 to 24 mm in an adult. The human crystalline lens grows throughout life by the deposition of new fibers. Figure 1 shows the growth of the human crystalline lens. The most rapid lens growth occurs from birth to 2 years of age. The mean diameter of the capsular bag is about 7.0 to 7.5 mm at birth, which increases to about 9.0 to 9.5 mm by the age of 2 years. Human crystalline lens growth is slower after the second decade. The lens does not increase much in size thereafter because of a relative loss of hydration and shrinkage of the lens nucleus, which offset some of the increase from new fiber deposition. Nuclear opacities (nuclear sclerosis) is the physiological change that occurs as the result of these changes in hydration and nuclear size. The lens nucleus may become sufficiently opaque to cause visual difficulties. Also, the lens capsule thickens with age and loses some of the inherent elasticity, which further decreases the capacity for accommodation, helping lead to presbyopia.

ANATOMY/HISTOLOGY OF THE HUMAN ADULT CRYSTALLINE LENS[19-21]

The adult crystalline lens measures approximately 9.6 ±0.4 mm in diameter with an approximate anterior-posterior diameter of 4.2 ±0.5 mm. The thickness of the lens decreases from the normal 4.5 mm to practically zero, whereas the equatorial circumference of the

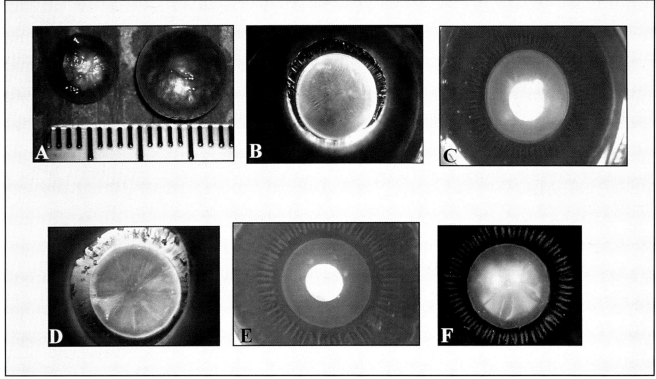

Figure 1. Growth of the human crystalline lens. A: Gross photo of a human crystalline lens taken from a 4-month-old child (left side). On the right, photo of a human crystalline lens from a 70-year-old adult. B: Gross photo of a pediatric human lens obtained postmortem, age 20 months, showing human crystalline, zonules, and ciliary body (anterior or surgeon's view). The diameter of human crystalline lens was 8.5 mm. C: Gross photo of a pediatric human lens obtained postmortem, age 20 months, showing human crystalline, zonules, and ciliary body (posterior view). D: Gross photo of a pediatric human eye obtained postmortem, age 3 years, showing crystalline lens zonules and ciliary body (anterior or surgeon's view). The diameter of human crystalline lens was 9.3 mm. E: Gross photo of a pediatric human eye obtained postmortem, age 3 years, showing crystalline lens zonules and ciliary body (posterior view). F: Gross photograph of an adult human eye obtained postmortem, age 60 years, showing crystalline lens, zonules, and ciliary body (posterior view). The diameter of human crystalline lens was 9.8 mm.

lens extends laterally, increasing from the normal diameter of 9.5 mm to a new diameter of approximately 10.5 mm. Figure 2 shows the empty capsular bag after removal of the crystalline lens. The diameter of ciliary sulcus is 11.1 ±0.5 mm according to studies performed at the Center for Research on Ocular Therapeutics and Biodevices, Storm Eye Institute, Charleston, SC. The anterior and posterior poles form the optical and geometrical axes of the lens. Although the normal lens is transparent and clear in vivo, it is seldom completely colorless; even in children, a slight yellowish tint is present and tends to intensify with age.

The crystalline lens is a unique transparent, biconvex intraocular structure that lies in the anterior segment of the eye, suspended radially at its equator by the zonular fibers and ciliary body between the iris and the vitreous body. Enclosed in an elastic capsule, the lens has no innervation or blood supply after fetal development. Its nourishment must be obtained from the surrounding aqueous and vitreous, and the same media must also remove metabolic waste products. Therefore, disturbances in circulation of these fluids or inflammatory processes in these chambers play a large role in the pathogenesis of lens abnormalities. The aqueous humor continuously flows from the ciliary body to the anterior chamber, bathing the anterior surface of the lens. Disturbances in permeability of the lens capsule and epithelium can occur, leading to the formation of cataracts. Posteriorly, the crystalline lens is supported by the vitreous (hyaloid) face and lies in a small depression called the *patellar fossa*. In younger eyes, the vitreous comes in contact with the posterior capsule in a circular area of thickened vitreous, the *ligamentum hyaloideocapsulare*. The potential space between the capsule and the circle of condensed vitreous is called *Berger's space*. The lateral border of the lens is the equator, formed from the joining of the anterior and posterior capsules, and is the site of insertion of the zonules.

The lens consists of three components: capsule, epithelium, and lens substance. The lens substance is a product of the continuous growth of the epithelium and consists of the cortex and nucleus. The transition between the cortex and nucleus is gradual. It does not reveal a concise line of demarcation when observed in histological sections. The lines of demarcation are often better visualized by slit-lamp microscopy.

LENS CAPSULE

The lens capsule is a basement membrane elaborated by the lens epithelium anteriorly and by superficial fibers posteriorly. By light microscopy, the lens capsule appears as a structureless, elastic membrane that completely surrounds the lens. It is a true periodic acid

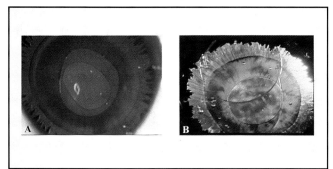

Figure 2. Gross photographs of pediatric and adult human eyes obtained postmortem showing the capsular bag, zonule shape, and status after phacoaspiration/phacoemulsification of the lens substance. Both photos were taken from an anterior (surgeon's) view; cornea and iris were excised to allow better visualization. A: Empty capsular bag of a pediatric (age 24 months) human eye obtained postmortem stained with 0.1% trypan blue. The diameter of the crystalline lens and empty capsular bag were 9.2 mm and 9.6 mm, respectively. The anterior and posterior capsulorrhexii are also visible. B: Empty capsular bag of an adult (age 44 years) human eye obtained postmortem stained with 0.5% indocyanine green dye. The diameter of human crystalline lens and empty capsular bag were 9.9 mm and 10.4 mm, respectively. Note that the zonules are stained in green and clearly visible.

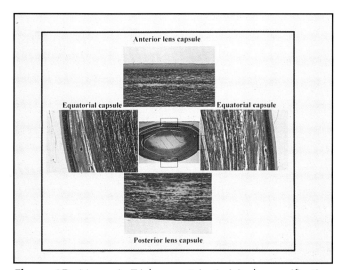

Figure 3B. Masson's Trichome stain (original magnification X100).

Schiff (PAS)-positive basement membrane, a secretory product of the lens epithelium. Figures 3A and 3B demonstrate histology of the anterior, equatorial, and posterior lens capsule using two different staining techniques. The capsule functions as a metabolic barrier and may play a role in lens shaping during accommodation. The lens capsule is of variable thickness in various zones. At its thickest regions, the lens capsule represents the thickest basement membrane in the body. The relative thickness of the anterior capsule compared with the much thinner posterior capsule may result from the fact that the former lies directly adjacent to and is actively secreted by the epithelium, whereas the lens epithelium is not present on the posterior surface. Local differences in capsular thickness

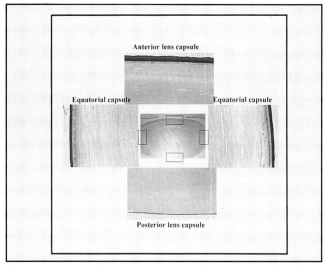

Figure 3A. Histological section of human crystalline lens showing anterior, equatorial, and posterior lens capsules. The section is stained with PAS stain, which imparts a brilliant red hue to the basement membranes. The anterior lens epithelium creates a basement membrane, which is thick anteriorly; it is the thickest basement membrane in the body (original magnification X100).

are important surgically, particularly because of the danger of tears or rupture of the thin posterior capsule during cataract surgery. Remnants of the tunica vasculosa lentis are common and appear as light gray opacities (Mittendorf dots) at or near the posterior pole. These opacities are rarely responsible for significant visual loss.

AGING OF THE HUMAN LENS CAPSULE

Human lenses undergo an age-dependent decrease in capsular elasticity with increasing age. These changes led to the suggestion that presbyopia is entirely attributable to changes in the lens, whereby the decreased molding pressure of the lens capsule fails to mold the increasingly resistant lens substance into an accommodated form. Some of the studies of the human lens capsule show an increased thickness up to age 75, followed by a decline thereafter. The human lens capsule becomes thicker, less extensible, and more brittle with aging. As accommodation is mediated by the capsule surrounding the lens, it is important to understand the relationship between the capsule and the lens. The general consensus is that the fully accommodated shape of the lens is achieved through elasticity of the capsule. These have been demonstrated by removing the capsule from isolated crystalline lenses. Measuring the profiles of lenses at different ages before and after removing the capsule is helpful in understanding how the capsule subserves accommodation. When younger, the human lens capsule ensures that the lens is in a maximally accommodated configuration, and any alteration in lens shape with decapsulation occurs to a lesser extent with increasing age. In the aged lenses of older individuals, removal of the capsule is without effect on lens shape.[22,23]

LENS EPITHELIAL CELLS

It is pertinent to discuss some details about the lens epithelial cells and their behavior after cataract surgery. Postoperative proliferation of these cells may lead to opacification of the posterior lens capsule, which in turn may contribute to failed accommodation after the use of accommodative intraocular lenses. The lens epithelium is confined to the anterior surface and the equatorial lens bow (Figure 4). It consists of a single row of cuboidal-cylindrical cells, which can biologically be divided into two different zones with two different types of cells:

1. *A-cells* are located in the anterior–central zone (corresponding to the central zone of the anterior lens capsule). They consist of relatively quiescent epithelial cells with minimal mitotic activity. When disturbed, they tend to remain in place and not migrate. However, in a variety of disorders (eg, inflammation, trauma), an anterior subcapsular epithelial plaque may form. The primary type of response of the anterior epithelial cells is to proliferate and form fibrous tissue by undergoing fibrous metaplasia.

   Recently, a new potential complication of A-cell proliferation has emerged in the field of refractive surgery. The anterior subcapsular opacities that have been described with various phakic posterior chamber (PC) intraocular lenses (IOLs) are based on A-cell proliferation. The fibrotic response of the anterior lens epithelium is what determines the degree of anterior capsular thickening following implantation of a phakic PC IOL in close proximity (or on) the anterior surface of the crystalline lens.

2. *E-cells* are located in the second zone as a continuation of the anterior lens epithelial cells around the equator, forming the equatorial lens bow with the germinal cells. These cells normally show mitotic capability, and new lens fibers are continuously produced at this site. Because cell production in this region is relatively active, the cells are rich in enzymes and have extensive protein metabolism. E-cells are responsible for the continuous formation of all cortical fibers, and they account for the continuous growth in size and weight of the lens throughout life. During lens enlargement, the location of older fibers becomes more central as new fibers are formed at the periphery.

   In pathologic states, the E-cells tend to migrate posteriorly along the posterior capsule. Instead of undergoing a fibrotic transformation, they tend to form large, balloon-like bladder cells (ie, Wedl cells). These are the cells that are clinically visible as "pearls." These equatorial cells are the primary source of classic secondary cataract, especially the pearl form of posterior capsule opacification (PCO). E-cells are responsible for the formation of a Soemmering's ring, which is a donut-shaped lesion composed of retained/regenerated lens cortex and cells that may form following any type of disruption of the anterior lens capsule. This lesion was initially described in connection with ocular trauma. It is the basic precursor of classic PCO. The E-cells have also been implicated in the pathogenesis of opacification between piggyback IOLs, also termed *interlenticular opacification*.

Lens Substance (Cortex and Nucleus)

The lens substance consists of the lens fibers themselves, which are derived from the equatorial lens epithelium. On cross-section, these cells are hexagonal and bound together by ground substance. After formation, the cellular nuclei of the lens fibers are present only temporarily. Subsequently, they disappear, leaving the lens center devoid of cell nuclei except in certain pathologic situations (eg, maternal rubella syndrome).

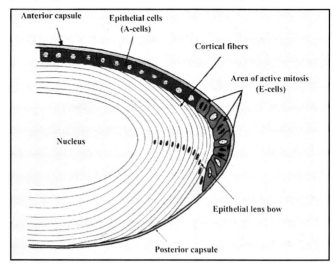

Figure 4. Schematic illustration of the microscopic anatomy of the lens, showing the "A" cells of the anterior epithelium and the "E" cells, the important germinal epithelial cells of the equatorial lens bow. These lens epithelial cells play a predominant role in the pathogenesis of various complications as postoperative opacification of the anterior and posterior capsules.

The original lens vesicle represents the primary embryonic nucleus; in later stages of gestation, the fetal nucleus encircles the embryonic nucleus. The various layers surrounding the fetal nucleus are designated according to stages of growth. The most peripherally located fibers, which underlie the lens capsule, form the lens cortex. The designation of *cortex* is actually an arbitrary term signifying a peripheral location within the lens, rather than specific fibers.

Aging of the Lens Substance (Nuclear Sclerosis)[24]

Classically, presbyopia has been attributed to increased sclerosis of the lens. The relationship between sclerosis and hardness is uncertain. Traditionally, the word *sclerosis* has been associated with decreased water content of the crystalline lens.[25-33] Although there is no consensus in the past literature about the extent to which the lens hardens, recent evidence has demonstrated more consistently that increased hardness of the crystalline lens occurs with age. Emery and Little[34] proposed a classification of lens nuclei depending on varying degree of hardness. Using postmortem human eyes, we have developed a model of inducing cataract of varying degree of hardness in a laboratory setting, shown in Figure 5.[8,35]

The crystalline lens in younger individuals is soft and offers little resistance to mechanical deformation, making it capable of large changes in optical power. On the other hand, crystalline lenses from increasingly aged globes show a reduced accommodative capacity and an exponentially increasing resistance to mechanical deformation. Although experimentally applied, compressive forces are very different from accommodative forces on the lens—they clearly demonstrate an increased hardness with age. This increase in hardness continues well beyond the age at which accommodation is lost and does not necessarily correlate with declining accommodative amplitude.

Mechanical compression and accommodation are profoundly different processes, but the end result (ie, loss of accommodation) is

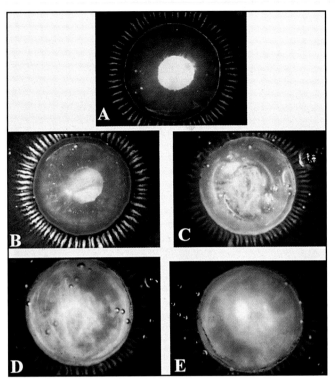

Figure 5. Aging of the lens substance (nuclear sclerosis). Emery and Little's classification was proposed for the hardness of nuclear cataract (varying from soft, semisoft, medium hard, hard, and rock-hard) in a clinical setting. Posterior view of a postmortem phakic human eye showing an experimental example of induction of different degrees of nuclear sclerotic cataract after injection of Karnovsky's solution in the lens substance. A: Posterior view from a 79-year-old male showing the crystalline lens. There is a grade 1 nuclear hardness (soft cataract according to the Emery-Little classification). B, C, D, and E: Same eye 5, 15, 20, and 30 minutes after the injection of Karnovsky's solution within the nucleus, with the creation of grades 2, 3, 4, and 5 nuclear hardness, respectively.

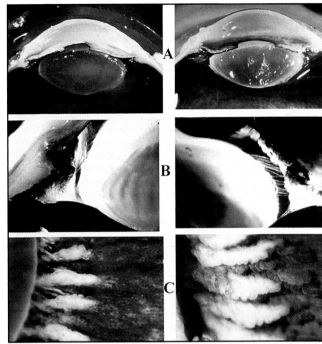

Figure 6. Parasagittal section of a phakic human eye obtained postmortem. Note the crystalline lens suspended by the ciliary zonules. A: Crystalline lens and zonules. B: Higher magnification of crystalline lens, ciliary body, and zonules from another case. C: Higher magnification of ciliary body and zonules from another case, posterior view.

certainly predictable from the degree of hardening of the lens. The continued increase in hardness suggests that the age at which the accommodation is lost may simply represent one point in time on a continuum that is reached when the capsule can no longer mold the hardened lens by use of the remaining ciliary muscle contraction. According to this theory, presbyopia is simply a consequence of the gradual age-change in lens hardness, the ultimate endpoint of which is advanced cataract near the end of one's life span. In this scenario, then, the question is no longer why humans develop presbyopia, but rather why the lens becomes hardened?

Changes in lenticular deformability could occur consequent to dehydration, the formation of various types of chemical or physical bonds between adjacent lens fibers, the hyperpolymerization of proteins, or myriad other events.[36,37] It is unknown whether these events happen causally or as a consequence of the development of presbyopia. Although lens hardening unequivocally occurs, the thesis that presbyopia is due to lens hardening, or loss of lenticular elasticity, is but one of many possible theories in the pathophysiology of presbyopia, each of which is supported by evidence. It is possible, for example, that lens hardening may occur as a consequence of

reduced accommodative effect on the lens, which is consequent to reduced ciliary muscle efficacy. Certainly, further study is required to ascertain the cause of presbyopia and whether the progression of presbyopia can be slowed, prevented, or reversed.

ANATOMY/HISTOLOGY OF THE HUMAN CILIARY MUSCLE AND CILIARY ZONULES

Figure 6 summarizes the anatomical relationship of the human crystalline lens, ciliary body, and zonules. The human ciliary body extends from the base of the iris to become continuous with the choroid at the ora serrata. On sagittal section, it appears as a right triangle with one side forming the lateral boundary of the posterior chamber. Two principal parts of the ciliary body include the pars plicata (corona ciliaris) and the pars plana (orbicularis ciliaris). The pars plicata forms the anterior 2 mm of the ciliary body and contains the ciliary processes. Because of the irregularity of the ciliary processes, the ordinary meridional sections of the eye reveal segments of several processes projecting into the posterior chamber. The orbicularis ciliaris (pars plana) is the posterior, flat part of the ciliary body measuring 4 to 4.5 mm in length. Posteriorly, the stroma of pars plana merges with the choroid, while the ciliary epithelium abruptly unites with the retina. The union presents a scalloped outline (the ora serrata), the convex projections of which are directed posteriorly. The serrations are more prominent and more numerous on the nasal side.

Histologically, the human ciliary body consists of seven layers (Figure 7):

1. The outermost lamina fusca or suprachoroidal tissue plane
2. The ciliary muscles
3. The layer of vessels
4. The basement membrane of the pigmented ciliary epithelium or external basement membrane, also known as the *lamina vitrea*
5. The pigmented ciliary epithelium
6. The nonpigmented ciliary epithelium
7. The basement membrane of the nonpigmented ciliary epithelium, or internal basement membrane

The lamina fusca or suprachoroidal tissue plane is a potential space between the sclera and the ciliary body. The ciliary muscle can be separated into three groups of fibers. The outermost, Brucke's muscle, forms the longitudinal portion that attaches anteriorly to the scleral spur and trabecular fibers. The innermost, Müller's muscle, forms the circular portion. The radial portion is formed by some of the anterior fibers of the longitudinal portion, which run obliquely to become continuous with the circular fibers. Posteriorly, the fibers end in branched stellate figures (muscle stars) in the suprachoroid at the equator and beyond. The major vascular circle of the iris lies in the ciliary body in front of the circular muscle. The connective tissue stroma of the ciliary muscle layer contains blood vessels, nerves, and melanocytes. In accommodation, contraction of the ciliary muscle lessens zonular tension on the crystalline lens, which allows the lens to assume a more spherical space, thereby increasing the diopter power of the eye.

The vessel layer of the ciliary muscle is a direct continuation from the vessel layer of the choroid. The stroma of this layer resembles that of the choroid but has fewer melanocytes and a denser connective tissue. Each ciliary process is a fold of connective tissue with a vascular core and is covered by two layers of epithelium. The posterior ciliary arteries traverse the suprachoroidal space to supply the major circle of the iris, from which branches pass to enter the ciliary processes.

Each process is supplied by a small arterial branch that breaks up into large capillaries, 20 to 30 μm in diameter, all of which are drained by a single vein. The walls of these capillaries are much more permeable than those elsewhere in the eye. Electron microscopy shows these capillaries have very thin walls that contain large pores. Occasionally, a ciliary process is continuous with the periphery of the iris.

Bruch's membrane splits at the ora serrata into an outer elastic layer and an inner cuticular layer, which are separated by a layer of avascular collagenous connective tissue. The elastic lamina gradually vanishes in the anterior part of the corona ciliaris, but the cuticular lamina reaches the iris root.

The epithelium consists of two layers of cells: the outer pigmented and the inner nonpigmented cell layers. In the adult, the two layers are firmly united at the ora serrata; thus, most separations of retinal layers stop at this site. In some instances, retinal separation extends into the pars plana and up to the ciliary processes. The innermost layer of the ciliary epithelium acquires pigment as it approaches the iris root.

The internal limiting membrane is a complicated meshwork that on electron microscopy is seen to contain homogenous material of low density. The membrane dips down to fill cleft-like spaces between adjacent epithelial cells. The zonular fibers of the lens are attached to this membrane and extend into the cells of the nonpig-

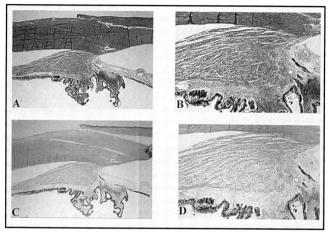

Figure 7. Histology of a normal ciliary body of the human eye showing corona ciliaris (pars plicata) and orbicularis ciliaris (pars plana). Pars plicata shows ciliary processes lined internally by the nonpigmented and pigmented ciliary epithelia, the vascular layer, and muscular layer composed of the circular, radial, and the longitudinal muscles. The longitudinal muscle inserts into the scleral spur. A, B: Masson's Trichome stain (original magnification X40, X100, respectively). C, D: PAS stain (original magnification X40, X100, respectively).

mented epithelium. The basement membrane of the pigmented ciliary epithelium is thicker and has a reticular pattern after removal of the epithelium.

Another important function of the ciliary body is the production of aqueous. The principal source of aqueous is the nonpigmented ciliary epithelium of the pars plicata. Production of vitreous mucopolysaccharide has been attributed to the nonpigmented ciliary epithelium of the pars plana.

The ciliary zonules consist essentially of a series of fibers passing from the ciliary body to the lens. They hold the lens in position and enable the ciliary muscle to act on the lens during accommodation. The lens and zonules form a diaphragm, which divide the eye into a smaller anterior portion and a larger posterior portion. The zonule forms a ring, which is roughly triangular in meridional section. The base of the triangle is concave and faces the equatorial edge of the lens.

AGING OF THE CILIARY MUSCLE AND ZONULES[38,39]

Main age-related changes in the ciliary body include the hyalinization of the ciliary processes and ciliary portions of the ciliary muscle. A nodular hyperplasia of the pigmented ciliary epithelium of the pars plana and of the pars plicata nonpigmented epithelium have been reported.

Concerning age-related changes in the zonules, the fetal and infantile zonular fibers are finer and less aggregated than in the adult. On the other hand, in the elderly, the zonular fibers are finer and more sparse, and they rupture more readily. The zonular attachments are narrow, especially in the first two decades of life. With aging, they broaden and move more centrally, both anteriorly and posteriorly.[40] The zonule-free zone of the anterior capsule reduces from 8 mm at age 20 years to 6.5 mm (or even as low as 5.5 mm) at about 80 years of age. During surgical intracapsular cataract extraction, most of the zonular complex is torn from the capsule.

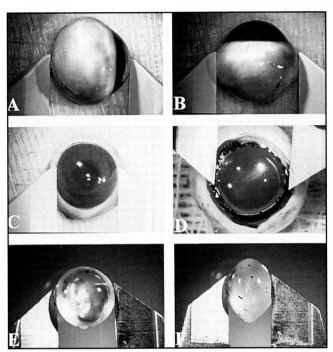

Figure 8. Ophthalmologists, researchers, and vision scientists commonly use the animal model for study of various types of implants (eg, IOLs, injection of silicone polymer in the capsular bag, etc). Rabbit is one of the commonly used animal models for evaluation of sizing, fitting of the new IOLs, and studying the postcataract surgery proliferation of the lens epithelial cells. A: Measurement of axial length of the eye. B: Measurement of equatorial diameter of the eye. C: Measurement of corneal diameter. D: Measurement of crystalline lens diameter. E, F: Measurement of crystalline lens thickness.

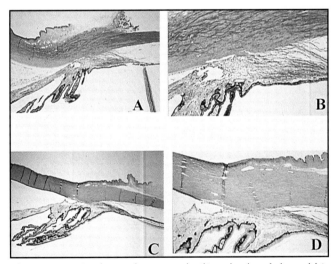

Figure 10. Histology of a normal ciliary body of the rabbit eye. The muscle layer is sparse or absent. The ciliary body is very poorly developed and comparatively flat due largely to the scarcity of muscle fibers. A, B: Masson's Trichome stain (original magnification X40, X100, respectively). C, D: PAS stain (original magnification X40, X100, respectively).

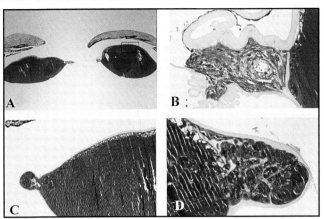

Figure 9. Rabbits have been commonly used for assessing the size and fit of the IOL in the capsular bag. These animals have also been used to study of posterior capsule opacification (PCO) and capsular bag fibrosis due to proliferation of lens epithelial cells (LECs). A: Photomicrograph from a rabbit capsular bag showing a massive Soemmering's ring formation in this model (Masson's Trichome, original magnification X20). B: Photomicrograph from a rabbit capsular bag showing anterior capsule fibrosis associated with Soemmering's ring formation (Masson's Trichome, original magnification X40). C, D: Photomicrograph from a rabbit capsular bag showing Soemmering's ring formation, residual cortical material (right and left sides of the capsular bag, Masson's Trichome, original magnification X100).

ANATOMY/HISTOLOGY OF THE RABBIT CRYSTALLINE LENS AND CILIARY BODY[41]

Researchers have attempted to inject a polymer lens into the capsular bag after phacoemulsification through a small capsulorrhexis in experimental animal models. Animals (eg, rabbits) have increasingly been used for experimental implantation and evaluation of recently manufactured IOLs. For the sake of comparison, we have provided a brief overview of the anatomy and histology of the rabbit crystalline lens and ciliary body (Figures 8 to 10).

RABBIT CRYSTALLINE LENS

The rabbit lens is a little larger than the human lens and is more spherical (see Figure 9). It, therefore, takes up relatively more space within the globe than does the human's. The rabbit lens weight has been assessed over a wide range, from 0.142 to 0.304 g in young rabbits and from 0.540 to 0.578 g in adult rabbits. The posterior surface curvature has a radius of 5.0 mm, while that of the anterior surface is 5.3 mm. It has an average anteroposterior dimension of 7.0 mm, and an equatorial diameter of 9 to 11 mm. Removal of the rabbit lens leaves the eye 10 diopters (D) hypermetropic. There are two single-line sutures, the anterior vertical suture and the posterior horizontal suture. The elastic lens capsule is thick anteriorly (varying from 10 to 25 μm without epithelium), with the maximum thickness a little closer to the equator than at the anterior pole. At the equator, it can be from 8 to 17.5 μm thick; and it thins gradually to a minimum thickness of 4 to 6 μm at the posterior pole. The lens nucleus is less sharply marked than that of the human lens, and the elongated lens cells are usually from 2 to 3 μm thick.

The anterior surface of the lens loses much of its curvature during the first 12 weeks of life, and there is even a slight continued flattening up to 80 weeks of age. The total flattening recorded is approximately 1.8 mm. Half of this flattening occurs during the first 13 weeks of life. A 0.6 mm deepening of the anterior chamber accompanies the lens flattening. After the first 20 weeks of life, the anterior chamber depth is relatively static at about 2.9 mm. Most of both these changes (ie, flattening and deepening) take place in the first 5 to 7 weeks; and over the entire growth span they synchronize with the corneal changes. As in humans, the nucleus of the rabbit lens scleroses with age and becomes hard and unresilient.

Rabbit Lens Capsule

The transparent elastic lens capsule, which is probably a secretory product of the epithelium beneath it, is like a basement membrane or Descemet's layer of the cornea. It appears to be structureless but with a faint suggestion of lamination. Rabbits have been commonly used for assessing the development of PCO and capsular bag fibrosis, as postcataract surgery proliferation of LECs is rapid in this model, as shown in Figure 9.

Rabbit Ciliary Body

The ciliary body is very poorly developed and comparatively flat due largely to the scarcity of muscle fibers. The circular fibers appear to be missing altogether and there are very few others, although there are many fine elastic fibers in the stromal tissue. The distance from the ora ciliaris retinae to the iris root is about 1.5 mm, and the ciliary body is only 0.3 mm thick at its thickest part. These findings support the repeated observations of negligible accommodative power in the rabbit. Figure 10 demonstrates the histopathology of the rabbit ciliary body. Some observers have separated the rabbit ciliary body into two parts: an iridic and a scleral portion, but there is no physical demarcation to show this unless one thinks of the posterior zone as scleral and the zone adjacent to the drainage angle as iridic. The few ciliary muscle fibers mentioned above are buried in dense connective tissue that contains fibroblasts and branching pigment cells. There are spindle-shaped smooth muscle fibers with oval nuclei, which are not as granular as in the cat and many primates. This is another detail that has been cited to account for the poor accommodative power of the rabbit. In animals having powerful accommodation, a large number of granules are present in these fibers. There is considerable pigmentation in the stroma of the ciliary body ordinarily, although in the white rabbit there is none and its structures are clearly visible.

Loss of Accommodative Ability of the Human Crystalline Lens

Excellent discussion has been provided concerning presbyopia versus age-related changes, changes in optical and biometric properties, and also about zones of discontinuity changes in refractive index distribution in the literature and in later chapters of this book.[1,42-54] We will briefly discuss the loss of accommodative ability of the human crystalline lens. Human lenses undergo an age-dependent increase in resistance to mechanical stretching forces applied through the ciliary body and zonule. Mechanical stretching experiments in conjunction with lens optical measurements have been performed to determine age-related changes in the accommodative performance of human lenses. These experiments take advantage of the fact that the young human lens becomes accommodated when zonular tension is released. Mechanical stretching then can be used to disaccommodate the lens to cause an increase in focal length. Young lenses undergo a 14 D decrease in focal power with stretching. With increasing age, the extent of the dioptric change following mechanical stretching is reduced such that lenses older than 60 years are unable to undergo any change in lens power with stretching. This age-related loss in ability of the human lens to accommodative optical changes very closely matches the age-related loss of accommodative amplitude. Cumulatively, this suggests that accommodation declines due at least in part to a gradual loss in the ability of the human lens to undergo optical change. The observation that lens accommodative change in thickness and diameter are both absent in presbyopes but that ciliary muscle function, although reduced, is still present also suggests that at its end point presbyopia involves the ability of the lens to undergo accommodative change within the remaining ciliary muscle contraction. This implies no causality for presbyopia, as each condition can be a consequence of the previous. But it does show that ultimately lens accommodation is completely lost even when some ciliary muscle function is still present.

Human Crystalline Lens and Surgical Restoration of Accommodation

Presbyopia may be caused by many different aging factors including changes in elasticity, thickness, and shape of the lens; efficiency of zonular tension; changes of properties in the ciliary body and scleral tissue, etc. Physiological changes, mechanism, and other details of presbyopia have extensively been discussed in the literature.[55-68] Consult Chapter 3 for physiology of presbyopia and accommodation. The existing techniques for the correction of presbyopia include scleral expansion band (SEB), sclera radial incision, and implantation of accommodative IOLs. Presbyopia patients may also be treated by a Ho:YAG or conductive keratoplasty for monovision correction. Laser presbyopia reversal (LAPR) using sclera ablation was also recently introduced.[69-73]

Scleral Expansion Surgery

Restoration of accommodation with the use of SEBs has been reported by several surgeons. However, this surgery for restoration of accommodation is not fully supported by recent experiments.[74] The SEB surgery is based on a different theory of accommodation that has been promulgated by Schachar and associates.[75-77] Interested readers should consult Section II of this book to learn more about principles and surgical details of SEB surgery.

Accommodative Intraocular Lenses

The stellar success and perfected results of modern small-incision cataract IOL surgery after phacoemulsification has provided motivation for cataract surgeons to restore accommodation. Several manufacturers, ophthalmologists, and vision research scientists are in the process of designing and evaluating accommodative IOLs for placement in the capsular bags of human and animal eyes to assess some degree of functional accommodation.[69,78] These approaches are based on replacing the presbyopic crystalline lens with an artificial IOL of fixed focal length that could, theoretically, be translated forward in the eye with an accommodative effort. One possible approach that has been explored experimentally in animals is injection of a polymer lens into the capsular bag through a small capsulorrhexis after phacoemulsification.[79] Some researchers have explored the surgical techniques required to inject a polymer into the capsular bag and the efficacy of this procedure to restore accommodation in monkeys.[80-87] Some of the currently available accommodative IOLs include the BioCom Fold IOL (Morcher, GmbH, Germany), Akkommodative 1CU (HumanOptics, Erlangen, Germany), and AT-45 IOL (C & C Vision, Aliso Viejo, Calif).

Despite an enormous effort by many investigators, many unanswered questions remain about the loss of accommodation with age. Also, restoration of normal accommodation with age in presbyopia or after cataract surgery remains just beyond the surgical technique available today. Ultimately, "the most common ocular affliction in the world," presbyopia, will be understood and cured. Much work remains but many are motivated to succeed. The frequency with which cataract surgery is performed in the growing population suggests that many more lenses of varying designs will be proposed as prosthetic devices to replace the human crystalline lens in an attempt to restore accommodation.

ACKNOWLEDGMENTS

The authors gratefully acknowledge the partial support of an unrestricted grant from Research to Prevent Blindness, Inc, New York, NY, and the editorial assistance of Luanna R. Bartholomew, PhD.

REFERENCES

1. Bito LZ, Miranda OC. Accommodation and presbyopia. In: Reinecke RD, ed. *Ophthalmology Annual*. New York, NY: Raven Press; 1989:103.
2. Cameron ME. Headaches in relation to the eyes. *Med J Aust*. 1976;1:292-4.
3. Coleman DJ, Fish SK. Presbyopia, accommodation, and the mature cataract. *Ophthalmology*. 2001;108:1544-51.
4. Coleman DJ. Unified model for accommodative mechanism. *Am J Ophthalmol*. 1970;69:1063-79.
5. Cook CA, Koretz JF, Pfahnl A, Hyun J, Kaufman PL. Aging of the human crystalline lens and anterior segment. *Vision Res*. 1994;4:2945-54.
6. Glasser A. On modeling the causes of presbyopia. *Vision Res*. 2001;41:3083-87.
7. Millodot M. The influence of age on the chromatic aberration of the eye. *Albrecht Von Graefes Arch Klin Exp Ophthalmol*. 1976;198:235-43.
8. Miyake K, Miyake C. Intraoperative posterior chamber lens haptic fixation in the human cadaver eye. *Ophthalmic Surgery*. 1985;16:230-6.
9. Weale R. Presbyopia toward the end of the 20th century. *Surv Ophthalmol*. 1989;34:15-30.
10. Weale R. Why does the human visual system age in the way it does? *Exp Eye Res*. 1995;60:49-55.
11. Weale RA. On potential causes of presbyopia. *Vision Res*. 1999;39:1263-72.
12. Weale RA. Human ocular aging and ambient temperature. *Br J Ophthalmol*. 1981;65:869-70.
13. Weale RA. The aging eye. *Sci Basis Med Annu Rev*. 1971;244-60.
14. Weale RA. The lens. In: Weale RA, ed. *The Aging Eye*. New York: Harper and Row;1963:69-102.
15. Weinstein MN. Accommodation reconsidered. *American Journal of Optometry and Archives of the American Academy of Optometry*. 1969;46:250-61.
16. Pandey SK, Wilson ME, Trivedi RH, et al. Pediatric cataract surgery and intraocular lens implantation: current techniques, complications and management. *Int Ophthalmol Clin*. 2001;41:175-96.
17. Wilson ME, Apple DJ, Bluestein EC, Wang XH. Intraocular lenses for pediatric implantation: biomaterials, designs and sizing. *J Cataract Refract Surg*. 1994;20:584-91.
18. Wilson ME, Pandey SK, Werner L, Ram J, Apple DJ. Pediatric cataract surgery: current techniques, complications and management. In: Agarwal S, Agarwal A, Sachdev MS, Mehta KR, Fine IH, Agarwal A, eds. *Phacoemulsification, Laser Cataract Surgery and Foldable IOLs*. New Delhi, India: Jaypee Brothers; 2000:369-388.
19. Vargas LG, Peng Q, Escobar-Gomez M, Apple DJ. Overview of modern foldable intraocular lenses and clinically relevant anatomy and histology of the crystalline lens. *Int Ophthalmol Clin*. 2001;41(3):1-15.
20. Werner L, Apple DJ, Pandey SK. Postoperative proliferation of anterior and equatorial lens epithelial cells: a comparison between various foldable IOL designs. In: Buratto L, Osher R, Masket S, eds. *Cataract Surgery in Complicated Cases*. Thorofare, NJ: SLACK Incorporated; 2000:399-417.
21. Werner L, Pandey SK, Escobar-Gomez M, et al. Anterior capsule opacification: a histopathological study comparing different IOL styles. *Ophthalmology*. 2000;107:463-471.
22. Abramson DH, Franzen LA, Coleman DJ. Pilocarpine in the presbyope. Demonstration of an effect on the anterior chamber and lens thickness. *Arch Ophthalmol*. 1973;89:100-2.
23. Adler-Grinberg D. Questioning our classical understanding of accommodation and presbyopia. *Am J Optom Physiol Opt*. 1986;63:571-80.
24. Roper KL. The aging lens. *Postgrad Med*. 1966;39:416-24.
25. Brown NP, Harris ML, Shun-Shin GA, et al. Is cortical spoke cataract due to lens fiber breaks? The relationship between fiber folds, fiber breaks, water-clefts and spoke cataract. *Eye*. 1993;7:672-9.
26. Fisher RF, Pettet BE. Presbyopia and the water content of the human crystalline lens. *J Physiol*. 1973;234:443-7.
27. Fisher RF. Presbyopia and the changes with age in the human crystalline lens. *J Physiol*. 1973;28:76.
28. Fisher RF. Proceedings: Some experimental studies of human accommodation and presbyopia. *Proc R Soc Med*. 1973;66:1037.
29. Fisher RF. The elastic constants of the human lens. *J Physiol*. 1971;212:147.
30. Fisher RF. The mechanics of accommodation in relation to presbyopia. *Eye*. 1988;2:646-9.
31. Fisher RF. The significance of the shape of the lens and capsular energy changes in accommodation. *J Physiol*. 1969;201:21-47.
32. Gilmartin B. The etiology of presbyopia: a summary of the role of lenticular and extralenticular structures. *Ophthalmic Physiol Opt*. 1995;15:431-7.
33. Nordmann J, Mack G. Nucleus of the human lens: III. Its separation, its hardness. *Ophthalmic Res*. 1974;6:216.
34. Emery JM, Little JH. *Phacoemulsification and Aspiration of Cataracts: Surgical Techniques, Complications, and Results*. St Louis, Mo: CV Mosby; 1979:45-8.
35. Pandey SK, Werner L, Escobar-Gomez M, et al. Creating cataracts of varying hardness to practice extracapsular cataract extraction and phacoemulsification. *J Cataract Refract Surg*. 2000;26:322-29.
36. Siebinga I, VrensenGF, De Mul FF, Greve J. Age-related changes in local water and protein content of human eye lenses measured by Raman microspectroscopy. *Exp Eye Res*. 1991;53 233-9.
37. Stevens MA, Bergmanson JP. Does sunlight cause premature aging of the crystalline lens? *J Am Optom Assoc*. 1989;60:660-3.
38. Strenk SA, Semmlow JL, Strenk LM, et al. Age-related changes in human ciliary muscle and the lens: a magnetic resonance imaging study. *Invest Ophthalmol Vis Sci*. 1999;40:1162-9.
39. Tamm S, Tamm E, Rohen JW. Age-related changes of the human ciliary muscle. A quantitative morphometric study. *Mech Aging Dev*. 1992;62:209-21.
40. Farnsworth PN, Shyne SE. Anterior zonular shifts with age. *Exp Eye Res*. 1979;28:291-7.
41. Prince JH, Eglitis I. The crystalline lens. In: Prince JH, ed. *The Rabbit in Eye Research*. Springfield, Ill: Charles C Thomas Publisher; 1964:342-51.
42. Beers AP, Van Der Heijde GL. In vivo determination of the bio-

mechanical properties of the component elements of the accommodation mechanism. *Vision Res.* 1994;34:2897-905.

43. Beers AP, Van der Heijde GL. Presbyopia and velocity of sound in the lens. *Optom Vis Sci.* 1994;71:250-3.

44. Blake J, Horgan T, Carroll P, et al. Effect of accommodation of the lens on ocular pressure. *Journal of Medicine and Science.* 1995;164:269-70.

45. Bron AJ, Vrensen GF, Koretz J, et al. The aging lens. *Ophthalmologica.* 2000;214:86-104.

46. Brown N. The change in lens curvature with age. *Exp Eye Res.* 1974;19:175

47. Glasser A, Campbell MC. Biometric, optical and physical changes in the isolated human crystalline lens with age in relation to presbyopia. *Vision Res.* 1999;39:1991-2015.

48. Glasser A, Campbell MC. Presbyopia and the optical changes in the human crystalline lens with age. *Vision Res.* 1998;38:209-29.

49. Glasser A, Croft MA, Kaufman P. Aging of the human crystalline lens and presbyopia. *Int Ophthalmol Clin.* 2001;41:1-15.

50. Glasser A, Kaufman PL. The mechanism of accommodation in primates. *Ophthalmology.* 1999;106:863-72.

51. Moffat BA, Landman KA, Truscott RJ, et al. Age-related changes in the kinetics of water transport in normal human lenses. *Exp Eye Res.* 1999;69:663-9.

52. Tester R, Pace NL, Samore M, Olson RJ. Dysphotopsia in phakic and pseudophakic patients: incidence and relation to intraocular type. *J Cataract Refract Surg.* 2000;26:810-6.

53. Willenkens B, Kappelhof J, Vrensen GF. Morphology of the aging human lens: I. biomicroscopy and biometrics. *Lens Research.* 1987;4:207.

54. Bron AJ, Vrensen GF, Koretz J, et al. The aging lens. *Ophthalmologica.* 2000;214:86-104.

55. Hodos W, Miller RF, Fite KV. Age-dependent changes in visual acuity and retinal morphology in pigeons. *Vision Res.* 1991;31:669-77.

56. Jungschaffer DA, Saber E, Zimmerman KM, et al. Refractive changes induced by electrocautery of the rabbit anterior lens capsule. *J Cataract Refract Surg.* 1994;20:132-7.

57. Koretz JF, Cook CA, Kaufman PL. Accommodation and presbyopia in the human eye. Changes in the anterior segment and crystalline lens with focus. *Invest Ophthalmol Vis Sci.* 1997;38:569-78.

58. Koretz JF, Handelman GH, Brown NP. Analysis of human crystalline lens curvature as a function of accommodative state and age. *Vision Res.* 1984;24:1141-51.

59. Koretz JF, Kaufman PL, Neider MW, Goeckner PA. Accommodation and presbyopia in the human eye—aging of the anterior segment. *Vision Res.* 1989;29:1685-92.

60. Koretz JF, Cook CA, Kuszak JR. The zone of discontinuity in the human lens: development and distribution with age. *Vision Res.* 1994;34:2955.

61. Koretz JF, Handelman GH. How the human eye focuses. *Sci Am.* 1988;92-99.

62. Krag S, Olsen T, Andreassen TT. Biomechanical characteristics of the human anterior lens capsule in relation to age. *Invest Ophthalmol Vis Sci.* 1997;38:357-63.

63. Kuszak JR, Sivak JG, Weerheim JA. Lens optical quality is a direct function of lens sutural architecture. *Invest Ophthalmol Vis Sci.* 1991;32:2119-29.

64. Lerman S, Kuck JF Jr, Borkman R, Saker E. Acceleration of an aging parameter (fluorogen) in the ocular lens. *Annals of Ophthalmology.* 1976;8:558-61.

65. Pointer JS. The presbyopic add. II. Age-related trend and a gender difference. *Ophthalmic Physiol Opt.* 1995;15:241-8.

66. Saka Y, Hara T, Yamada Y, Hayashi F. Accommodations in primate eyes after implantation of refilled endocapsular balloon. *Am J Ophthalmol.* 1996;121:210-2.

67. Saladin JJ, Stark L. Presbyopia: new evidence from impedance cyclography supporting the Hess-Gullstrand theory. *Vision Res.* 1975;15:537-41.

68. Scammon R, Hesdorffer M. Growth in mass and volume of the human lens in postnatal life. *Arch Ophthalmol.* 1937;17:104.

69. Murthy SK, Ravi N. Hydrogels as potential probes for investigating the mechanism of lenticular presbyopia. *Curr Eye Res.* 2001;22:384-93.

70. Myers RI, Krueger RR. Novel approaches to correction of presbyopia with laser modification of the crystalline lens. *J Refract Surg.* 1998;14:136-9.

71. Nishi O, Hara T, Saka Y, et al. Refilling the lens with an inflatable endocapsular balloon: surgical procedures in animal eyes. *Graefes Arch Clin Exp Ophthalmol.* 1992;230:47-55.

72. Nishi O, Hara T, Hayashi F, et al. Further development of experimental techniques for refilling the lens of animal eyes with a balloon. *J Cataract Refract Surg.* 1989;15:584-8.

73. Nishi O, Nishi K. Accommodation amplitudes after lens refilling with injectable silicone by sealing the capsule with a plug in primates. *Arch Ophthalmol.* 1998;116:1358-61.

74. Mathews S. Scleral expansion surgery does not restore accommodation in human presbyopia. *Ophthalmology.* 1999;106:873-7.

75. Schachar RA, Tello C, Cudmore DP, et al. In vivo increase of the human lens equatorial diameter during accommodation. *Am J Physiol.* 1996;271:670-6.

76. Schachar RA. Cause and treatment of presbyopia with a method for increasing the amplitude of accommodation. *Annals of Ophthalmology.* 1992;24:445-7.

77. Schachar RA. Theoretical basis for the scleral expansion band procedure for surgical reversal of presbyopia. *Compr Ther.* 2001;27:39-46.

78. Pandey SK, Werner L, Apple DJ, et al. Evaluation of an accommodative intraocular lens in human and rabbit eyes. Presented at: ASCRS Symposium on Cataract, IOL and Refractive Surgery; June 2002; Philadelphia, Pa.

79. Parel JM, Gelender H, Trefers WF, Norton EW. Phaco-Ersatz: cataract surgery designed to preserve accommodation. *Graefes Arch Clin Exp Ophthalmol.* 1986;224:165-73.

80. Bito LZ, DeRousseau CJ, Kaufman PL, Bito JW. Age-dependent loss of accommodative amplitude in rhesus monkeys: an animal model for presbyopia. *Invest Ophthalmol Vis Sci.* 1982;23:23-31.

81. Bito LZ, Kaufman PL, DeRousseau CJ, Koretz J. Presbyopia: an animal model and experimental approaches for the study of the mechanism of accommodation and ocular aging. *Eye.* 1987;1:222-30.

82. Croft MA, Kaufman PL, Crawford KS, et al. Accommodation dynamics in aging rhesus monkeys. *Am J Physiol.* 1998;275:R1885-97.

83. Haefliger E, Parel JM. Accommodation of an endocapsular silicone lens (phaco-ersatz) in the aging rhesus monkey. *J Refract Corneal Surg.* 1994;10:550-5.

84. Hara T, Saka Y, Sakanishi K, et al. Complications associated with endocapsular balloon implantation in rabbits eyes. *J Cataract Refract Surg.* 1994;20:507-12.

85. Hemenger RP, LaMotte JO, Occhipinti JR. Is accommodative amplitude correlated with lens fluorescence? *Optom Vis Sci.* 1990;67:860-2.

86. Hettlich HJ, Lucke K, Asiyo-Vogel MN, et al. Lens refilling and endocapsular polymerization of an injectable intraocular lens: in vitro and in vivo study of potential risks and benefits. *J Cataract Refract Surg.* 1994;20:115-123.

87. Lucke K, Hettlich HJ, Kreiner CF. A method of lens extraction for the injection of liquid intraocular lenses. *Ger J Ophthalmol.* 1992;1:342-5.

BIBLIOGRAPHY

Al-Ghoul KJ, Nordgren RK, Kuszak AJ, et al. Structural evidence of human nuclear fiber compaction as a function of ageing and cataractogenesis. *Exp Eye Res.* 2001;72:199-214.

Apple DJ, Auffarth GU, Peng Q, Visessook N. *Foldable Intraocular Lenses.* Thorofare, NJ: SLACK Incorporated; 2000.

Apple DJ, Lim E, Morgan R, et al. Preparation and study of human eyes obtained postmortem with the Miyake posterior photographic technique. *Ophthalmology.* 1990;97:810-6.

Assia EI, Castaneda VE, Legler UFC, et al. Studies on cataract surgery and intraocular lenses at the Center for Intraocular Lens Research. *Ophthalmology Clinics North America.* 1991;4:251-266.

Atchison DA. Accommodation and presbyopia. *Ophthalmic Physiol Opt.* 1995;15:255-72.

Fisher RF. The force of contraction of the human ciliary muscle during accommodation. *J Physiol*. 1977;270:51.

Fisher RF. Presbyopia and the changes with age in the human crystalline lens. *J Physiol*. 1973;228:765-79.

Green WR. The uveal tract. In: Spencer WH. *Ophthalmic Pathology: An Atlas and Textbook*. Philadelphia, Pa: WB Saunders; 1986:1364-70.

Hibbert FG, Goldstein V. Defective accommodation in members of one family with an account of an apparatus for recording electrical potential changes. *Transactions of the Ophthalmological Society UK*. 1975;95:455-61.

Milder B. Prescribing glasses for myopia. *Ophthalmology*. 1979;86:706-12.

Obstfeld H. Crystalline lens accommodation and anterior chamber depth. *Ophthalmic Physiol Opt*. 1989;9:36-40.

Pandey SK, Cochener B, Apple DJ, et al. Intracapsular ring sustained 5-fluorouracil delivery system for prevention of posterior capsule opacification in rabbits: a histological study. *J Cataract Refract Surg*. In press.

Pau H, Kranz J. The increasing sclerosis of the human lens lens with age and its relevance to accommodation and presbyopia. *Graefes Arch Clin Exp Ophthalmol*. 1991;229:294-6.

Pierscionek B. Presbyopia-effect of refractive index. *Clinical and Experimental Optometry*. 1990;73:23.

Pierscionek B. What we know and understand about presbyopia. *Clinical and Experimental Optometry*. 1993;76:83.

Pierscionek BK. Age-related response of human lenses to stretching forces. *Exp Eye Res*. 1995;60:325-32.

Pierscionek BK, Weale RA. The optics of the eye-lens and lenticular senescence. A review. *Doc Ophthalmol*. 1995;89:321-35.

Pointer JS. Broken down by age and sex. The optical correction of presbyopia. *Ophthalmic Physiol Opt*. 1995;15:439-43.

Stark L. Presbyopia in light of accommodation. *Am J Optom Physiol Opt*. 1988;65:407-16.

Wyatt HJ. Application of a simple mechanical model of accommodation to the aging eye. *Vision Res*. 1993;33:731-8.

Chapter 3

Physiology of Accommodation and Presbyopia

Leonardo P. Werner, MD; Liliana Werner, MD, PhD;
Suresh K. Pandey, MD; and David J. Apple, MD

INTRODUCTION

Accommodation is a dioptric change in power of the eye that occurs to allow near objects to be focused on the retina. Presbyopia is one of the earliest universal signs of aging, and the basic pathophysiology involved in its development has been a matter of controversy for centuries. Studying the basic mechanism of accommodation and presbyopia is fundamental to understanding the pathophysiology of the eye. The normal, young human eye can easily focus on near and distant objects (ie, it can change focus or accommodate). The word *accommodation* has a relatively recent origin, introduced by Burow in 1841.[1,2] Certain standard textbooks before that time used the term *adaptation*, now accepted as connoting the changes in the sensitivity of the retina to varying intensities of light. Explanations of how accommodation occurs have been speculated upon for centuries.

Scientists have studied the change in the eye's ability to focus (amplitude of accommodation) in relationship to age. They have found that the amplitude of accommodation declines in a linear fashion with age and that this decline occurs universally and predictably (Figure 1).[1] If a patient is properly corrected for distance, his or her age can be determined within 1.5 years by measuring his or her amplitude of accommodation. Therefore, an adequate theory of the mechanism of accommodation and presbyopia in man must take into account the changes observable in the human eye during the effort of accommodation and provide a reasonable explanation for the decline in this function with age. This chapter discusses many aspects of presbyopia by reviewing the literature on the multitude of age-related changes that occur in the eye, which were previously described by many authors worldwide. In viewing the great number of theories proposed in years past, we have found that the mechanism and interrelationship of these have not yet been completely clarified, and some analyses have been attempted to provide a more accurate understanding of accommodation and presbyopia.

THE MECHANISM OF ACCOMMODATION

HISTORICAL BACKGROUND[2-4]

Reflex accommodation is modeled routinely as a closed-loop negative feedback system that operates to maximize or optimize luminance contrast of the retinal image. Whenever fixation changes from a distant to a near target, each eye accommodates and both eyes converge in the interest of clear single binocular vision. The character of this synkinesis, the variables which affect it, and the means by which it may be altered have not ceased to arouse interest. Historically, the existence of an accommodative mechanism was first demonstrated by Scheiner (1619). In his experiment, two pinholes were made in a card at a distance apart that was less than the diameter of the pupil. The eye, looking through them, was focused on a needle held at right angles to a line joining the two holes: the needle appeared single. If, however, the eye was focused on some other object nearer or further away, the needle appeared double. If three holes were made, three needles were seen, and so on (Figure 2). This experiment shows that in the eye there is a mechanism controlling the adjustment of focus. Scheiner proved that accommodation occurred as a result of a change in the optical power of the eye and that the eye obeyed the laws of optics. However, the true explanation of this classical experiment was offered by William Porterfield (1759), who suggested that accommodation was affected by a change in the lens. Other possible hypotheses have been put forward to explain the rationale of accommodation. Albrecht von Haller (1763) considered that the contraction of the pupil diminished the blur circles sufficiently to account for the phenomenon, which is present in some animals and is a mechanism that resembles a camera obscura. Some authors suggested that an elongation of the eyeball caused by contraction of the extraocular muscles was responsible for the phenomenon. The orig-

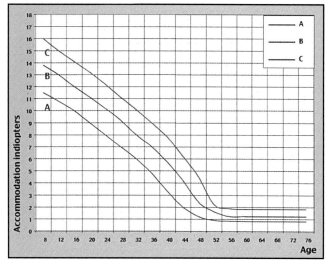

Figure 1. Duane's standard curve of accommodation in diopters in relation to age. A: Lowest values; B: average values; C: highest values (courtesy of Beau B. Evans, Center for Research on Ocular Therapeutics and Biodevices, Storm Eye Institute, Medical University of South Carolina, Charleston, SC).

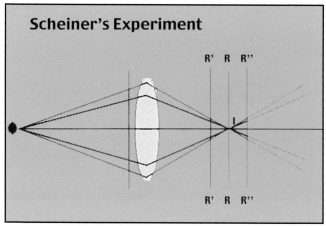

Figure 2. Schematic drawing showing Scheiner's experiment (1619). If the card is perforated at E and E, the object, O, is brought to a focus on a screen, R, at I, where one image will appear. If the screen is held at R' or R'', however, two images appear (E'F' and E''F'') (courtesy of Beau B. Evans, Center for Research on Ocular Therapeutics and Biodevices, Storm Eye Institute, Medical University of South Carolina, Charleston, SC).

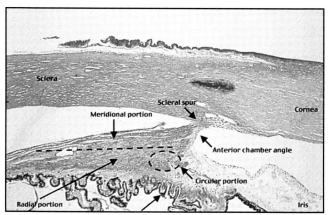

Figure 3. Photomicrograph from a human globe obtained postmortem showing the anterior segment. These histological sections are stained with Masson's Trichrome, which stains collagen fibers in blue and smooth muscle fibers in red (courtesy of Beau B. Evans, Center for Research on Ocular Therapeutics and Biodevices, Storm Eye Institute, Medical University of South Carolina, Charleston, SC).

inal theory of Kepler (1611) stating that changes in focus were attained by forward and backward movements of the lens (as occurs in some fish) received support from other investigators until it was demonstrated that an impossible excursion would be required in order to obtain the requisite change in focus: it would, indeed, require the lens to move forward by 10 mm.

Another possibility, that accommodation was accomplished by a change in the shape of the lens, was suggested at a very early date by Descartes (1677). Lobé (1742) postulated that the shape of the cornea changed. Later, Helmholtz (1853-1856) was able to demonstrate that the action of accommodation provided by the ciliary muscle was accompanied by an increase in curvature of both surfaces of the lens and an increase in its thickness. The histology of the anterior segment and the ciliary muscle of the human eye is reviewed in Figure 3.

HELMHOLTZ'S THEORY

In 1965, the American Committee on Optics and Visual Physiology adopted the slogan: "Put Helmholtz Back into Ophthalmology." Hermann von Helmholtz (1821-1894) trained as a physician, became a professor of physiology and physics, then spent his life studying physiologic optics.[2] In 1855, he observed that the center of the human lens thickened during accommodation. Based on this observation, he theorized that when the eye accommodates, the ciliary muscle contracts, reducing the tension on the zonules that span the circumlental space extending between the ciliary body and the lens equator. This releases the outward-directed equatorial tension on the lens capsule and allows this elastic capsule to contract, causing an increase in the anterior-posterior diameter of the lens and resulting in an increase in its optical power. Thus, the act of accommodation should result from a contraction of the ciliary muscle, which reduces the ciliary body diameter and releases the resting zonular tension. This allows young lenses to undergo elastic recovery, which causes an increase in the lens curvatures and lens power to enable near objects to be focused on the retina. When

accommodation ceases, the ciliary muscle relaxes and returns to its unaccommodated configuration, the zonular tension is once again increased, and the lens is pulled back into a relatively flattened state to increase the focal length.[4] The movement of the equatorial edge of the lens is, thus, away from the sclera during accommodation (Figure 4A) and toward the sclera during unaccommodation.

Although the influence of the capsule in determining the shape of the lens is undisputed, Helmholtz's theory cannot stand in its original form since it does not explain the shape assumed by the anterior surface of the lens. At a later date, Fincham[5] suggested that the peculiar form taken in this molding might be due to the structure of the capsule. It is much thicker in front than behind, and the anterior and posterior portions are thicker laterally just within the attachment of the zonular fibers than at the poles. The variations of its thickness in different parts suggest that on the application of ten-

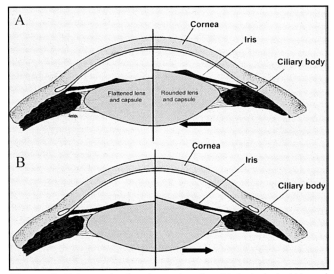

Figure 4. Schematic drawings showing Helmholtz's (A) and Schachar's (B) theories of accommodation. The arrows indicate the movement of the equatorial lens edge away from the sclera (A) and toward the sclera (B) during accommodation. A: The left side of the drawing shows the unaccommodated state. On the right side, the ciliary muscle has contracted during accommodation; the lens is thicker and more steeply curved. B: The left side is the same as in A. On the right side, note the flattening of the peripheral lens surfaces while the central anterior lens surface curvature increases (courtesy of Beau B. Evans, Center for Research on Ocular Therapeutics and Biodevices, Storm Eye Institute, Medical University of South Carolina, Charleston, SC).

sion, a flattening of the lens would occur preferentially in the periphery where the capsule is thickest and strongest, and a bulging in the axial region where it is weakest. At the posterior pole the capsule is very thin, and here the maximal curvature of the lens occurs even in the unaccommodated state.[6] It is this difference in the thickness of the central and lateral parts of the anterior capsule that Fincham believed was responsible for the hyperbolic form of the anterior surface of the lens during accommodation.

New Theories

For many years, there was a consensus of opinion on the mechanism of accommodation derived from the theory of Helmholtz. However, Schachar et al[7] recently proposed an alternative accommodative mechanism for the primate eye that is similar to a theory originally proposed by Tscherning.[8] Both theories[8-13] state that the equatorial zonules insert into the anterior ciliary muscle at the root of the iris, and the anterior and posterior zonules insert into the posterior ciliary body. Schachar and Anderson[13] allege that during ciliary muscle contraction, through the action of the radial and longitudinal fibers, the anterior portion of the ciliary muscle curls toward the sclera at the iris root. This movement increases tension on the equatorial zonular fibers while releasing tension on the anterior and posterior zonular bundles. Schachar believes that this provides a net outward-directed force at the lens equator through the equatorial zonular fibers. This force, putatively, would pull the lens equator toward the sclera during accommodation and, together with the

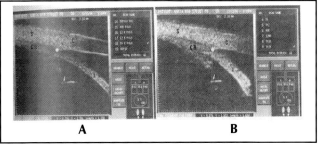

Figure 5. Ultrasound biomicroscope images of the human lens equator in relation to the scleral spur during an unaccommodated state induced by tropicamide (1%) and an accommodated state induced by pilocarpine (2%). The probe is positioned over the temporal ciliary region. Cornea, sclera, iris, and ciliary body can be identified in both pictures. A: In the unaccommodated state, the distance between the lens equator and the scleral spur is 1.568 mm. B: In the accommodated state, the distance between the lens equator and the scleral spur is 1.721 mm (courtesy of Fernando Trindade, MD, São Geraldo Eye Hospital, Federal University of Minas Gerais, São Paulo, Brazil).

concurrent relaxation of the anterior and posterior zonular bundles, would cause a flattening of the peripheral lens surfaces while increasing the central anterior and posterior lens surface curvatures. The movement of the equatorial edge of the lens is thus toward the sclera during accommodation (Figure 4B) and away from the sclera during unaccommodation. From a theoretical standpoint, pulling on the lens equator could cause an increase in the central lens curvatures depending on the viscoelastic properties of the lens. Schachar's theory, however, differs from that of Tscherning because it does not depend on the vitreous to explain the changes in lens shape that occur during accommodation.[14] The background of Schachar's theory is that the lens equatorial diameter increases with accommodation. However, a group of recent studies showed, using various imaging techniques, that the crystalline lens diameter decreases with accommodation, as the classical literature maintains and contrary to Schachar's contention (Figure 5). Wilson[15] has also shown lens equatorial movements away from the sclera during accommodation using transilluminated infrared light in a young human subject with ocular albinism. Glasser and Kaufman[14] studied the movements of the lens equator and the ciliary body using ultrasound biomicroscopy and goniovideography during accommodation and unaccommodation. They found that despite the systematic eye movement occurring with electrical stimulation and the nonsystematic eye movements occurring with pharmacological stimulation, in all instances the ciliary body and the lens equator moved away from the sclera during accommodation. Another study conducted by Glasser and Campbell[16] showed that mechanically stretching the zonule of the human lens increases lens focal length in accordance with classic teachings from Helmholtz. In addition, there has been no independent confirmation of the anatomic arrangements of the ciliary region, the accommodative mechanism, or the causes of presbyopia described by Schachar. The localized posterior or outward movement of the anterior portion of the ciliary muscle toward the sclera, as suggested by this author from histological analysis, was not visible by imaging techniques.[14] Also, his description concerning the insertion of the zonule conflicts with evidence provided by analyses of fresh human tissues and from scanning electron microscopic studies.[16,17] They show no insertion of equatorial bundles or any other zonular fibers at the iris root and anterior ciliary muscle (Figure 6).

By scanning electron microscopy, the zonules appear to attach to the lens capsule in three distinct sets. The fibers destined for the anterior and equatorial lens capsule have been shown to be strongly adherent to the valleys of the ciliary processes. They part company with the posterior zonules by continuing in an almost straight course to their insertion. Both the anterior and posterior zonules exit from the pars plicata in ribbonlike swaths, lining up parallel to the ciliary processes. The few zonules attaching 1.5 mm anterior and posterior to the equator of the lens arise from the midsides of the processes or from the valleys and usually derive from anterior or posterior zonular bundles.[6]

PRESBYOPIA

Presbyopia is the most common refractive disorder of later life, related to decrease of accommodative amplitude.[18] In emmetropes and hyperopes, it is usually manifested at 40 years of age by the need for reading glasses or contact lenses. Although normal myopes benefit at this age because of their shortsightedness, their accommodative amplitude also diminishes with age in a more or less regular manner. The number of presbyopes dramatically increases every year due to longer life expectancy. The symptoms begin with an annoying inertia of focus when gazing from far to near objects and advances to an inability to carry out prolonged near work without stinging, smarting, or tearing, which eventually leads to disinterest in reading. Fine print and small targets can no longer be resolved at the customary reading distance, and when the object is habitually brought nearer, the blur strangely increases. Soon even ordinary print begins to blur, smudge, smear, run together, and disappear. These symptoms are intensified under inadequate light, amplified by poor contrast, and exaggerated at the end of the day.[19]

Many studies based on Helmholtz's theory have attempted to explain the loss of accommodation in the aging eye. By considering many possibilities, any proposed theory must take into account the known decline in the ability of the eye to alter its focus as age advances. Some suggest a loss of zonules or capsule elasticity with aging; thus, when the zonules are relaxed, the lens is not able to change its shape.[20] There are some conflicting reports on whether the ciliary muscle atrophies with age.[21] There is also continued deposition of the lens fibers within the lens as it ages, causing the lens to become more compact and stiff. A major factor in the loss of accommodation may be the increased stiffness of the aging lens with inability to respond to accommodative stimuli.[22] In general, the multitude of changes that occur in the eye resulting in presbyopia can be broadly grouped into three categories:[16]

1. Lens and capsule-based theories, which consider changes in the elasticity and compliance of the lens and capsule
2. Extralenticular theories, which consider changes in the ciliary muscle and choroid
3. Geometric theories, which consider changes in the geometry of the zonular attachments to the lens

Fincham[23] added additional experiment support to Helmholtz's accommodative theory and also offered evidence that presbyopia was caused by the inability of the lens capsule to mold the hardened lens substance into the accommodated form. Fischer[24] and Pau and

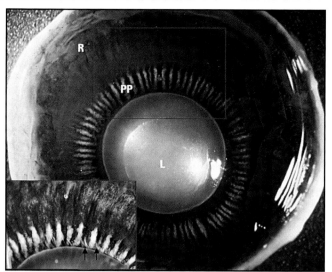

Figure 6. Photograph of a human globe obtained postmortem taken from an operating microscope after sectioning the globe at the equator to show the inner surface of the anterior segment from a posterior view. The crystalline lens (L) is in the center, surrounded by a series of radial lines, which are the ciliary processes, the pars plicata (PP). This latter portion is surrounded by the pars plana, which terminates in a scalloped edge, the ora serrata, where the retina (R) begins. Viewing with higher magnification, note the zonules (arrows) attaching the crystalline lens to the pars plicata of the ciliary body (courtesy of Beau B. Evans, Center for Research on Ocular Therapeutics and Biodevices, Storm Eye Institute, Medical University of South Carolina, Charleston, SC).

Kranz[25] also supported Fincham's theory of presbyopia by attributing accommodative loss to changes in the elastic properties of the lens. In addition, Fischer[26] found that Young's modulus of elasticity of the lens capsule decreases by half between youth and 60 years of age. Based on such evidence, we can assume that reduced capsular elasticity alone cannot explain presbyopia, only diminished capacity to change curvature. Furthermore, by evaluating capsular molding pressure versus lenticular strain, Fischer[24] concluded that decreased amplitude can be accounted for reduced elasticity of the capsule, changes in the elasticity of the lens substance, and flattening of the lens. This finding supports Fincham's theory of presbyopia because a less elastic lens capsule would exert less force on the hardening substance of the aging lens. When the capsule is stripped off (in young monkeys), the lens becomes thinner and flatter.[3] These observations suggest that the lens substance houses restoring forces, which tend to maintain it in the unaccommodated form. These forces are in turn antagonized by capsular elasticity. Weale[27] proposed that in the young eye, elastic capsular forces are dominant, while restoring forces predominate in presbyopia.

The lens and capsule-based theories accept indirect evidence that ciliary muscle is capable of providing the same magnitude of force in presbyopic as in prepresbyopic eyes. Impedance cyclography has been used to measure ciliary muscle contraction and to show that it remains normal up to the age of 60 years, supporting lens or capsule-based theories of presbyopia.[28] However, these findings have been criticized because of the uncertainties of exactly what impedance cyclography measures. This stems, in part, from the observation that a given accommodative demand does not consistently produce the same impedance.[29] Also, in the rhesus monkey, which has an accommodative apparatus similar to that of the human and develops presbyopia on a comparable time scale relative to its lifespan,[30] the ability of the ciliary muscle to alter its configuration in response to topical cholinomimetic drugs or electrical stimulation of the Edinger-Westphal nucleus clearly declines with age.[31-33] These potentially confounding results may suggest a possible loss of ciliary muscle function concurrent with the development of presbyopia. Supporting this concept in agreement with extralenticular theories, Fuchs first reported that cycloplegia is more effective in young eyes than old, and Duane[1] found the onset of cycloplegia to be more rapid in early presbyopes than nonpresbyopes. Moreover, if ciliary muscle wasting was significant, its vigorous exercise (eg, hyperopia, prolonged near work) should postpone presbyopia, and there is no evidence that this occurs.[16,34]

Brown[35] has suggested that presbyopia is associated with liquefaction of the vitreous, since the two processes occur at about the same point in the human life span. However, this theory does not explain why the age-related decline in accommodative amplitude begins so early in life.[36] Another possibility may support the concept of geometric theories, because it arises from the observation that the location of the zonulolenticular attachments relative to the lens equator and the ciliary muscle change with age, as the lens increases in size.[37] Such an alteration in the anterior segment geometry would result in greater retention of zonular force applied to the lens during ciliary muscle contraction without necessarily requiring other changes in the anterior segment properties.[38-40] The observations also provided by Brown[41] of an increase in lens size with age changing its curvatures and by Farnsworth and Shyne[37] of an anterior shift of the zonular attachments onto the lens led to the suggestion that distinct factors may be interacted to contribute to the failure of the older lens to accommodate, as it becomes retained in an unaccommodated state.

More recently, presbyopia has been described as a geometric disorder only attributed to changes in the size and volume of the lens. Schachar[7] proposed that zonular tension is increased during accommodation in young subjects, in contrast with the classic Helmholtz's theory, as described. In support of his hypothesis, Schachar and colleagues[9] believe that presbyopia results from a decrease in zonular tension caused by the normal growth of the crystalline lens with age. Until recently, lens diameter could be measured only in isolated lenses from donor eyes. Recently, however, magnetic resonance imaging (MRI) has been used for the first time to measure lens diameter in vivo. The lens is of ectodermal origin and continues to grow throughout life, and the equatorial diameter increases at approximately 0.02 mm/year. However, except for the progressive myope, the dimensions of the scleral shell do not change significantly after 13 years of age. The distance between the ciliary muscle and the equator of the lens decreases throughout life. Therefore, the effective force that the ciliary muscle can apply to the lens equator is reduced in a linear fashion with age. The amplitude of accommodation decreases linearly with age, resulting in presbyopia, and is a consequence of normal lens growth.[9-13] According to Schachar,[11] surgical expansion of the sclera surrounding the ciliary body can restore accommodation as a remedy for presbyopia. Scleral expansion surgery involves the implantation of a plastic ring or arches of plastic (scleral expansion bands) in the sclera surrounding the ciliary body to increase the space between the ciliary body and the lens equator. Restoration of accommodation with the use of scleral expansion bands is based on a revisionist theory of accommodation that is not supported by recent experiments.

In four patients operated in our department of ophthalmology, we found that the near vision improved in two patients, while the amplitude of accommodation remained stable in all cases after surgery. Based on such findings by other authors,[14,42] we can presume that the efficacy of scleral expansion surgery in the treatment of presbyopia was not completely determined and there is some evidence accumulating that the improvement obtained in some patients may represent a consequence of lenticular aberrations resulting in a multifocal optical system, rather than true accommodation.

This concept of age-related loss of accommodation related to decreased zonular tension resulting from continued growth of the lens throughout life, rather than lenticular sclerosis, was also described by Weale[27] and Bito and Miranda.[43] Tscherning[8] also postulated that there is increased zonular tension during accommodation, as described by Schachar and previously mentioned. However, he thought the lens equator moved posteriorly during accommodation and he attributed presbyopia to enlargement of the lens nucleus. Such lenticular contribution to presbyopia was suggested because of a change in the ratio of the lens capsular and also lens matrix elasticity. The continuous equatorial growth of the lens claimed by Schachar and other authors is without experimental support and is no longer generally accepted due to the fact that Farnsworth and Shyne[37] showed that the distance from the ciliary body to the zonular insertion onto the lens does not change with increasing age. Furthermore, Weale[27] and Bito and Miranda[43] provided no experimental evidence to support their claim that lenticular sclerosis does not occur, and their contention is not consistent with subsequent experimental finding.

Although many theories on the causes of presbyopia have invoked changes in the make-up of the lens (such that it would be concurrent with a change in the refractive index of the lens), relatively few studies have directly measured the age-related optical changes in the lens. Glasser and Campbell[16] used an in vitro scanning laser technique to measure the optical properties of crystalline lenses from 27 human eyes that ranged in age from 10 to 87 years. They found that crystalline lenses beyond 58 years of age would not change focal length when increasing and decreasing radial stretching forces were applied through the ciliary body-zonular complex. Schachar's theory proposes that presbyopia is due purely to lens growth and that the lens remains pliable with increasing age. Contrary to Schachar's theory, Glasser and Campbell's study strongly supports the classical theories of presbyopia based on the crystalline lens becoming unmalleable with age.

CONCLUSION

The eye ages in structure and function and, although part of the physiological aging process, presbyopia has until now been considered an irreversible optical failure, an intriguing evolutionary blunder that comes as a psychological shock. However, its diagnosis and treatment with spectacles are probably the most common, if not the simplest, refractive problem. We have seen that none of the experiments that tried to explain the loss of accommodation with age are crucially conclusive, and certainty of the results may be influenced by training the subject. By reviewing many theories proposed since early times, the dispute is still unresolved, but the mechanism of the lens itself appears to be the most important factor in the determination of presbyopia. The human lens undergoes profound optical and physical changes with increasing age. To date, Helmholtz generated the most widely accepted theory of the physical mechanism of accommodation. However, further experimental work is still necessary to dispel many of the incorrect notions about the development of presbyopia and to identify those age-related changes in the eye that contribute to the loss of accommodative ability with increasing age.

REFERENCES

1. Duane A. Normal values of the accommodation at all ages. *JAMA*. 1912;59:1010-1013.
2. Michaels DD. Accommodation, vergences, and heterophorias. In: Michaels DD, eds. *Visual Optics and Refraction*. 3rd ed. St. Louis, Mo: CV Mosby; 1985.
3. Duke-Elder S. Adjustments to the optical system: accommodation. In: Duke-Elder S, ed. *System of Ophthalmology: Ophthalmic Optics and Refraction*. Vol V. St. Louis, Mo: CV Mosby; 1970.
4. von Helmholtz H. *Physiological Optics*. Vol I. New York: Dover; 1962:143-172,375-415.
5. Fincham EF. The mechanism of accommodation. *Br J Ophthalmol*. 1937;8(Suppl):5-80.
6. Last RJ. The eyeball. In: Wolff E, ed. *The Anatomy of the Eye and Orbit*. 6th ed. Philadelphia, Pa: WB Saunders; 1968.
7. Schachar RA, Cudmore DP, Black TD. Experimental support for Schachar's hypothesis of accommodation. *Annals of Ophthalmology*. 1993;25:404-409.
8. Tscherning M. *Physiologic Optics: Dioptrics of the Eye, Functions of the Retina, Ocular Movements, and Binocular Vision*. 2nd ed. Philadelphia, Pa: Keystone; 1904:160-189.
9. Schachar RA, Black TD, Kash RL, Cudmore DP, Schanzlin DJ. The mechanism of accommodation and presbyopia in the primate. *Annals of Ophthalmology*. 1995;27:58-67.
10. Schachar RA, Cudmore DP, Torti R, Black TD, Huang T. A physical model demonstrating Schachar's hypothesis of accommodation. *Annals of Ophthalmology*. 1994;26:4-9.
11. Schachar RA. Cause and treatment of presbyopia with a method for increasing the amplitude of accommodation. *Annals of Ophthalmology*. 1992;24:445-452.
12. Schachar RA, Tello C, Cudmore DP, Liebmann JM, Black TD, Ritch R. In vivo increase of the human lens equatorial diameter during accommodation. *Am J Physiol*. 1996;271:670-676.
13. Schachar RA, Anderson DA. The mechanism of ciliary muscle function. *Ann Ophthalmol*. 1995;27:126-132.
14. Glasser A, Kaufman PL. The mechanism of accommodation in primates. *Ophthalmology*. 1999;106:863-872.
15. Wilson RS. Does the lens diameter increase or decrease during accommodation? Human accommodation studies: a new technique using infrared retro-illumination video photography and pixel unit measurements. *Trans Am Ophthalmol Soc*. 1997;95:261-270.
16. Glasser A, Campbell MCW. Presbyopia and the optical changes in the human crystalline lens with age. *Vision Res*. 1998;38:209-229.
17. Rohen JW. Scanning electron microscopic studies of the zonular apparatus in human and monkey eyes. *Invest Ophthalmol Vis Sci*. 1979;18:133-144.
18. Milder B, Rubin ML. Progressive power lenses. *Surv Ophthalmol*. 1987;32:189-198.
19. Eichenbaum JW, Simmons DH, Velazquez C. The correction of

20. presbyopia: a prospective study. *Annals of Ophthalmology*. 1999;31:81-84
21. Brown N. The change in shape and internal form of the lens of the eye on accommodation. *Exp Eye Res*. 1973;15:441-459.
22. Fischer RF. The force of contraction of the human ciliary muscle during accommodation. *J Physiol*. 1977;270:51-74.
23. Van Heyningen R. What happens to the human lens in cataract? *Sci Am*. 1975;233:70-72, 77-81.
24. Fincham EF. The mechanism of accommodation. *Br J Ophthalmol*. 1937;8:5-80.
25. Fischer RF. Elastic constants of the human lens. *J Physiol*. 1971;212:147-180.
26. Pau H, Kranz J. The increasing sclerosis of the human lens with age and its relevance to accommodation and presbyopia. *Graefes Arch Clin Exp Ophthalmol*. 1991;229:294-296.
27. Fischer RF. Presbyopia and the changes with age in the human crystalline lens. *J Physiol*. 1973;228:765-779.
28. Weale RA. Presbyopia. *Br J Ophthalmol*. 1962;46:660-668.
29. Swegmark G. Studies with impedance cyclography on human ocular accommodation at different ages. *Acta Ophthalmologica*. 1969;46:1186-1206.
30. Sladin JJ, Stark L. Presbyopia: new evidence from impedance cyclography supporting the Hess-Gullstrand theory. *Vision Res*. 1975;15:537-541.
31. Bito LZ, DeRousseau, CJ, Kaufman PL, Bito JW. Age-dependent loss of accommodative amplitude in rhesus monkeys: an animal model for presbyopia. *Invest Ophthalmol Vis Sci*. 1982;23:23-31.
32. Neider MW, Crawford K, True B, Kaufman PL, Bito LZ. Functional studies of accommodation and presbyopia in rhesus monkeys. *Invest Ophthalmol Vis Sci*. 1986;27(S):81.
33. Bito LZ, Kaufman PL, Neider M, Miranda OC, Antal P. The dynamics of accommodation (ciliary muscle contraction, zonular relaxation and lenticular deformation) as a function of stimulus strength and age in iridectomized rhesus eyes. *Invest Ophthalmol Vis Sci*. 1987;28(Suppl):318.
34. Lutjen-Drecoll E, Tamm MD, Kaufman PL. Age-related loss of morphologic responses to pilocarpine in rhesus monkey ciliary muscle. *Arch Ophthalmol*. 1988;106:1591-1598.
35. Koretz JF, Kaufman PL, Neider MW, Goeckner PA. Accommodation and presbyopia in the human eye-aging of the anterior segment. *Vision Res*. 1989;29:1685-1692.
36. Brown NP. In the human lens in relation to cataract. *CIBA Foundation Symposium*. 1973;19:65-78.
37. Duane A. Studies in monocular and binocular accommodation with their clinical applications. *Am J Ophthalmol*. 1922;5:867-877.
38. Farnsworth PN, Shyne SE. Anterior zonular shifts with age. *Exp Eye Res*. 1979;28:291-297.
39. Handelman GH, Koretz JF. A mathematical representation of lens accommodation. *Vision Res*. 1982;22:924-927.
40. Koretz JF, Handelman GH. A model of the accommodative mechanism in the human eye. *Vision Res*. 1982;22:917-924.
41. Koretz JF, Handelman GH. A model for accommodation in the young human eye. *Vision Res*. 1983;23:1679-1686.
42. Brown NP. The change in lens curvature with age. *Exp Eye Res*. 1974;19:175-183.
43. Mathews S. Scleral expansion surgery does not restore accommodation in human presbyopia. *Ophthalmology*. 1999;106:873-877.
44. Bito LZ, Miranda OC. Accommodation and presbyopia. In: Reinecke RD, ed. *Ophthalmology Annual*. New York: Raven Press; 1989:103-128.

Chapter 4

The Mechanism of Accommodation and Presbyopia

The Scleral Expansion Band Procedure

Ronald A. Schachar, MD, PhD

INTRODUCTION

Presbyopia, age-related loss of accommodation, is universal and manifests between 40 and 45 years of age.[1,2] It is one of the first signs of aging. Since 1855, Helmholtz's theory of accommodation[3] and its modifications[4-9] have attributed accommodation to a decrease in zonular tension (Figure 1) and presbyopia to lens sclerosis and/or ciliary muscle atrophy. However, as late as 1950 in the textbook edited by the famous American ophthalmologist Conrad Berens, MD, William H. Luedde, MD stated, "For nearly fourscore years textbooks and teachers have routinely repeated an imaginary mechanism of accommodation without basis in fact."[10]

In 1992, I proposed a unique theory stating that during accommodation, equatorial zonular tension is increased.[11-19] My theory attributes presbyopia to a continuous age-related increase in the equatorial diameter of the lens with a subsequent decrease in the effective working distance of the ciliary muscle. As a direct deduction from this theory, scleral expansion successfully treats presbyopia,[18,20] ocular hypertension, and primary open-angle glaucoma.[21,22]

SCHACHAR'S THEORY OF ACCOMMODATION

The lens zonules can be divided into three groups: anterior, posterior, and equatorial.[12,23,24] The equatorial zonules play the most active role in accommodation.[11,12,14] The anterior and posterior zonules serve primarily to stabilize the lens when not accommodating. During accommodation, there is increased equatorial zonular tension and relaxation of the anterior and posterior zonules. This increased equatorial zonular tension causes central steepening, an increase in central thickness (anterior-posterior diameter), and peripheral flattening of the human crystalline lens[11] (Figure 2). The surface changes are similar to the induced central corneal steepening that occurs when a tight suture is placed in the peripheral cornea.[25] This phenomenon has been demonstrated in bovine lenses,[17] in constant volume, deformable, water-filled[26] and gel-filled[27] lenses, and is readily demonstrated by equatorially stretching an air-filled mylar balloon (Figure 3). It is the increased central steepening that occurs secondary to equatorial zonular tension that results

in accommodation.[11-19,28] This is in contrast to Helmholtz's theory, which states that the lens is under decreased zonular tension during accommodation.

The loss of accommodative amplitude occurs because of equatorial crystalline lens growth. The crystalline lens grows from the equatorial region.[29] At birth, the lens is fairly round; and as the crystalline lens grows, it becomes flatter in its periphery and its shape changes from spherical to hyperboloid.[29] This age-related shape change of the lens can only occur if the equatorial diameter is increasing with age, as has been observed histologically.[30-35] Like other ectodermal structures, the lens continually grows at approximately 20 microns/year.[30] Except for the progressive myope, the dimensions of the scleral shell remain unchanged after 13 years of age.[36] As a result, the distance between the ciliary body muscle and the equator of the lens decreases, which reduces the effectiveness of the ciliary muscle in a linear age-related fashion and ultimately leads to presbyopia.[11-19] By stretching the sclera in the region of the ciliary body, the effective working distance of the ciliary muscle is increased and accommodation is restored in the presbyope.[18,20,37,38]

SCLEROSIS OF THE CRYSTALLINE LENS OR CAPSULE IS *NOT* THE CAUSE OF PRESBYOPIA

Crystalline lens sclerosis cannot be the basis for presbyopia. No tissue in the human body becomes uniformly hard in an age-related linear fashion. The crystalline lens consists of 35% protein and 65% water.[39] The crystalline lens can only become harder by losing water or by calcifying. No relationship between crystalline lens water content and age has been found.[40] If the crystalline lens were calcifying or becoming harder by some other mechanism, then the speed of ultrasound in the crystalline lens would increase in a linear fashion. No such relationship to the speed of ultrasound in the crystalline lens has been found.[41]

Careful statistical analysis of both experiments performed by Kruger et al[42,43] and Fisher,[44] in which cadaver crystalline lenses of different ages were exposed to a constant centrifugal force, demonstrate that the elasticity of the crystalline lens is not related to age. The correlation coefficients of the relationship of polar strain versus age in both experiments were $r \leq 0.45$ and therefore $r^2 \leq 0.20$.

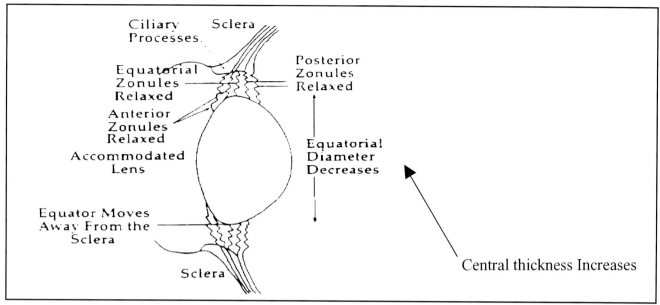

Figure 1. Helmholtz's theory of accommodation. All of the zonules relax and the crystalline lens "rounds up" because of its elasticity.

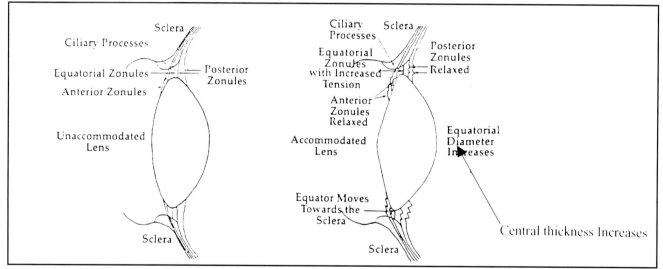

Figure 2. Schachar's theory of accommodation. In the unaccommodated state, all of the zonules are under tension. During accommodation, there is increased tension on the equatorial zonules, and the anterior and posterior zonules relax. As a result of the increased equatorial zonular tension, there is steepening of the central surfaces, an *increase* in the central thickness (anterior/posterior diameter), and simultaneous flattening of the peripheral surfaces.

The ratio of the standard error of the prediction for including or omitting age as a variable for both experiments is:[45]

$$\text{ratio of standard error of the prediction} = \sqrt{1 - r^2}$$
$$\geq 0.89$$

Since this ratio is very close to 1, age has very little effect ($\leq 11\%$) on the value of the polar strain (ie, both experiments demonstrate that there is *no* clinically important association between age and polar strain [elasticity] of the crystalline lens).

Clinical experience from cataract removal clearly demonstrates that a linear relationship between age and crystalline lens hardness does not exist. The amount of ultrasound power used for phacoemulsifying the crystalline lens nucleus is unrelated to the patient's age. In fact, even with a hard nucleus, the cortex of the crystalline lens is soft. There is no need to increase the irrigation/aspiration (I/A) power for removal of the cortex even when a very hard nucleus is present. The *sine qua non* of a cortical cataract is water clefts[46] (ie, there is increased water content and, therefore, the cortex of the crystalline lens is getting softer with age and *not* harder).[47] The crystalline lens is made up of interconnected epithelial cells; however, these connections are weak and do not offer any significant mechanical resistance.[48]

Since lens hardness cannot explain the age-related decline in accommodative amplitude, it has been proposed that the crystalline lens capsule stiffens in a linear fashion with age. Examination of the stress-strain curves of the capsule for different ages reveals that only if the capsule were stretched more than is physiologically possible is

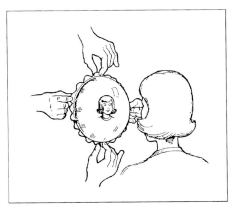

a. Look at your reflection in the center of an air-filled mylar balloon.

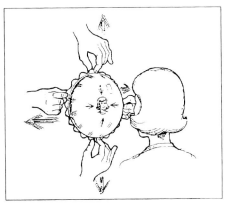

b. Note that your reflection in the center of the balloon minifies when the balloon equator is stretched. This demonstrates that the center of the balloon is steepening with equatorial stretching.

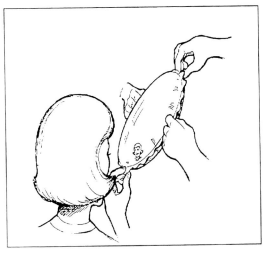

a. Then look at your reflection in the periphery of the mylar balloon.

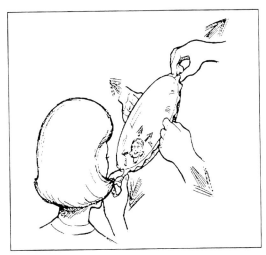

b. Note that your reflection from the periphery of the balloon enlarges when the balloon's equator is stretched. This demonstrates that the periphery of the balloon is flattening, while the center is steepening, when the balloon's equator is stretched.

Figure 3. Pulling on the equator of an air-filled mylar balloon while observing the changes in the size of a reflected image from its surface readily demonstrates Schachar's theory.

there a relationship of capsular stiffness to age.[49] Change in capsular stiffness cannot account for the linear age-related decline in accommodative amplitude.

CILIARY MUSCLE ATROPHY OR FIBROSIS IS *NOT* THE CAUSE OF PRESBYOPIA

Ciliary muscle atrophy and/or fibrosis of the connections of the posterior portions of the ciliary muscle have been proposed to account for the age-related decline of accommodation.[4,50] The ciliary muscle does atrophy and posterior fibrosis is apparent in older

patients;[51] however, impedance cyclography has demonstrated that the ciliary muscle reacts normally in presbyopes.[52]

EVALUATION OF PREVIOUS EXPERIMENTS

One of the major supporting arguments for the Helmholtz theory of accommodation is the observation made by Graves in 1925[53] of the changes in the perfectly clear anterior and posterior capsules during accommodation of a patient who had no vestige of lens matter between the capsules. Graves noted that when the patient accommodated, the anterior and posterior capsules wrinkled (Figure 4).

He concluded, in support of Helmholtz's theory, that the anterior and posterior zonules must relax during accommodation in order

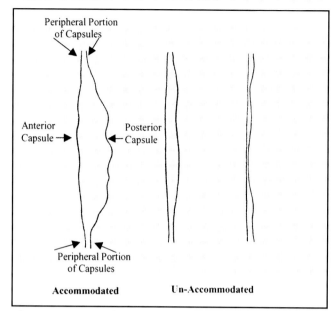

Figure 4. Graves' drawings of the crystalline lens capsule in the accommodated and unaccommodated states. Note how the peripheral portions of the crystalline lens capsule are straight in the accommodated state.

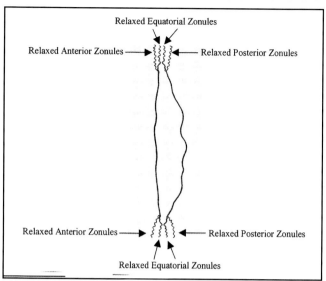

Figure 5. If all the zonules were relaxed during accommodation, then the peripheral portions of the capsule should be wrinkled.

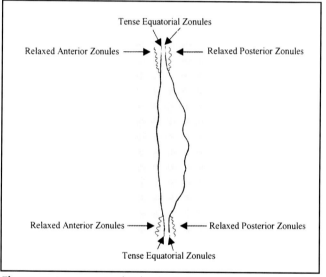

Figure 6. In support of Schachar's theory, the only way that the peripheral portion of the capsules can be straight during accommodation is if the equatorial zonules are under tension while the anterior and posterior zonules are relaxed.

to account for the wrinkling of the anterior and posterior capsules. Careful examination of his drawings reveals that his observations actually support Schachar's theory of accommodation. If all the zonules—anterior, equatorial, and posterior—relax, then the peripheral portions of the capsules must wrinkle during accommodation, as shown in Figure 5.

The only way that the peripheral portions of the capsules can be straight, as shown in Figure 4, is if the equatorial zonules are under tension while the anterior and posterior zonules are relaxed (Figure 6).

Careful examination of other experiments in support of Helmholtz's theory involving both human and primate eyes reveals that there is a systematic error. There is movement between the imaging device and the eye.[8,28,54-58] Measurement of the thickness and/or diameter of the cornea in the unaccommodated and accommodated states during these experiments revealed a change in corneal thickness or corneal diameter.[28,59,60] These experiments are flawed and cannot be used to reveal the mechanism of accommodation because none had proper controls,[59,60] and neither corneal curvature, thickness, nor diameter change during accommodation.[61]

OBJECTIVE WAVEFRONT SUPPORT FOR THE SCHACHAR THEORY OF ACCOMMODATION

According to Helmholtz's theory, all the zonules relax and the crystalline lens rounds up during accommodation (ie, both the central and peripheral surfaces of the crystalline lens steepen [see Figure 1]). According to Schachar's theory, during accommodation the central surfaces steepen and the peripheral surfaces flatten (see Figure 2). Reflection of light from the anterior central and periph-

eral surfaces of the crystalline lens during accommodation demonstrates that the central surface does steepen while the peripheral surface flattens.[8,62] The Helmholtz theory predicts that spherical aberration will move in the positive direction during accommodation (Figure 7A), and Schachar's theory predicts that it would move in the negative direction (Figure 7B).

Wavefront measurements made optically[63-66] with a Hartman-Shack wavefront sensor (Bausch & Lomb Zywave)[67,68] and by retinal imaging aberrometry[69,70] demonstrate that during accommodation spherical aberration of the human eye moves in the *negative* direction.

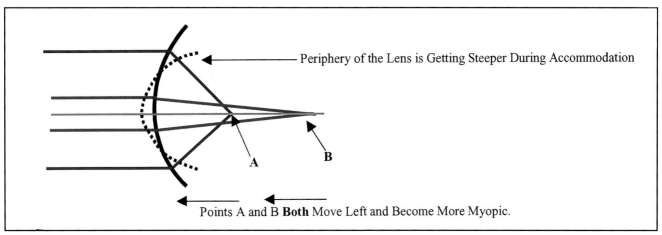

Figure 7A. Direction of the spherical aberration change predicted by each theory—Helmholtz's theory during accommodation. The lens rounds up, both the center and periphery of the lens get steeper (dotted line); points A and B will move in the *same* direction; both points A and B will move left and become more myopic; point A will be more myopic than point B. Spherical aberration will be in the *positive* direction during accommodation.

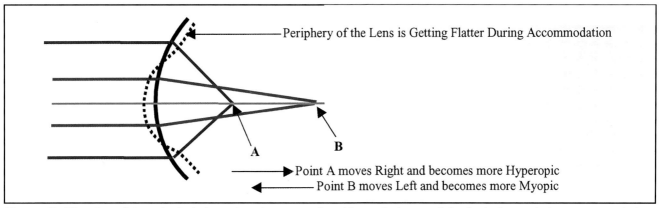

Figure 7B. Direction of the spherical aberration change predicted by each theory—Schachar's theory during accommodation. The center of the lens gets steeper while the periphery gets flatter (dotted line); points A and B will move in *opposite* directions; point A will move to the right and point B will move to the left; point B becomes more myopic, while point A becomes more hyperopic; spherical aberration will move in the *negative* direction during accommodation.

GRAVITY DOES NOT AFFECT ACCOMMODATIVE AMPLITUDE

Since the crystalline lens is denser than aqueous and vitreous, according to Helmholtz's theory gravity should displace the crystalline lens as all the zonules relax during accommodation. No change in the amplitude of accommodation of young subjects placed in the supine and prone positions while accommodating has been demonstrated.[71] Measurements of the accommodative amplitude of astronauts on Earth and in the microgravity environment of the Space Shuttle have not demonstrated a difference in accommodative amplitude.[72] Glasser and Kaufman have noted that the primate crystalline lens appeared to move in the direction of gravity when accommodating.[54] However, they were viewing the monkey crystalline lens through a contact lens and did not account for the optical effects of contact lens movement. Neider et al noted similar rhesus monkey crystalline lens displacements with gravity.[55]

A review of Neider's data reveals that the photographs they used to prove monkey crystalline lens displacement also demonstrate a change in corneal thickness. Since primate and human corneas do not change thickness or curvature during accommodation,[61] their observations were flawed because they did not use a proper reference system.

THE ULTIMATE PRACTICAL TEST OF A THEORY

DOES IT LEAD TO IMPROVED PATIENT CARE?

From a clinical point of view, a theory is only important if it has practical implications for patient care. The scleral expansion band procedure (SEB) does objectively increase the accommodative amplitude of presbyopes[20] and successfully treats ocular hypertension and primary open-angle glaucoma.[22]

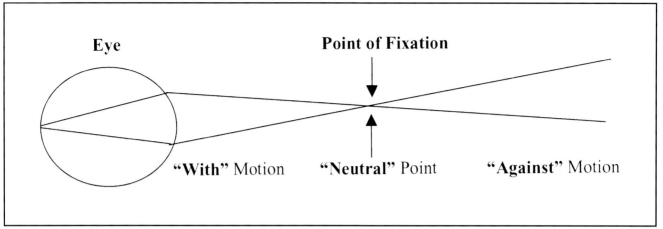

Figure 8. The subject fixates a near acuity target, the point of fixation. The working distance of the retinoscope is varied so that the retinal reflex changes from "against" to "neutral" to "with" motion. The "neutral" point defines the accommodative response.

OBJECTIVE MEASUREMENTS OF PHYSIOLOGICAL ACCOMMODATION FOLLOWING SEB IN THE PRESBYOPE

Video Dynamic Retinoscopy

Dynamic retinoscopy, where the working distance is varied to obtain a "neutral" reflex, has been demonstrated to be the "method of choice for the clinical assessment of the accommodative response."[73]

Retinoscopy has been the gold standard for all objective refractions for over 150 years. Dynamic retinoscopy, as described by Cross in 1911,[74] is a simple modification of retinoscopy. While the subject monocularly fixates a near acuity target, the working distance of the retinoscope is varied to obtain a "neutral" reflex. The distance of the retinoscope at which the "neutral" reflex is observed determines the optical power of the eye (Figure 8). Because of the potential error of measuring the distance of the retinoscope from the eye, three modifications of the Cross method of dynamic retinoscopy have been introduced.

In 1920, Sheard modified Cross's technique by using plus lenses to determine the "neutral" point.[75,76] The problem with Sheard's technique is that the plus lens reduces the accommodative response with a resulting underestimation of the accommodative amplitude. The monocular estimate method (MEM) involves trying to avoid the decrease in accommodative response by only briefly introducing the plus lens to determine the "neutral point."[77] The problem with the MEM modification is that the accommodative reaction time is approximately 350 ms,[78] which makes it extremely difficult for the examiner to move a plus lens in front of the subject without altering the accommodative response. The use of crossed cylinders to assess the "neutral" point is fraught with the same problems as the Sheard and MEM techniques. The reason that the Sheard, MEM, and crossed cylinder techniques are performed binocularly is to try to have the unexamined eye hold the accommodative level required for fixation on the near target while the plus lenses are placed in front of the examined eye. The presumption is that the unexamined eye will hold the accommodative level in spite of the inhibitory effect of the plus lenses being placed in front of the examined eye.

Video dynamic retinoscopy (VDR) is a modification of Cross's method. A video camera and a laser are attached to a retinoscope in order to videographically record the changes that occur in the dynamic retinoscopic images and to accurately measure the distance of the retinoscope from the eye (Figures 9 and 10). The video images of the retinoscopic retinal reflexes and the distance that the retinoscope is from the eye are objectively evaluated by computer image recognition software.[79] A comparison of the VDR technique to the standard "push-up" technique[80] for measuring accommodative amplitude in 15 normal patients found an accuracy of ±10% (Figure 11).

VDR objectively demonstrates that presbyopic eyes, post-SEB procedure, have accommodative amplitudes greater than the contralateral unoperated eye and the untreated eyes of age-matched presbyopes. In addition, the SRP patients have dynamic retinoscopic accommodative amplitudes that exceed the reported extreme upper limit for their ages[79] (Figures 12 to 14).

Infrared Optometer: PowerRefractor

The PowerRefractor (Multichannel Systems, Reutlingen, Germany) utilizes infrared LEDs to objectively measure the accommodative amplitude, pupil size, and vergence of patients.[81] The PowerRefractor video camera is placed 1 meter from the patient's eye. The patient views a near acuity target through his or her distance correction while the PowerRefractor takes 25 readings per second (Figure 15). In order to ensure accuracy, measurements are only taken when the subject's gaze is within ±10 degrees horizontally and ±5 degrees vertically of the line of sight of the PowerRefractor video camera. By placing the near acuity chart at multiple distances from the eye, the PowerRefractor can demonstrate whether the patient's accommodative mechanism is tracking the target.

The PowerRefractor was used to measure the accommodative response of a nonpresbyope, a normal presbyope, and an SEB patient. The SEB patient was able to track the near acuity chart at each distance (Figure 16), similar to the nonpresbyope (Figure 17). The normal presbyope had essentially no accommodative response and was unable to track the near acuity target (Figure 18). The PowerRefractor demonstrates that following SEBs the accommodative mechanism is active, the improvement in near vision is due to an active physiological process and is not a result of multifocal changes in the crystalline lens.

Wavefront Measurements

The Hartman-Shack wavefront sensor was used to compare the changes in the wavefront that occur during pharmacologically

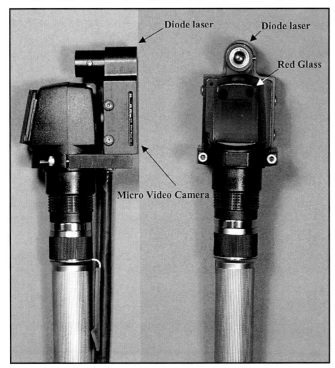

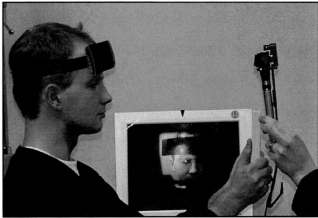

Figure 10. A black card is attached to the forehead of the patient in order to provide a minimal scattering surface for reflecting the laser spot. The subject fixates on a near acuity target while the working distance of the retinoscope is varied. The video camera records the images of the retinal reflexes and laser spot. Image recognition software objectively determines the "neutral" point, the distance of the retinoscope, and calculates the amplitude of accommodation from the video images.

Figure 9. Photograph of the VDR with its attached laser and microcamera. The red glass in front of the retinoscope decreases pupillary miosis during the video dynamic retinoscopy.

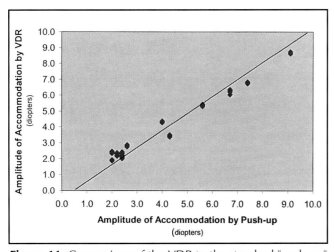

Figure 11. Comparison of the VDR to the standard "push-up" technique for measuring the amplitude of accommodation.

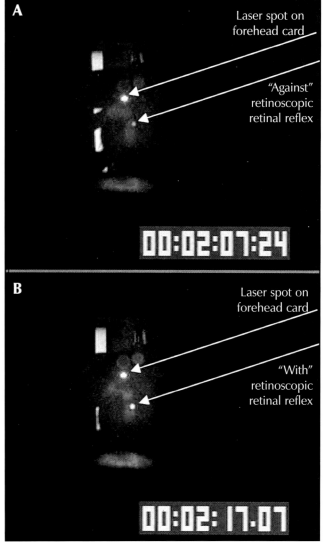

Figure 12. VDR images 1.5 years after the SEB procedure of the right eye of a 49-year-old female who has a plano distance refraction, while focusing on a near acuity target set at 23 cm from the eye. The distance of the video retinoscope from the eye as determined by the image recognition software of the laser spot size of image A ("against" motion) is 25 cm and 22 cm for image B ("with" motion). Therefore, the amplitude of accommodation is objectively >4 D. The mean accommodative amplitude for a 49-year-old is 2.2 D and the extreme upper limit is 3.4 D.[1]

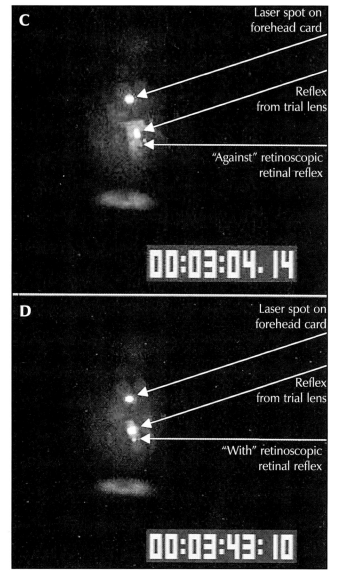

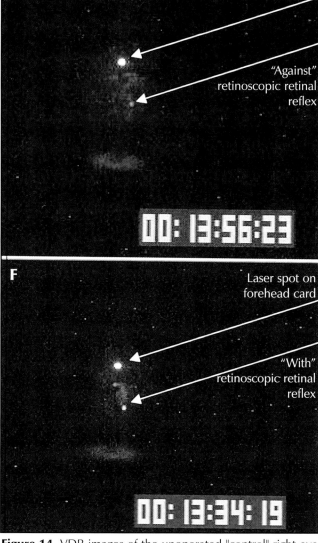

Figure 13. VDR images 1 year after the SEB procedure of the left eye of a 54-year-old female with a distance refraction of 1.00 -0.50 at 90 degrees in place while focusing on a near acuity target set at 30 cm from the eye. The distance of the video retinoscope from the eye as determined by the image recognition software of the laser spot size of image C ("against" motion) is 30 cm and 28 cm for image D ("with" motion). Therefore, the amplitude of accommodation is objectively >3.3 D. The mean accommodative amplitude for a 54-year-old is 1.4 D and the extreme upper limit is 2.0 D.[1]

Figure 14. VDR images of the unoperated "control" right eye of the patient in Figure 13 without the distance refraction of 0.50 -0.25 at 90 degrees in place while focusing on a near acuity target set at 30 cm from the eye. The distance of the video retinoscope from the eye as determined by the image recognition software of the laser spot size of image E ("against" motion) is 43 cm and 40 cm for image F ("with" motion). Therefore, the amplitude of accommodation is objectively >2.3 D.

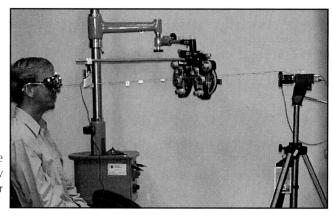

Figure 15. This patient has his distance refraction in place. The PowerRefractor video camera is set at 1 meter. The near acuity chart is placed at multiple distances while the PowerRefractor measures the refraction.

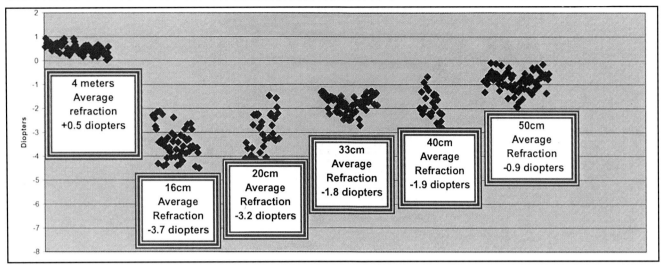

Figure 16. PowerRefractor measurements of the right eye of a 64-year-old male 7 months after the SEB procedure while focusing on a near acuity target placed at multiple distances. He was able to track the target and had a maximum average accommodative response of 3.7 D. The mean accommodative amplitude for a 64-year-old is 1.1 D and the extreme upper limit is 1.5 D.[1]

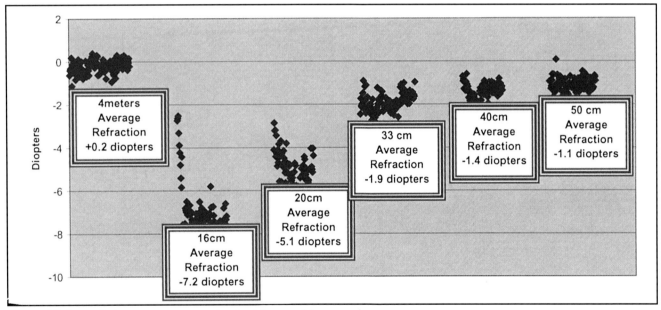

Figure 17. PowerRefractor measurements of a 32-year-old nonpresbyope.

induced accommodation in a nonpresbyope, a presbyope, and an SEB patient.[20] Wavefront measurements were made with the patient looking at distance and then 15 minutes after the administration of pilocarpine 6%. All measurements were made at the same 4 mm pupil size using the same wavefront height scale. Following the pilocarpine, the wavefronts of both the nonpresbyope and the SRP patient demonstrated central myopia with rounding-up of the general topography of the wavefronts. The peripheral portions of the wavefronts following the pilocarpine demonstrated a shift toward hyperopia consistent with spherical aberration shifting in the negative direction (Figure 19B and F). On the other hand, following the pilocarpine there was essentially no change in the wavefront of the normal presbyope (Figure 19D).

These Hartman-Shack wavefront sensor measurements objectively demonstrate that the post-SEB presbyope undergoes the same optical changes as a nonpresbyope during pharmacologically induced accommodation and that the SEB physiologically increases the accommodative amplitude.

SEB TREATMENT FOR OCULAR HYPERTENSION AND OPEN-ANGLE GLAUCOMA

Pilocarpine reduces intraocular pressure (IOP) by inducing contraction of the longitudinal ciliary muscle that is inserted on the

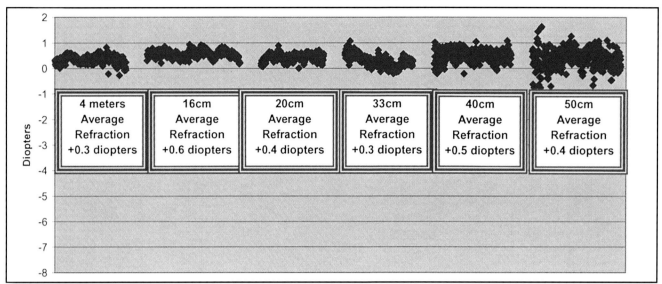

Figure 18. PowerRefractor measurements of a 48-year-old normal presbyope. The subject's refraction remains hyperopic independent of the distance of the near acuity target.

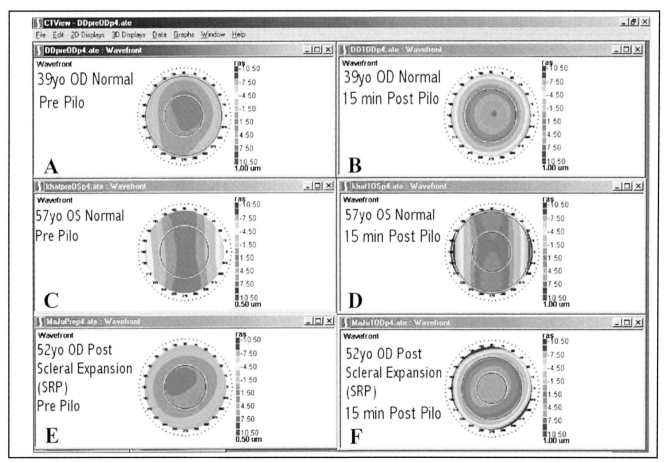

Figure 19. Hartman-Shack wavefront sensor images of a nonpresbyope, presbyope, and SEB presbyope while viewing distance (A, C, E) and 15 minutes after pilocarpine 6% (B, D, F), respectively. Following the pilocarpine, the wavefront demonstrates a central myopic shift with a peripheral hyperopic shift (consistent with spherical aberration shifting in the negative direction) in the nonpresbyope (B) and the SEB presbyope (F). There is minimal change in the wavefront of the presbyope (D) (courtesy of Jay S. Pepose, MD, PhD).

scleral spur.[82,83] The increased tension on the scleral spur opens the trabecular meshwork, reducing aqueous outflow resistance. Loss of tension on the scleral spur is related to the development of abnormally elevated IOP in some aging populations. The tone of the ciliary muscle decreases with age, just as it does with presbyopia, reducing the facility of aqueous from the eye. The scleral expansion band procedure increases ciliary muscle tone and, therefore, dramatically decreases IOP in ocular hypertensives and primary open-angle patients, but only minimally decreases IOP of normotensive patients.[21]

A prospective, nonrandomized, controlled, comparative human trial has been performed in Canada under a precisely defined and monitored protocol approved by Health Canada and an ethics committee. One glaucoma specialist, Aaron W. Rifkind, MD performed all the SEB procedures. Michael E. Yablonski, MD independently evaluated the patients. Following the scleral expansion band procedure both ocular hypertensives and primary open angle patients had a 7 mmHg median decrease in IOP that remained stable during the 1-year follow-up. The IOP decrease was equal to or better than that obtained from preoperatively physician-prescribed glaucoma medication. In addition, the patients had an improvement in their uncorrected near vision. Patient satisfaction was extremely high. One hundred percent of the patients at the 6-month gate elected to have the SEB procedure on the control eye. Fluorophotometry demonstrated that the mechanism for the decrease in IOP is due to an increase in aqueous outflow.[84]

The SEB procedure offers first-line continual reversible therapy for the treatment of ocular hypertension and primary open-angle glaucoma without the local or systemic side effects, adverse reactions, and compliance problems of medication. The scleral expansion band procedure may prevent or delay the onset of primary open-angle glaucoma in genetically predisposed patients.

SEB AND OTHER REFRACTIVE PROCEDURES

The SEB procedure has been successfully performed after laser-assisted in situ keratomileusis (LASIK), photorefractive keratotomy (PRK), and radial keratotomy (RK). LASIK has been performed after the SEB procedure; however, to simplify application of the suction ring it is easier to perform LASIK before the SEB procedure. The SEB procedure has been performed as early as 6 weeks post-LASIK.[85,86]

SUMMARY

The SEB procedure effectively and physiologically treats presbyopia, ocular hypertension, and primary open-angle glaucoma. Because of the counterintuitive nature of Schachar's theory and the systematic error that has been made in previous experiments, it is difficult for many to accept the theory as unequivocally correct. However, once the realization occurs that when tension is applied to the crystalline lens equator there is central steepening of its surfaces and an increase in central thickness (anterior/posterior diameter) with simultaneous flattening of the peripheral surface, everything falls into place.[19,28] All of the clinical observations of accommodation, presbyopia, and the results of scleral expansion can be easily and simply explained. In addition, the theory satisfies Occam's razor, which states that the simplest theory that explains all observed phenomena must be the correct theory.[87]

REFERENCES

1. Donders FC. *On the Anomalies of Accommodation and Refraction of the Eye*. London: The New Sydenham Society; 1864:204-214.
2. May CH, Perera CA. *Manual of the Diseases of the Eye for Students and General Practitioners*. 17th ed. Baltimore, Md: William Wood & Co; 1941:365-366.
3. von Helmholtz H. Über die akkommodation des auges. *Albrecht von Graefes Arch Ophthalmol*. 1855;1:1-89.
4. Tamm E, Drecoll L, Jungkunz, Rohen JW. Posterior attachment of ciliary muscle in young, accommodating old, presbyopic monkeys. *Invest Ophthalmol Vis Sci*. 1991;32:1678-1692.
5. Rohen JW. Scanning electron microscopic studies of the zonular apparatus in human and monkey eyes. *Invest Ophthalmol Vis Sci*. 1979;18:133-144.
6. Fisher RF. Presbyopia and the changes with age in the human crystalline lens. *J Physiol (Lond)*. 1973;228:765-779.
7. Coleman DJ. Unified model for accommodative mechanism. *Am J Ophthalmol*. 1970;69:1063-1079.
8. Fincham RF. The mechanism of accommodation. *Br J Ophthalmol*. 1937;8(Suppl):5-80.
9. Stuhlman O. *An Introduction to Biophysics*. New York: John Wiley and Sons; 1948:106-107.
10. Luedde WH. Accommodation. In: Berens C. *The Eye and Its Diseases*. Philadelphia, Pa: WB Saunders; 1950:140-141.
11. Schachar RA, Bax AJ. Mechanism of accommodation. *Int Ophthalmol Clin*. 2001;41(2):17-32.
12. Schachar RA. Histology of the ciliary muscle-zonular connections. *Annals of Ophthalmology*. 1996;28:70-79.
13. Schachar RA, Tello C, Cudmore DP, et al. In vivo increase of the human lens equator diameter during accommodation. *Am J Physiol (Regulatory Integrative Comp Physiol 40)*. 1996;271:R670-R676.
14. Schachar RA, Anderson DA. The mechanism of ciliary muscle function. *Annals of Ophthalmology*. 1995;27:126-32.
15. Schachar RA, Black TD, Kash RL, et al. The mechanism of accommodation and presbyopia in the primate. *Annals of Ophthalmology*. 1995;27:58-67.
16. Schachar RA. Zonular function: a new hypothesis with clinical implications. *Annals of Ophthalmology*. 1994;26:36-8.
17. Schachar RA, Cudmore DP, Black TD. Experimental support for Schachar's hypothesis of accommodation. *Annals of Ophthalmology*. 1993;25:404-9.
18. Schachar RA. Cause and treatment of presbyopia with a method for increasing the amplitude of accommodation. *Annals of Ophthalmology*. 1992;24;445-52.
19. Schachar RA. Is Helmholtz's theory of accommodation correct? *Annals of Ophthalmology*. 1999;31:10-17.
20. Pepose JS. Scleral expansion surgery. Presented at: American Academy of Ophthalmology Annual Meeting; Nov 9, 2001; New Orleans, La.
21. Schachar RA. The scleral expansion band procedure: therapy for ocular hypertension and primary open angle glaucoma. *Annals of Ophthalmology*. 2000;32:87-89.
22. Rifkind AW, Yablonski ME, Shuster JJ. Effect of scleral expansion band on ocular hypertension: Canadian phase I study. *Compr Ther*. 2001;27:333-340.
23. Farnsworth PN, Burke P. Three-dimensional architecture of the suspensory apparatus of the lens of the rhesus monkey. *Exp Eye Res*. 1977;25:563-76.
24. Streeten BW. Zonular apparatus. In: Jakobiec FA, ed. *Ocular Anatomy Embryology and Teratology*. Philadelphia, Pa: Harper & Row; 1982:331-353.
25. Emory JM, Paton D. *Current Concepts in Cataract Surgery*. St Louis, Mo: Mosby; 1976:182-189.
26. Schachar RA, Cudmore DP, Black TD. A revolutionary variable focus lens. *Annals of Ophthalmology*. 1996;28:11-18.
27. Schachar RA, Cudmore DP, Torti R, et al. A physical model demonstrating Schachar's hypothesis of accommodation. *Annals of Ophthalmology*. 1994;26:4-9.
28. Schachar RA, Bax AJ. Mechanism of human accommodation as analyzed by nonlinear finite element analysis. *Compr Ther*. 2001;27:122-132.
29. Tripathi RC, Tripathi BJ. Anatomy, orbit and adnexa of the

human eye. In: Davson H, ed. *The Eye*. Vol 1A. 3rd ed. Orlando, Fla: Academic Press; 1984: 55-60.

30. Rafferty NS. Lens morphology. In: Maisel H, ed. *The Ocular Lens*. New York, NY: Marcel Dekker Inc; 1985:2-6.

31. Sakabe I, Oshika T, Lim SJ, Apple DJ. Anterior shift of zonular insertion onto the anterior surface of human crystalline lens with age. *Ophthalmology*. 1998;105:295-299.

32. Lim SJ, Shin JK, Kim HB, Kurata Y, Sakabe I, Apple DJ. Analysis of zonular-free zone and lens size in relation to axial length of eye with age. *J Cataract Refract Surg*. 1998;24:390-396.

33. Coulombe JL, Coulombe AJ. Lens development. IV. Size, shape and orientation. *Invest Ophthalmol Vis Sci*. 1969;8:251-257.

34. Marshall J, Bauconsfield M, Rothery S. The anatomy and development of the human lens and zonules. *Trans Ophthalmol Soc UK*. 1982;102:423-440.

35. Kleinman NJ, Worgul BV. The Lens. In: Tasman W, ed. *Duane's Foundations of Clinical Ophthalmology*. Vol 1. Philadelphia, Pa: JB Lippincort; 1994.

36. Duke-Elder S, Waybar KD. Anatomy of the visual system. In: Duke-Elder S, ed. *System of Ophthalmology*. Vol. 2. London: Henry Kimpton; 1961:80-81.

37. Cross WD, Zdenek GW. Surgical reversal of presbyopia. In: Agarwal S, Agarwal A, Pallikaris IG, Neuhann TH, Knorz MC, Agarwal A. *Refractive Surgery*. New Delhi, India: Jaypee Brothers Medical Publishers, Ltd; 2000:592-608.

38. Zdenek GW. Clinical results. In: Schachar RA, Roy HF, eds. *Presbyopia: Cause and Treatment*. The Hague, Netherlands: Kugler Publications; 2001:81-90.

39. Duke-Elder S, Gloster J, Weale RA. The physiology of the eye and of vision. In: Duke-Elder S, ed. *System of Ophthalmology*. Vol. 4. London: Henry Kimpton; 1968:365-3581-89.

40. Fisher RF. Presbyopia and the water content of the human crystalline lens. *J Physiol*. 1973;234:443-447.

41. Beers APA, van der Heijde GL. Presbyopia and velocity of sound in the lens. *Optom Vis Sci*. 1994;71:250-253.

42. Kruger RR. Sun XK, Stroh J, Myers R. Experimental increase in accommodative potential after neodymium: Yttrium-aluminum-garnet laser photodisruption of paired cadaver lenses. *Ophthalmology*. 2001;108:2122-2129.

43. Schachar RA. Polar strain and crystalline lens age. Letter to the editor. *Ophthalmology*. Submitted.

44. Fisher RF. The elastic constants of the human lens. *J Physiol*. 1971;212:147-180.

45. Neter J, Wasserman, Kutner MH. *Applied Statistical Models*. 3rd ed. Homewood, Ill: Irwin Publication; 1990:444-445.

46. Hogan MJ, Zimmerman LE. *Ophthalmic Pathology*. 2nd ed. Philadelphia, Pa: WB Saunders; 1962:666-668.

47. Vajpayee RB, Bansal A, Sharma N, Dada T, Dada VK. Phacoemulsification of white hypermature cataract. *J Cataract Refract Surg*. 1999;25:1157-1160.

48. Hogan MJ, Alvarado JA, Weddell JE. *Histology of the Human Eye*. Philadelphia, Pa: WB Saunders; 1971:667-673.

49. Krag S, Olsen T, Andreassen TT. Biomechanical characteristics of the human anterior lens capsule in relation to age. *Invest Ophthalmol Vis Sci*. 1997;38:357-363.

50. Atchison DA. Accommodation and presbyopia. *Ophthalmic Physiol Opt*. 1995:15:255-272.

51. Tamm S, Tamm E, Rohen JW. Age-related changes of the human ciliary muscle. A quantitative morphometric study. *Mechanism of Aging and Development*. 1992;62:201-221.

52. Swegmark G. Studies with impedance cyclography on human ocular accommodation at different ages. *Acta Ophthalmol*. 1969; 47:1186-1206.

53. Graves B. The response of the lens capsules in the act of accommodation. *Transactions of the American Ophthalmology Society*. 1925;23:184-198.

54. Glasser A, Kaufman PL. The mechanism of accommodation in primates. *Ophthalmology*. 1999;106:863-72.

55. Neider MW, Crawford K, Kaufman PL, et al. In vivo videography of the rhesus monkey accommodative apparatus. *Arch Ophthalmol*. 1990;108:69-74.

56. Koretz JF, Bertasso AM, Neider MW, True-Gabelt BA, Kaufman

PL. Slit-lamp studies of the rhesus monkey eye: II. Changes in crystalline lens shape, thickness and position during accommodation and aging. *Exp Eye Res*. 1987;45:317-326.

57. Wilson RS. Does the lens diameter increase or decrease during accommodation? Human accommodation studies: a new technique using infrared retroillumination video photography and pixel unit measurements. *Transactions of the American Ophthalmology Society*. 1997;95:261-70.

58. Strenk SA, Semmlow JL, Strenk LM, et al. Age-related changes in human ciliary muscle and lens: a magnetic resonance imaging study. *Invest Ophthalmol Vis Sci*. 1999;40:1162-9.

59. Levy NS. The mechanism of accommodation in primates. *Ophthalmology*. 2000;107:625.

60. Levy NS. Comparing MRIs with movement artifact [letter]. *Invest Ophthalmol Vis Sci*. Available at: http//www.iovs.org/cgi/eletters/40/6/1162#EL1. Accessed Feb. 2, 2000.

61. Young T. On the mechanism of the eye. *Phil Trans Soc Lond B Biol Sci*. 1901;92:23-88.

62. Tscherning M. *Physiological Optics*. Philadelphia, Pa: Keystone; 1904:160-189

63. Koomen M, Tousey R, Scolnic R. The spherical aberration of the eye. *J Opt Soc Am A*. 1949;39: 370-6.

64. Van den Brink G. Measurements of the geometrical aberrations of the eye. *Vision Res*. 1962;2:233-244.

65. Jenkins TCA Aberrations of the eye and their effects on vision: Part 1. *Brit J Physiol Optics*. 1963;20:59-91.

66. He JC, Burns SA, Marcos S. Monochromatic aberrations in the accommodated human eye. *Vision Res*. 2000;40:41-48.

67. Artal P, Hoffer H, Williams DR, Aragon JL. Dynamics of ocular aberration during accommodation. Presented at: Optical Society of America Annual Meeting; 1999.

68. Williams DR, Yoon G-Y, Guirao A, Hofer H, Porter J. How far can we extend the limits of human vision? In: MacRae SM, Krueger RR, Applegate RA, eds. *Customized Corneal Ablation: The Quest for Supervision*. Thorofare, NJ: SLACK Incorporated; 2001:25-25.

69. Schachar RA. Retinal imaging aberrometry. *Ophthalmology*. 2002;109:3-4.

70. Krueger RR, Mrochen M, Kaemmerer M, Seiler T. Understanding refraction and accommodation through retinal imaging aberrometry. *Ophthalmology*. 2001;108:674-678.

71. Schachar RA, Cudmore DP. The effect of gravity on the amplitude of accommodation. *Annals of Ophthalmology*. 1994;26:65-70.

72. Vanderploeg JM. Near visual acuity measurements of space shuttle crewmembers. *Aviat Space Environ Med*. 1985;57:492.

73. Rosenflied M, Potello JK, Blustein GH, Jangs C. Comparison of clinical techniques to assess the near accommodative response. *Opt Vis Sci*. 1996;73:382-388.

74. Cross AJ. *Dynamic Skiametry in Theory and Practice*. New York: A. Jay Cross Optical Co; 1911:80-99.

75. Sheard C. *Dynamic Skiametry and Methods of Testing the Accommodation and Convergence of Eyes*. Chicago, Ill: Cleveland Press; 1920.

76. Sheard C. Dynamic retinoscopy. *Am J Optom*. 1929;6:609-23.

77. Hayes HM. Clinical observations with dynamic retinoscopy. *Optometry Weekly*. 1960;51:2243-2246, 2306-2309.

78. Alpern M. Accommodation. In: Davson H, ed. *The Eye*. Vol 3. New York: Academic Press; 1969:217-218.

79. Schachar RA, Wastalu MR, Cudmore, DP. Objective evidence of an increase in the amplitude of accommodation in presbyopes following the scleral expansion band procedure. *Compr Ther*. Submitted.

80. Birnbaum MH. *Optometric Management of Nearpoint Vision Disorders*. Boston, Mass: Butterworth-Heinemann; 1993:229-230.

81. Choi M, Weiss S, Schaeffel F, et al. Laboratory, clinical, and kindergarten test of a new eccentric infrared photorefractor (PowerRefractor). *Optom Vis Sci*. 2000;77:537-548.

82. Noyes HD. *Diseases of the Eye*. New York: William Wood & Co; 1894:241.

83. Kolker AE, Hetherington J. *Becker-Shaffer's Diagnosis and Therapy of the Glaucomas*. 3rd ed. St Louis, Mo: CV Mosby Co; 1970:303-305.

84. Rifkind AW, Yablonski ME, Shuster JJ. Health Canada phase I study to determine the effect of scleral expansion band (SEB) on

ocular hypertension and primary open angle glaucoma. Presented at: American Academy of Ophthalmology Annual Meeting; Nov 13, 2001; New Orleans, La.

85. Roy FH. Surgical reversal of presbyopia. Personal experience of three ophthalmologists. In: Schachar RA, Roy FH, eds. *Presbyopia:* *Cause and Treatment.* The Hague, Netherlands: Kugler Publications; 2001:111-113.

86. Roy FH. Mechanism of accommodation in primates. *Ophthalmology.* 2001;108:1369-1370.

87. Thorburn WM. Occam's razor. *Mind.* 1915;24:287-288.

Chapter 5

Presbyopia and Accommodation

Anatomy, Physiology, and Optics

Luis Alberto Carvalho, PhD; Odemir Martinez Bruno, PhD; Luiz Antonio Vieira de Carvalho, PhD;
Jarbas Caiado Castro, PhD; Wallace Chamon, MD; and Paulo Schor, PhD, MD

This chapter will discuss the anatomy, physiology, and optics involved in the process of accommodation and presbyopia. In the first section we will discuss fundamental concepts of geometrical optics such as Snell's law and the law of reflection; in the second section we will discuss traditional eye models (such as the Helmholtz-Gullstrand schematic eye) and more recent models that include nonspherical surfaces. At the end of this section we present a simple optical model of presbyopia. The third section deals with general characteristics of the lens, and the fourth section explains the optical principle of important instrumentation for anterior segment analysis. Sections five and six explain the different theories of accommodation and presbyopia; and section seven discusses the current clinical approaches for the surgical correction of presbyopia. Finally, in section eight we have included an up-to-date discussion of the controversial and polemic topic of the causes of presbyopia and possible future research approaches.

INTRODUCTION TO GEOMETRIC OPTICS AND BASIC FEATURES OF THE EYE

Light presents itself as an ambiguous phenomenon, behaving in certain occasions as particle (geometric optics or quantum optics) and at other times as waves (physical optics). This makes its study a diverse field of research made up of several areas. For the comprehension of the optics of the eye and the process through which we acquire presbyopia, it is sufficient to study the light through its particle behavior (ie, field of geometric optics). In this section we will present basic concepts in geometrical optics, intended to make a brief revision of the subject (for a complete description of optical geometry we recommend the textbook *Fundamentals of Physics*[1]). These concepts allow us to, at the end of this section, present the eye as an optical device and, furthermore, understand the optical principles underlying accommodation and presbyopia.

RAY TRACING, REFLECTION, AND SNELL'S LAW

If light encounters no other medium through its path it will always propagate in a straight line. If light from a translucent medium encounters an opaque barrier, for example, the phenomenon of *diffuse* reflection occurs. If this barrier has a sufficiently well-pol-

ished surface (such as a mirror), reflection is said to be *specular* and the law of reflection applies to its rays (Figure 1). Note that any given surface may present a combination of both specular and diffuse reflection. In Figure 1 we present a diagram of a perfect specular reflection. The law of reflection states that if an incoming ray (ray 1 in Figure 1) intersects the surface at an angle θ_1 (called angle of incidence, measured relative to the normal vector to this surface [n̂]), the angle between the surface and the outgoing ray (ray 2), θ_2 (called angle of reflection), should be equal.

If the barrier of impact is not an opaque medium, light experiences a phenomenon called *refraction*. To understand the principle of refraction it is essential to understand the concept of *index of refraction*. The index of refraction is a property specific to each material in nature and is simply a measure of the speed of light in vacuum (approximately c = 300,000 km/s) divided by the speed of light in that medium (v). It is usually represented in physics texts by the letter n:

$$n = \frac{c}{v}$$
(equation 1)

A light ray, in order to maintain its energy (associated with its frequency), changes direction when traveling through mediums of different indices of refraction. The mathematical formula that describes this phenomenon is called *Snell's law* and can be written as:

$$n_1\sin\theta_1 = n_2\sin\theta_2$$
(equation 2)

where n_1 and n_2 are the indices of refraction of the anterior (medium 1) and posterior (medium 2) surfaces, respectively; and θ_1 and θ_2 are the angles of the incident ray with the anterior surface normal and the angle of the refracted ray with the negative of the posterior surface normal, respectively (Figure 2). A ray that has an angle of incidence equal to zero ($\theta_1 = 0$) should not experience refraction (ie, $\theta_2 = 0$). This is very typical when studying paraxial optical systems, such as rays entering the eye though the apex of the cornea. These rays do not experience refraction inside the eye. This is why placing very small pin holes in front of a myopic eye seems to correct for myopia. The marginal rays, in this case, do not enter the eye, causing a sensation of ametropy correction to the patient.

As the angle of incidence (θ_1) increases, equation 2 tells us that

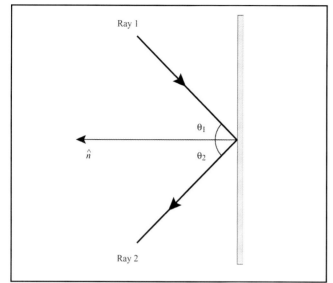

Figure 1. The simple principle of specular reflection. Although a simple phenomenon, it is used in certain ophthalmic equipment, such as keratometers[2-4] and corneal topographers.[5]

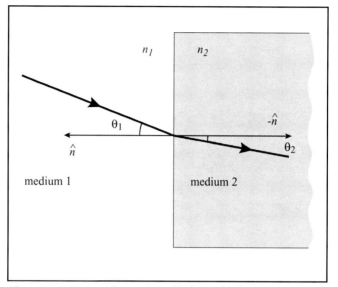

Figure 2. Diagram showing Snell's law of refraction.

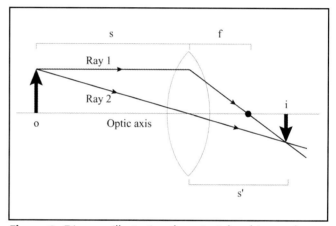

Figure 3. Diagram illustrating the principle of image formation for a thin lens.

$$\frac{1}{f} = \frac{1}{s} + \frac{1}{s'},$$
(equation 3)

the angle of refraction (θ_2) should also increase. In a limiting situation, the angle of refraction becomes a right angle ($\theta_2 = 90°$) and, in this case, the angle of incidence is called the *critical angle* (θ_c). When $n_2 < n_1$ and the angle of incidence reaches the critical angle value (θ_c), the phenomenon of refraction ceases and the *total internal reflection* of the incoming rays may be observed. Snell's law is essential to the visual process. It is the difference in refraction index of our eye components, especially the difference between cornea and the air, that allows our eyes to function as an optical system, "bending" light rays toward the retina. Interestingly, nature designed our optical system to perform optimally in the medium of air. A practical example of this may be experienced by diving and opening our eyes inside a swimming pool. Since water and the cornea have very similar refraction indices, our eyes greatly lose their dioptric power, and images become very blurred. Divers do not experience this because of the thin layer of air inside their masks. Following we will discuss why the shape between mediums is also important to the phenomenon of refraction.

THE THIN LENS

The concept of *thin lens* is important to understand how the eye works as an optical device. As in the first section, the difference in refractive indices promotes the refraction between surfaces, but this is not the only parameter that controls how light "bends" when entering the eye. The curvature of the different eye components is also important. Because the eye components behave essentially as thin lenses, we'll introduce its concept here and the mathematical formula that describes its dioptric power as a function of the refractive indices and curvature.

A lens may be considered thin when its focusing distance is much greater than its diameter. Figure 3 is a diagram of a thin lens and incident and refracted rays. The most basic mathematical equation, which governs the image formation property of a thin lens, is given by:

where f is the distance from the intersection of the marginal ray (ray 1) with the optical axis of the lens, called the *focus distance*; s is the distance from the object to the lens, called *object distance*; and s' is the distance from the image to the lens, called *image distance*. Although Figure 5 is not in scale, these distances should be interpreted as much greater than lens thickness in order for equation 3 to hold. Equation 3 may be deduced by using simple geometry and Snell's law, but it has limited use in the practical sense because it does not use quantities with which visual optics scientists are used to dealing. A more practical approach would be to associate the refractive index and lens curvature to the dioptric power of the lens. This may be accomplished by the well-known (and well-designated, in terms of practical use) *lens maker equation*, given by:

$$\frac{1}{f} = (n_2 - n_1)\left(\frac{1}{r_1} - \frac{1}{r_2}\right)$$
(equation 4)

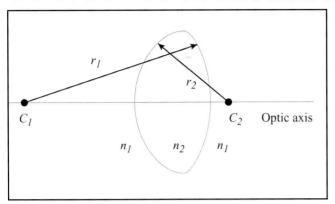

Figure 4. Diagram illustrating the principle of thin lenses according to the parameters of the lens maker equation.

TABLE 1	GULLSTRAND'S REFRACTIVE INDICES*
Eye Component	Refractive Index
Cornea	1.376
Aqueous humor	1.336
Lens	1.409
Vitreous humor	1.336

*Refractive indices of different eye media, as described in Gullstrand's model of the eye.

where the parameters may be seen in Figure 4 (n_1), f is the focal distance, n_2 is the refractive index of the lens, and n_1 is the refractive index of the surrounding media; and r_1 and r_2 are respectively the anterior and posterior radii of curvature of the lens, where the minus sign depends on the sign convention used. Equation 4 is what most texts on geometric optics present for a thin lens embedded in a uniform medium. When considering sequential surfaces separating different media, such as the surfaces of the different components of the eye, a simpler equation may be used, which considers one radius of curvature at a time (Table 1).

This equation is actually derived from equation 4 and is more suitable for description of the human eye. By making the value of the second refractive surface to infinity ($r_2 \to \infty$), equation 4 becomes:

$$\frac{1}{f} = (n_2 - n_1)\left(\frac{1}{r_1}\right)$$

(equation 5)

which describes the focal properties of the each interface and may be applied to each surface successively. Note here that if we write the focal distance in meters, the quantity 1/f becomes the well-known *dioptric power*, more popular in the visual sciences. Also observe that the quantity 1/r is the inverse of the radius of curvature, which is called *curvature* (for a precise and thorough definition of curvature based on rigorous integral and differential calculus please refer to Thomas et al[6]). From this definition of curvature and equation 5 it is possible to conclude that the dioptric power of a refracting surface is directly proportional to the curvature of the surface (the inverse of the radius of curvature) and the difference in refractive indices separating it from the surrounding medium. From this conclusion, one may notice (and even perform some basic algebra) from equation 5 and Table 1 that the greatest difference in ($n_2 - n_1$) among interfaces of the eye will happen between air ($n_1 = 1$) and the cornea ($n_2 = 1.376$). This is basically why the cornea is such an important component of the eye and also why refractive surgeries may correct very high ametropes even with minimal tissue ablation. Equation 5 also tells us why corneal topography is such an important tool for pre- and postanalysis of the net amount of change in the refractive power of the eye. In the next section we will describe many of the current eye models used for calculation of total and partial eye refraction properties. We shall then be able to analyze quantitatively the individual importance of each optical component to the overall refraction of the eye and also understand how, using the thin lens model, the crystalline focuses, as well as the geometric optics involved in presbyopia.

THE HUMAN EYE AS AN OPTICAL SYSTEM

As we saw in the previous section, a simplification of the lens maker equation (equation 5) may be used to explain the refractive power between single refracting interfaces. Although it was not demonstrated quantitatively, this simple "thin lens model" explains the importance of the cornea to the overall refraction of the eye. In this section we'll introduce several schematic eye models (some of them more than a century old and some very recent). The purpose of doing so is to give us a solid understanding of the basic parameters for modeling each surface of each component of the eye. In turn, this will furnish tools that may be used to quantitatively determine the refractive contribution of each surface and, therefore, the optical importance of each one to the total dioptric power of the globe. It will also allow us to understand how the geometric shape of the crystalline may be changing during accommodation and give us insight for better understanding the different theories that coexist for presbyopia, which will be discussed later in the chapter.

SCHEMATIC MODELS OF THE EYE

The modeling of eye components is an important field for the study of vision. It allows us, among other things, to understand the importance of each component in the overall quality of the retinal image. Historically, after Gauss (1841) established the basic laws that govern the formation of images, many theoretical models of the eye have been proposed. The first model was proposed by Moser (1844). Nevertheless, as Moser assumed a value of 1.384 for the effective refractive index of the lens, the focal point was localized behind the retina. This under-refracted model was corrected by Listing, who calculated a very realistic theoretical eye that was modified later by Helmholtz and Gullstrand.[7] In the following subsections, we present some of the most popular schematic eye models to date.

Helmholtz-Laurence Schematic Eye

The Helmholtz-Laurence eye model is one of the most precise models available[8] because it contains all optical surfaces found in the biological eye (Figure 5). Table 2 lists all the parameters of this eye model. This model designates refractive indices to the different eye components that do not necessarily correspond to the true measured values, but the overall properties of this model resemble very closely those of the human eye.

The schematic eye shown in Figure 5 corresponds to the eye in its relaxed state (ie, with the crystalline lens in its greatest focusing distance). For the lens in its shortest focusing distance, the curvature of the anterior surface of the crystalline increases considerably (ie, the radius of curvature decreases [from 9 to 6 mm]).

TABLE 2 — PARAMETERS FOR THE HELMHOLTZ-LAURENCE SCHEMATIC EYE

Optical Surface/ Element	Defining Symbol	Distance From Corneal Vertex (mm)	Radius of Curvature of Surface (mm)	Refractive Index	Refractive Power (D)
Cornea	S_1	-	+8	-	+41.6
Lens	L	-	-	1.45	+30.5
Anterior surface	S_2	+3.6	+10	-	+12.3
Posterior surface	S_3	+7.2	-6	-	+20.5
Eye	-	-	-	-	+66.6
Front focal plane	F	-13.04	-	-	-
Back focal plane	F'	+22.38	-	-	-
Front principle plane	H	+1.96	-	-	-
Back principle plane	H'	+2.38	-	-	-
Front nodal plane	N	+6.96	-	-	-
Back nodal plane	N'	+7.38	-	-	-
Anterior chamber	AC	-	-	1.333	-
Vitreous chamber	VC	-	-	1.333	-
Entrance pupil	E_nP	+3.04	-	-	-
Exit pupil	E_xP	+3.72	-	-	-

Gullstrand's Schematic Eye

The Swedish ophthalmologist Allvar Gullstrand (1862-1930) conducted important research in the field of physiology and in 1911 received the Nobel prize for his work regarding the eye as an optical element. A simplified version of his schematic eye, well known and used today, is described below.

Figure 6 shows that in this model the cornea is treated as a single refracting surface, just as the previous model from Helmholtz-Laurence. In Gullstrand's nonsimplified model, the cornea is considered to have two surfaces. The crystalline lens in Figure 5 has a refraction index of 1.413, and the distance from cornea to macula is fixed at 24.17 mm, which guarantees a perfect image formation on the retina. This model has special application to the calculation of intraocular lenses (IOLs) for cataract patients or calculation of corrective spectacles for aphakic (no crystalline lens) patients. This happens because although it treats the cornea, vitreous humor, and aqueous humor with simplicity, it maintains the anterior and posterior surface of the crystalline lens.

Emsley Schematic Eye

This is one of the simplest eye models available because it involves a single refractive surface. Due to its simplicity, it is widely used in undergraduate courses in optometry, ophthalmology, and the visual sciences in general. Parameters of this model are illustrated in Figure 7.

The axial distance for this eye is 22.22 mm. The principle points H and H' and the nodal points N and N', previously separated in Gullstrand's schematic eye, are now fused into the principle points H and N, with H fixed where the cornea intersects the optic axis. The net dioptric power of the eye is due to the single corneal surface and has value of 60 D. The refractive index of the entire eye is 1.33.

Schwiegerling Schematic Eye

With the improvement of corneal topography techniques starting in the 1990s, the inclusion of corneal surface data into schemat-

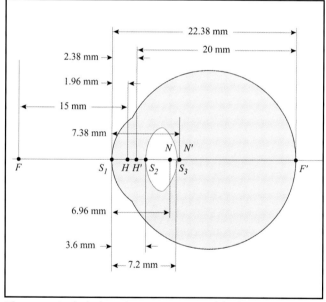

Figure 5. Helmholtz schematic eye model after modification by Laurence.

ic eye models became possible. This is an important step in the development of more precise eye models since the cornea contributes to approximately two-thirds of the overall refractive power. In 1995, Greivenkamp and colleagues[9] proposed a model that uses four refracting, nonspherical surfaces. The parameters of this model, used by Sarver and colleagues[10] for implementing a computer simulation of visual acuity tests, is shown in Table 3.

The Complete Theoretical Eye

Figure 8 shows the complete theoretical eye proposed by Le Grand and El Hage[7] in their article in *Physiological Optics*.

The dioptric power of the cornea is D_c = 42.36 D and the abscis-

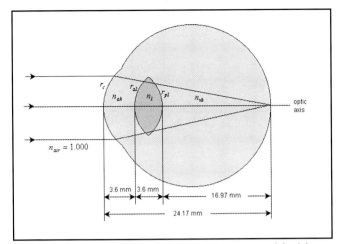

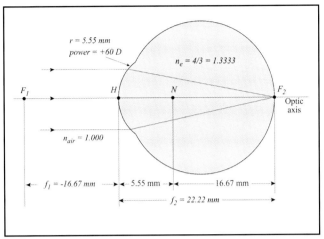

Figure 6. Gullstrand's schematic model in its simplified form. The axial length is chosen such that paraxial rays focus on the retina for the emmetropic eye. r_c = radius of curvature of the cornea = 7.8 mm; r_{al} = anterior radius of curvature of the crystalline = 10 mm; r_{pl} = posterior radius of curvature of the crystalline = -6 mm; n_{ah} = refractive index of aqueous humor = 1.336; n_l = refractive index of crystalline lens = 1.413; n_{vh} = refractive index of vitreous humor = 1.336.

Figure 7. Emsley's schematic eye.

TABLE 3	PARAMETERS FOR THE SCHWIEGERLING EYE MODEL			
Surface	Radius (mm)	Conic, p	Length (mm)	Refraction Index
Anterior cornea	7.8	0.75	0.55	1.3771
Posterior cornea	6.5	0.75	3.05	1.3374
Anterior lens	11.03	-3.30	4.0	1.42
Posterior lens	-5.72	-1.17	16.60	1.336

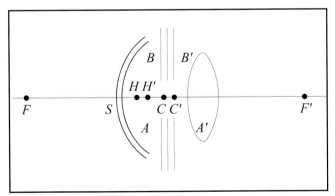

Figure 8. Diagram of the complete theoretical eye. C: center of entrance pupil AB; C': center of the exit pupil A'B'; between them, the real pupil.

sa of its image $\overline{SH}_1$ = -0.06 mm. The power of the crystalline lens is D_1 = 21.78 D and the abscissa of its object is $\overline{SH}_1$ = -0.06 mm. We have then the reduced distance δ = (6.02 + 0.06). $10^{-3}/1.3374$ = 4.55 mm and the overall eye power of D = D_c + D_1 + δD_1 = 59.94 D. In this model the cornea contributes to approximately two-thirds of the overall eye power.

The focal distances may be deduced from the total power as:
Object: HF = -n/D = -1/59.94 = 16.68 mm
Image: H'F' = n'/D = 1.3336/59.94 = 22.29 mm
The positions of the principle points may be given by:
Object: $\dfrac{H_1H}{n}$ = $\dfrac{\delta D_2}{D}$, where n = 1 e D_2 = D_1,
H_1H = 1.65 mm such that $\overline{SH}$ = 1.59 mm
Image: $\dfrac{H'_2H'}{n'}$ = $\dfrac{\delta D_1}{D}$, where n' = 1.336 e D_1 = D_c
H'_2H' = 4.29 mm, consequently $\overline{SH}$ = 1.91 mm,
Finally, the abscissa of the focal points may be written as:
Object: $\overline{SF}$ = -15.09 mm
Image: $\overline{SF'}$ = 24.20 mm
Each of the eye models presented here has its own advantages and disadvantages. The simpler models are useful for didactic purposes and for simple calculations of eye correction lenses, although they serve very little in terms of the analysis of the specific contribution of individual components to image quality; the more complex models are hard to explain to students and require more elaborate algebra, but on the other hand they may work well to model higher-order optical aberrations of the eye,[10] the contribution of different surfaces, and the inclusion of surfaces that do not necessarily have to be spherical or even symmetrical, and so forth. Recent

eye models have become so sophisticated that one may use wavefront aberration data[11] to computationally model the retinal image and other parameters (point spread function [PSF], optical transfer function [OTF]). In is not in the scope of this chapter to introduce these interesting topics related to advanced optics. For this purpose, please refer to Born et al.[12]

In general terms, eye models became sufficiently sophisticated to model all basic low-order aberrations (eg, myopia, hyperopia, astigmatism) and some of the higher-order aberrations (eg, coma). Although these are common aberrations, they are all considered to be static aberrations (ie, the eye is considered to be unaccommodated). Consequently, they do not include the aberrations induced by accommodation. Furthermore, they do not include the various stages of accommodation of the eye.

A SIMPLE OPTICAL MODEL OF PRESBYOPIA

As mentioned, the crystalline lens may be considered a thin lens and therefore will obey the relation in equation 5. Let's analyze this relation more carefully. Equation 5 states that the dioptric power of a surface is directly proportional to the difference in refractive index of the separating media and inversely proportional to the radius of curvature of the surface. If we consider that the aqueous humor and the vitreous humor have approximately the same index of refraction (~1.336), then the refractive properties of the crystalline lens may be described by equation 4 (ie, the crystalline may be interpreted as a thin lens with index of refraction 1.413 situated inside a media of uniform index of refraction 1.336).

If we substitute these values in equation 5 plus the values for radius of curvature of anterior and posterior surfaces of the Gullstrand unaccommodated eye model, we'll get:

$$D_{ul} = \frac{1}{f} = (n_2 - n_1)\left(\frac{1}{r_1} - \frac{1}{r_2}\right) = 10^3(1.413 - 1.336)\left(\frac{1}{10} + \frac{1}{6}\right) = 20.53\,D$$

(equation 6)

For the completely accommodated eye we have:

$$D_{ul} = \frac{1}{f} = (n_2 - n_1)\left(\frac{1}{r_1} - \frac{1}{r_2}\right) = 10^3(1.413 - 1.336)\left(\frac{1}{5.33} + \frac{1}{5.33}\right) = 28.89\,D$$

(equation 7)

By subtraction of 6 from 7, we may conclude that for the Gullstrand eye model the crystalline lens has an amplitude of accommodation of 8.36 D. If we consider the dioptric power of the simplified Gullstrand cornea:

$$D_c = \frac{1}{f} = (n_2 - n_1)\left(\frac{1}{r_c}\right) = 10^3(1.336 - 1.000)\left(\frac{1}{7.8}\right) = 43.074\,D$$

(equation 8)

Therefore, the total power for the unaccommodated eye is $D_{u\_eye} = 20.53 + 43.07 = 63.6\,D$, and for the accommodated eye $D_{a\_eye} = 28.89 + 43.07 = 71.96\,D$.

Notice that these are only approximate calculations for a theoretical eye; even so, they resemble quite closely the mean values for the real biological eye.

There is an important definition based on the amplitude of accommodation of the eye: the *near point* and the *far point*. The near point is the closest point that the totally accommodated eye can focus, and the far point is the furthest point that the totally unaccommodated eye can focus. Of course, the location of these points depends on the ametropia and amplitude of accommodation of the

Age	Accommodation Amplitude (D)
10	11
15	10.3
20	9.5
25	8.6
30	7.6
35	6.5
40	5.3
45	3.5
50	2.1
55	1.5
60	1.2
65	1.1
70	1.0

TABLE 4 ACCOMMODATION AMPLITUDE*

*Accommodation amplitude for different ages. Mean values from 2000 subjects by Duane.[13]

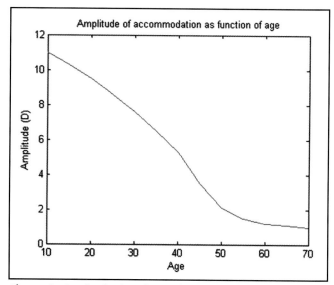

Figure 9. Graph of values from Table 4.

eye. For the very young and emmetropic, the far point is farther than 6 m and the near point may be as close as 25 cm.

Although the calculations here were made for a schematic eye, our amplitude of accommodation value (8.36 D) very closely resembles the mean value for a subject of age 25 from measurements made in 2000. Subjects by Duane in 1912[13] are listed in Table 4 and Figure 9.

These models do not account for presbyopia. Schematic eyes that include the crystalline lens and that account for accommodation[14] only include values for anterior and posterior lens radii for both the totally unaccommodated and totally accommodated eye. None of them tell us what is happening with the curvature in between the minimum and maximum accommodation ranges and do not precisely describe the changes in indices of refraction of the different layers of the crystalline, as postulated by Koretz.[15]*

---

*Although Koretz has theoretically suggested the change in refractive index of the lens with age, recent direct measurements[16] along the optic axis using an invasive optic fiber sensor have shown no significant age-dependent changes.

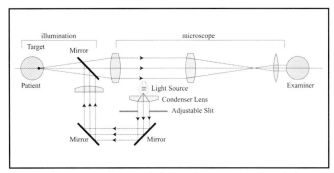

Figure 10. General view of the optical system of a slit lamp.

We can construct a simple optical model of presbyopia using Gullstrand's simplified eye. This can be done by fixing the value of the posterior radius of curvature of the lens, which is known in practice to vary little during accommodation[17] and let only the anterior lens curvature vary. Using the same equations (4 to 8) we could find each value of anterior radius of curvature for each age between 10 and 70 (in steps of 5 years) that fit to the dioptric power values given by Duane's measurements (see Table 4). We can then interpolate this curve and therefore have a theoretical model of how the anterior lens curvature behaves throughout age, accounting for the progressive loss in power.

To understand the principles that may explain presbyopia, we must look into the forces that act over the crystalline lens to make it flatter or more curved, the mechanism through which these forces are applied, the physiological and physical changes of the crystalline and its different layers throughout life, and so forth. These and other subjects will be explored in more detail later in the chapter.

OPTICAL INSTRUMENTS FOR THE ANALYSIS OF THE CRYSTALLINE LENS

Some of the basic ophthalmic equipment used in eye diagnosis for collecting information from the anterior segment is discussed below. This is an important subject because it gives the vision science student knowledge of the optical and mechanical principles behind many instruments in daily use and also because these are the current tools used to investigate the lens and causes of presbyopia.

THE CONVENTIONAL SLIT LAMP

The conventional slit lamp (SL) is one of the most commonly used instruments in any eye clinic, hospital, or vision research lab. The optical system of the SL is composed of two parts (Figure 10): an amplification system (microscope) and an illumination system. The illumination system is composed of a white, high-intensity light, a condenser for light diffusion, and a slit with mechanical adjustment of width. Depending on brand and model, the illumination may also have several filters of different colors that allow different applications, such as the excitation of fluorescein with blue light. The magnification system is composed of a set of magnifying lenses that normally provide magnifications between 15 and 40 times.

When compared to other traditional magnifying instruments, such as the surgical microscope, the moveable illumination in the form of a slit is what makes the slit lamp a perfect microscope for

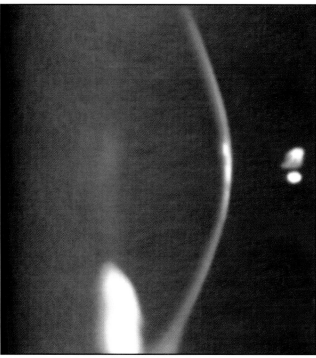

Figure 11. Keratoconus, as seen from a conventional slit lamp. A typical characteristic is a very fine, stromal, oblique striae (Vogt's lines) that disappears when submitted to an external pressure on the globe.

studying the eye. By varying the width of the slit and the angle of illumination it is possible to see details of the eye that would be impossible without these features. For this reason, the SL is an essential instrument for the vision professional.

As an example of application of the conventional SL, Figure 11 shows a photograph taken on a Zeiss SL of a cornea with keratoconus. The SL examination, together with the usual corneal topography and keratometry exams, helps in the early diagnosis of keratoconus.

Although the traditional SL is an excellent tool for the general diagnosis of the human eye, its optical design does not allow visualization of transversal sections of components of the eye other than the cornea. A modification of the SL that allows for this type of examination is described below. This instrument is an important tool for lens diagnosis.

THE SCHEIMPFLUG SLIT LAMP

The Scheimpflug SL is named after the inventor of the optical method for which it is used, Theodore Scheimpflug, an Austrian general. Scheimpflug invented this optical principle for adaptation in cameras that were hung in balloons and used to take landscape photographs from war fields. After careful analysis of the photographs, Scheimpflug could decide on better strategies of attack and invasion. The invention was patented in 1904[18] and since then has been used in several applications of photography, especially those that require a great depth of field. These cameras are still used for documentation of skyscrapers.

The principle of the Scheimpflug camera is illustrated in Figure 12. The diagram illustrates the optical principle defined by Scheimpflug, known as the *Scheimpflug rule*. In conventional cam-

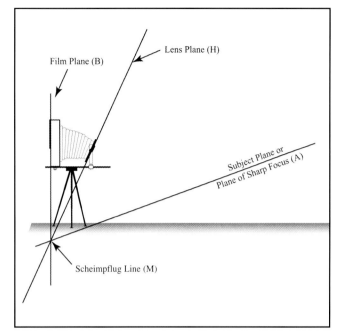

Figure 12. Principle of the Scheimpflug camera.

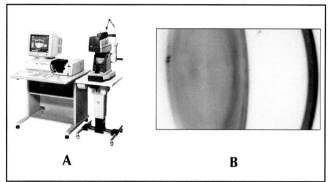

Figure 13. A: Commercial version (Nidek EAS 1000). B: Photograph obtained with this instrument; the lens and cornea can be seen. In such digitized images, it is possible to amplify and process the internal region of the lens, allowing for the analysis of internal structures like the embryonic nucleus.

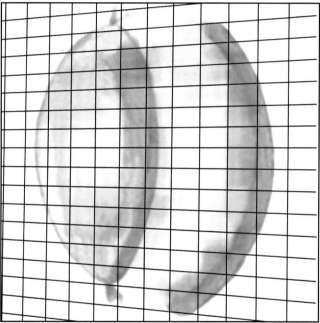

Figure 14. Typical illustration of photographs obtained from Brown using the Scheimpflug SL. Notice that the grid is distorted because of the Scheimpflug optical set-up. Brown empirically calibrated his images and used this information to correct distortions. In this way, he could determine the width, curvature, diameter, and other properties of the lens during accommodation for targets at different distances from the nonexamined eye.

eras, the object (photographic film) plane, lens plane, and subject plane are always parallel to each other, whereas in the Scheimpflug camera these planes intersect in a straight line. When the film plane and the subject plane intersect at a right angle, a 1:1 image to subject plane is achieved. As we have pointed out, one of the advantages of the Scheimpflug camera when photographing the eye is that one can take pictures along the optical axis. For a deeper understanding of the Scheimpflug principle, please refer to the work of Mayer.[19]

It was only in the 1970s that researchers specialized in cataract under the leadership of professor Otto Hockwin (Germany) in collaboration with an optical manufacturer to develop the first system for ophthalmic imaging based on the Scheimpflug principle. Because this system also uses the Scheimpflug principle, it became known as the Scheimpflug slit lamp. The first prototypes used conventional photographic films, which were recently replaced by digital imaging devices, allowing a great amount of images to be stored on computer disks.

The advantage of Scheimpflug SL compared to the conventional SL is that it yields clear images of the anterior segment, along with precise images of the corneal and lens profiles (Figure 13).

From the available instruments for anterior segment analysis (magnetic resonance, phakometry), the one that provides greater resolution is the Scheimpflug SL. Brown[17] was one of the pioneer researchers in the extraction of quantitative information about the process of accommodation from Scheimpflug images.

Brown used a projecting system together with Scheimpflug's principle to acquire images of the lens with a scaled grid (Figure 14). Due to unavoidable distortions caused by the Scheimpflug optics, Brown had to make empirical corrections on his images. Upon doing so, he could precisely determine lens position and geometry as a function of age and accommodation. This information has provided important clues about the aging of the crystalline lens and the process of presbyopia, discussed later in this chapter.

Since Brown's first experiments with conventional photographic techniques in the early 1970s, many other researchers have applied digital imaging and computational processing techniques to construct mathematical models for the process and geometry of accommodation.[20] A recent work by Cook et al[21] used digitized images provided by a frame grabber installed on a Scheimpflug SL. Although this hardware configuration is not new, Cook used sophisticated image-processing techniques to find the analytic expressions for the profile of anterior and posterior lens surfaces.

Other researchers[22] used processing techniques that depend on pixels (gray level) to define a region of interest on the image. Koretz argues that such techniques fail when applied to lens images due to typical noise. He used a transform, the *Hough transform* (a very well-known technique among computational vision scientists), which does not "break-up" or "lose" itself in the presence of local irregularities. There are several descriptions of this technique in the literature. For indepth information on algorithms, please refer to Gonzalez et al.[23]

Cook obtained the parameters of analytic curves that describe the profile of the lens. These analytic curves are of the form:

$$y = v + \frac{(x - \tau)^2}{\vartheta}$$

(equation 9)

which are parabolas of the form $y(x)$, where (τ, v) is the vertex location (the lens apex) and ϑ is a parameter equal to twice the radius of curvature, ranging from 300 to 3000 pixels. Angular orientation could be eliminated because images were aligned to the Cartesian plane. Precision, using this technique to obtain anterior and posterior lens, was 0.7% and 0.6%, and rays of curvature could be obtained with a precision of 0.6%. It is important to note that these results were only possible after careful correction of the inherent Scheimpflug image distortions.

DISCUSSION

The process through which the eye focuses images from distant and close range onto the retina is quite well understood from the optical engineering perspective. The cornea has a fixed dioptric power because neither its shape nor refractive index changes during the visual process; on the other hand, the lens is the optical component responsible for adjusting the focus for objects located at different distances, a process that became known as accommodation. When it comes to the accommodation process, the analogies of the human eye with optical instruments become less accurate. Human optically engineered instruments, such as cameras, contain moveable optical parts (lenses, mirrors, prisms) that all act together in order to change the focusing distance. The human eye is different. It has a deformable lens, the crystalline, a genially engineered lens that changes power by varying its shape and refractive index, a process that we humans cannot yet imitate or understand well. Nature probably "designed" the best solution for a static system (ie, an optical organ that had to have varying focus but no moveable pieces), indeed a very interesting approach toward an "unbreakable" system with minimum maintenance requirements.

From the physiological point of view, the process of accommodation is still a topic of discussion. In other words, we know why the lens changes its shape and optical power, but we really do not understand how. We do not know all the forces that are acting upon the lens in order to change its shape, although there are many clues. Helmholtz viewed the capsule as a deformable "bag," hung up by the zonule fibers with the function of simply holding an elastic lens and transmitting the tensions from the zonule to the lens. As the zonules relax as a consequence of less ciliary muscle tension, the "bag" would release the tension upon the inner lens, which in turn would return to its relaxed, more curved, thicker state. This is a beautiful and simple theory that explains a lot about the process of accommodation; and presbyopia theories may be built upon it. Nevertheless, it is important to notice that it is an old theory which, in principle, is irrelevant, but we have to take into account that the

materials and methods available in those days were much less accurate than what we have had for the past decades and today. This means that we may have the ability to look more carefully into the anatomy, physiology, and optics of the entire accommodation process in order to confirm or refute Helmholtz's theory. This is what some researchers like Glasser, Koretz, and Schachar have done and have found interesting information that was unavailable in Helmholtz's time.

Koretz and colleagues found an interesting phenomenon that occurs with the zonule fibers as we grow older. In young people, these fibers are attached at the equator of the capsule; and when they contract, the tension is parallel to the equator of the lens (ie, the capsule is pushed from its edges, causing a compression force in a perpendicular direction on the lens. The lens is "squeezed" inside the capsule). With aging, the position of attachment of the zonule fibers changes toward an unexpected direction, the center of the capsule. This seems surprising because in this configuration the transmission of tension from fibers to capsule becomes inefficient when the lens is unaccommodated (more tension). On the other hand, when the ciliary body becomes more tense, the zonule fibers should release their tension upon the capsule. This doesn't occur efficiently, since the zonules are in a overtensed positioning. Given these facts, Koretz and colleagues propose that presbyopia may be due essentially to a geometrical disorder in which the prevalent causes would be the change in size and angular relations between the lens and zonules.

Schachar's theory completely opposes that of Helmholtz's and similar theories. He argues that the tension of the zonule fibers increases lens power instead of decreasing it. Although a more recent theory, the complications seen in surgical cases in an attempt to correct presbyopia and lack of evidence indicate that this theory, in order to survive, must undergo further research. In this sense, we may affirm that Helmholtz is the most accepted theory to date.

Glasser and colleagues, in a recent and very methodic work,[24] measured lens hardness as a function of age. Their results show the importance of lens hardening with age as a main factor in the progression of presbyopia, contradicting other researchers that had even discarded lens hardening as a major factor. Another important result from this research is that they did not find evidence of considerable change in refraction index with aging, as the lens paradox theory states, although measurements were made in in vitro lenses.

A thin lens may well approximate the crystalline lens, and geometric optics show us where the focal points are for different lens powers and object distances. Although simple schematic eye models serve us for IOL and other calculations, they do not include physiological, anatomical, or optical properties of the inner lens, such as variation of index of refraction with age, different layers, and during accommodation itself. These are only factors regarding the optical properties of the lens. Other factors such as capsule function, viscoelastic properties, zonule function and geometry, and ciliary muscle function are all major components in the "puzzle" of accommodation and presbyopia, and they are not completely understood yet. We believe that understanding the causes of presbyopia will come from a theory that explains the dynamics of the interaction of all these components, as well as a theory based on the observation of real-time, in vivo human eyes during accommodation. Perhaps we will see this happening in a near future when magnetic resonance instrumentation will have resolutions that allow even zonule fibers to be distinguishable.

SUMMARY

In this chapter we have presented certain basic concepts that allow us a better comprehension of the optical, physiological, and anatomical principles that are related to presbyopia. Principles of geometrical optics, eye modeling, lens anatomy and instrumentation, and surgical procedures for a possible correction of presbyopia were presented. The overall conclusion is that the subject of presbyopia and its causes is still an intricate theme, far from being a consensus among researchers in the field.

ACKNOWLEDGMENTS

We would like to thank the Instituto de Fisica de São Carlos SP, Brazil; Escola Paulista de Medicina, UNIFESP, São Paulo, Brazil; FAPESP (Fundação de Apoio à Pesquisa do Estado de São Paulo), process number 01/03132-8.

REFERENCES

1. Halliday D, Resnick R, Walker J. *Fundamentals of Physics*. 6th ed. New York: John Willey & Sons; 2001.
2. Bicas HEA. *Sobre um Novo Princípio de Ceratometria (e da sua Aplicação através de um Instrumento Servindo também a outras Finalidades, adaptável aos Biomicroscópios)*. Brazil: Departamento de Oftalmologia; 1967.
3. Carvalho L, Tonissi SA, Castro JC. Preliminary tests and construction of a computerized quantitative surgical keratometer. *J Cataract Refract Surg*. 1999;25:821-826.
4. Schor P. *Idealização, Desenho, Construção e Teste de um Ceratômetro Cirúrgico Quantitativo, Tese Apresentada à Universidade Federal de São Paulo*. São Paulo, Brazil: Escola Paulista de Medicina para obtenção do título de Doutor em Medicina; 1997.
5. Klyce SD. Computer-assisted corneal topography, high resolution graphics presentation and analyses of keratoscopy. *Invest Ophthalmol Vis Sci*. 1984;25:426-435.
6. Thomas GB, Finney RL. *Calculus and Analytic Geometry*. 7th ed. Boston, Mass: Addison-Wesley; 1988.
7. Le Grand Y, El Hage SG. *Physiological Optics*. New York: Springer-Verlag; 1980.
8. Pedrotti LS, Pedrotti FL. *Optics and Vision*. New York: Prentice Hall; 1998.
9. Greivenkamp JE, Schwiegerling J, Miller JM, Mellinger MD. Visual acuity modeling using optical raytracing of schematic eyes. *Am J Ophthalmol*. 1995;120,227-240.
10. Sarver EJ, Applegate RA. Modeling and predicting visual outcomes with VOL-3D. *J Refract Surg*. 2000;16:611-616.
11. Liang J, Grimm B, Goelz S, Bille JF. Objective measurement of wave aberrations of the human eye with the use of a Hartmann-Shack wave-front sensor. *J Opt Soc Am*. 1994;14(11):1949-1957.
12. Born M, Wolf E. *Principles of Optics*. 6th ed. London: Pergamon Press; 1975.
13. Duane A. Normal values of the accommodation at all ages. *JAMA*. 1912;59:1010-1013.
14. Glasser A, Campbell MCW. Presbyopia and the optical changes in the human lens with age. *Vision Res*. 1998;38:209-229.
15. Koretz JF, Handelman GH. How the human eye focuses. *Sci Am*. 1998;256(7):92-99.
16. Pierscionek BK. Refractive index counters in the human lens. *Exp Eye Res*. 1997;64:887-893.
17. Brown N. The change in shape and internal form of the lens of the eye on accommodation. *Exp Eye Res*. 1973;15:441-459.
18. Scheimpflug T. Improved method for the systematic alteration or distortion of plane pictures and images by means of lenses and mirrors for photography and other purposes. Patent #1196. England: British Office of Patents; 1904.
19. Mayer H. Theodor Scheimpflug. *Ophthalmic Res*. 1994;26:S3-9.
20. Koretz JF, Handleman GH. Modeling age-related accommodative loss on the human eye. *Mathematical Modeling*. 1986;7:1003-1014.
21. Cook CA, Koretz JF. Methods to obtain quantitative parametric descriptions of the optical surfaces of the human crystalline lens from Scheimpflug slit-lamp images. *J Opt Soc Am A*. 1998;15(6):1473-1485.
22. Hachiha A, Simon S, Samson J, Hanna K. The use of gray level information and fitting techniques for precise measurements of corneal curvature. *Comput Vis Graph Image Process*. 1989;47:131-164.
23. Gonzalez RC, Woods RE. *Digital Image Processing*. Menlo Park, Calif: Addison-Wesley; 1992.
24. Glasser A, Campbell MCW. Biometric, optical and physical changes in the isolated human crystalline lens with age in relation to presbyopia. *Vision Res*. 1999;38:209-229.

BIBLIOGRAPHY

Augusteyn RC, Koretz JF. A possible structure for crystalline. *Federation of European Biomedical Societies (FEB)*. 1987;222(1):1-5.

Beers APA, Van der Heijde GL. In vivo determination of the biochemical properties of the component elements of the accommodative mechanism. *Vision Res*. 1994;34:2897-2905.

Burd JH, Judge SJ, Flavell MJ. Mechanics of accommodation of the human eye. *Vision Res*. 1999;9:1591-1595.

Fincham EF. The mechanism of accommodation. *Br J Ophthalmol*. 1937;8(Suppl):5-80.

Fisher RF. The elastic constants of the human lens. *J Physiol*. 1971;212:147-180.

Fisher RF. Elastic constants of the human lens capsule. *J Physiol*. 1969;201:1-19.

Greivenkamp JE, Schwiegerling J, Miller JM, Mellinger MD. Visual acuity modeling using optical raytracing of schematic eyes. *Am J Ophthalmol*. 1995;120:227-240.

Hachiha A, Simon S, Samson J, Hanna K. The use of gray level information and fitting techniques for precise measurements of corneal curvature. *Comput Vis Graph Image Process*. 1989;47:131-164.

Helmholtz von HH. Handbuch der physiologishen optik. In: Southall, JPC, trans. *Helmholtz's Treatise on Physiological Optics*. New York: Dover; 1962.

Nordmann J, Mack G, Mack G. Nucleus of the human lens III. Its separation, its hardness. *Ophthalmic Res*. 1974;6:216-222.

Pau H, Kranz J. The increasing sclerosis of the human lens with age and its relevance to accommodation and presbyopia. *Graefe's Arch Clin Exp Ophthalmol*. 1991;229:294-296.

Schachar RA. Cause and treatment of presbyopia with a method for increasing the amplitude of accommodation. *Annals of Ophthalmology*. 1992;4,445-452.

Schachar RA, Black TD, Kash RL, Cudmore DP, Schanzlin DJ. The mechanism of accommodation and presbyopia in the primate. *Annals of Ophthalmology*. 1995;27:58-67.

Schachar RA, Huang T, Huang X. Mathematic proof of Schachar's hypothesis of accommodation. *Annals of Ophthalmology*. 1993;25(1):5-9.

Schachar RA, Tello C, Cudmore DP, Liebmann JM, Black TD, Ritch R. In vivo increase of the human lens equatorial diameter during accommodation. *Am J Physiol*. 1996;271:R670-R676.

Tamm E, Croft M, Jungkunz W, Lütjen-Drecoll E, Kaufman PL. Age-related loss of ciliary muscle mobility in the rhesus monkey. Role of the choroid. *Arch Ophthalmol*. 1992;110:871-876.

Tamm E, Lütjen-Drecoll E, Jungkunz W, Rohen JW. Posterior attachment of ciliary muscle in young, accommodating old, presbyopic monkeys. *Invest Ophthalmol Vis Sci*. 1991;32:1678-1692.

Tamm S, Tamm E, Rohen JW. Age-related changes of the human ciliary muscle. A quantitative morphometric study. *Mechanisms of Aging and Development*. 1992;62:209-221.

Weale RA. Presbyopia toward the 20th century. *Surv Ophthalmol*. 1989;34:15-30.

Chapter 6

The New Mechanism for Laser Presbyopia Reversal and Accommodation

J.T. Lin, PhD and Vivek Kadambi, MD

INTRODUCTION

Accommodation is the ability to focus on near objects through controlled changes in the shape and thickness of the crystalline lens and is mediated by ciliary muscle contraction. To correct presbyopia, it is a fundamental necessity to understand how accommodation occurs and how it changes the optical and tissue parameters of an aged eye. The effectiveness of ciliary body contraction for lens relaxation (or accommodation) may be influenced by the combined aging factors, including lens property changes (index, size, thickness, and curvature), tissue elastic changes (in sclera and ciliary), and the zonular tension change. We note that all the methods using scleral expansion techniques (scleral expansion band [SEB], silicone expansion plug [SEP], anterior ciliary sclerotomy [ACS], supraciliary segment implant [SCI]) suffer from major regression due to tissue healing, whereas the laser method (laser presbyopia reversal [LAPR]) presented here showed a minimum regression even after 24 months follow-up. There is a fundamental difference between the mechanism behind LAPR and those behind nonlaser methods. The Lin-Kadambi hypothesis proposing increasing elasticity of the subconjunctival tissue fills in the gap of laser-ablated sclera area. This filling process also prevents the scleral tissue from healing, which closes the gap and leads to regression. We also present the two tension components that contribute to lens accommodation (curvature changes) and anterior movement of the lens.

AGING EFFECTS

It was found by Scheimpflug techniques that lens thickness increased steadily and linearly with increasing age, whereas anterior chamber depth decreased linearly with age. Lens paradox was reported by the radii curvature decreases of the lens by aging[1] and the anterior shift of the zonules.[2]

Many theories have been proposed for the age-related loss of accommodation, including:

+ Lens-based theories
+ Geometric theories
+ Lenticular theories
+ Multifactor theory

The factors that may contribute to changes in overall refractive power include the corneal shape and thickness, lens shape and thickness, anterior and vitreous chamber depth, and globe axial length.

The correlations between lens shape and lens placement (anterior chamber depth, lens thickness, and anterior segment length) were recently reported.[3] The anterior chamber depth decreases while lens thickness increases with increasing age. However, the sum of the two (anterior segment length) appeared to remain approximately constant with increasing age. The change in lens thickness with age was due almost entirely to an increase in anterior and posterior cortical thickness. This lens growth is due to the addition of lens fiber cells to the superficial cortex, and the volume of the lens nucleus remains constant.

Fisher[4] showed that the elasticity of the human lens capsule decreases with aging. He also showed that the human lens becomes increasingly resistant to the effects of stretching forces applied through the ciliary body/zonular complex. A geometric disorder attributed to changes in the size and volume of the lens, and the angle of zonular insertion onto the lens was proposed by Koretz and Handelman.[5] Weale[6] introduced a multifactorial basis for presbyopia in which the age-related loss of accommodation was attributed to decreased zonular tension resulting from the continuing growth of the lens, which changed the lens capsule and lens matrix elastic properties.

A change in the refractive index gradient of the lens cortex has been suggested[5,7] to be a substantial factor contributing to the progression of presbyopia. Pierscionek and Weale[8] proposed that because of the increased thickness of the lens and the anterior shift of the zonular attachments, presbyopia is a failure of the lens to maintain a flattened state. Cross-sectional studies of age-related changes in resting refraction show a drift toward hyperopia from about age 30 to 65 years, and then a drift toward myopia after age 65[9,10] attributed to growth and forward movement of the lens.

Table 1 summarizes the possible aging factor that may cause the patient's vision to be myopic or hyperopic (competing processes). We note that the "lens paradox" showing myopic shift with aging (due to lens curvature changes) may be counter-balanced by all those factors that may cause a hypershift, including the decreases of lens equivalent index and globe axial length with age. In addition, the increase of lens power due to radii decrease is a weaker age dependence than that of the equivalent refractive index change;

TABLE 1	THE AGING EFFECTS ON PRESBYOPIC EYES	

Eye Condition Change Due to Aging	Effects on Vision or Accommodation
Eye axial length decreases	Myopic (1)
Lens equivalent refractive index decreases	Hyperopic (2)
Lens anterior radius decreases	Myopic (3)
Lens cortex thickness increases	Myopic (4)
Lens capsule rigidity	Less accommodation (4)
Zonule-lens coupling weakness	Less accommodation (5)
Anterior zonular shift	Myopic (6)
Decrease of chamber depth	Myopic
Decrease of globe axial length	Hyperopic
Gravitation effects	Myopic
Sclera/ciliary muscle rigidity	Less accommodation
Age-altered alpha crystalline is sticky	Reduced accommodation capacity
Accumulated accommodative efforts	Reduced accommodation capacity (7)
Hypermetropia	Less accommodation than myopia (8)
UV radiation and high temperature	Earlier onset of presbyopia (9)
Reduction of pupil diameter	Smaller subjective accommodation (10)

Notes: (1) reduction of eye axial length by age was published by Grosvenor;[28] (2) the lens nucleus refractive index may increase with age but the net equivalent index may decrease, combining the effects of lens nucleus and lens capsule;[29,30] (3) the lens curvatures steepen with age, causing myopic shift that may be counterbalanced by the lens net index decrease or hyperopic shift;[1] (4) reported by Koretz et al;[31] (5) reported by Kaufman;[32] (6) reported by Farnsworth;[2] (7) proposed by Pierscioneck;[33] (8) reported by Lavinsky;[34] (9) reviewed by Bullimore and Gilmartin;[35] (10) reported by Miege.[36]

therefore, the "net effects" cause a hypershift by aging. These competing effects may be described by our calculations as follows:

The lens radii changes (R_1, R_2) and the lens refractive power (DL) change by aging (A) is given by (using a constant index of the lens, n = 1.413 and of the humors, n_1 = 1.336):

$$DL = (n - n_1)(1/R_1 + 1/R_2) = 16.17 + 0.0347 A$$
(equation 1)

With the age dependence equivalent refractive index of the lens (neg) = 1.441 – 0.00039 A, we obtain the lens power:

$$DL = 22.10 - 0.035 A$$
(equation 2)

Note that equation 2 has a sign change for the age dependence (ie, the overall power becomes hypershifted with age when the negative effect is included). Figure 1 shows these two competing effects with age.

PRESBYOPIA TREATMENTS

The effectiveness of ciliary body contraction for lens relaxation (or accommodation) may be reduced by the combined aging factors, including lens property changes (index, size, thickness, and curvature), tissue elastic changes (in sclera and ciliary), and the zonular tension change. Therefore, the treatment of presbyopia involves methods that may change one or more of these factors. Progressive additional spectacle lenses; monovision, bifocal, or multifocal contact lenses; monovision, bifocal, or multifocal corneal refractive surgery; multifocal and diffractive intraocular lenses (IOLs); and accommodative IOLs have been used for the correction of presbyopia by changing the corneal refractive power.

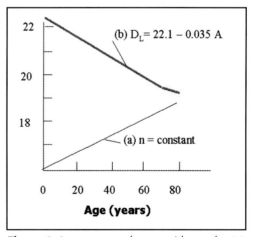

Figure 1. Lens power change with age for (a) constant index (n = 1.413), (b) age dependence equivalent index.

S. Thornton[11] attempted to cause scleral expansion through the ACS procedure, which was shown to have major regression due to the tissue healing postoperatively. R. Schachar[12] has proposed an SEB procedure with the help of scleral implants. H. Fukasaku[13] performed ACS in combination with SEP wedged into the incision in the hope of achieving greater effect and greater stability. Fukasaku and Schachar believe that presbyopia is the result of crowding in the posterior chamber due to continuous growth of the lens throughout life. The SEP technique improved the 24-month postoperative regression from about 94% (in a simple ACS) to about 39% (in SEP) according to Fukasaku's report at the ESCRS meet-

TABLE 2	COMPARISON OF PRESBYOPIA CORRECTION METHODS AND SEB

Method	Technique	Mechanism
SEB (1)	Scleral expansion band	Lens equatorial diameter expansion with increased zonule tension for accommodation
ACS (2)	Radial incision of sclera	Scleral tissue incision for the expansion of "crowding" chamber and lens
SEP (3)	Silicone expansion plugs	Same as ACS but with implant for reduced regression
SCI (4)	Band implanted in ciliary body	Based on Helmholtz's theory that lens diameter decreases during accommodation
LAPR (5)	Infrared laser sclera ablation	Based on Lin-Kadambi's elastic theory, the laser-ablated scleral gap is filled with subconjunctival tissue with increased elasticity for effective accommodation; regression caused by tissue healing is minimized by the laser "excision"

Notes: (1) method first proposed by R. Schachar; (2) proposed by Cramer in 1860, see also S. Thornton;[11] (3) first proposed by H. Fukasaku;[13] (4) proposed by G. Baikoff;[14] (5) proposed in 1988 and patented by J.T. Lin of SurgiLight.[37,38]

ing in 2001. G. Baikoff[14] used a technique to position the segments in front of the ciliary body in order to release the tension on the zonule and modify the shape of the crystalline lens.

The most recent method LAPR, proposed and patented by J.T. Lin,[37,38] is to use an infrared laser to ablate the scleral tissue and increase its elastic properties for accommodation after the treatment. Comparison of presbyopia correction methods and the mechanisms using SEB, ACS, SEP, SCI, and LAPR are listed in Table 2. Other methods to treat presbyopia using a monovision hyperopic correction are not included in Table 2.

Presbyopia, as traditionally accepted by Helmholtz,[15] is due to progressive weakening or atrophy of the ciliary muscles. However, Schachar believes that the ciliary muscle does not really become weak but rather "functionally less efficient." This inefficiency, he proposes, can be attributed to a progressive increase in the diameter of the lens during middle age, which causes a "crowding effect." Consequently, the ciliary muscle is left with no space to contract. Thus, with the idea of giving the muscle more room for contraction, Helmholtz's and Schachar's hypotheses explain how accommodation occurs in a normal person. Helmholtz says that the ciliary muscles contract, which relaxes the zonules, causing the lens capsule to become lax. Hence, the jelly-like lens material bulges in the center. In the process, there is a decrease in the equatorial diameter. Schachar, on the other hand, postulates that when the ciliary muscles contract, the equatorial zonules tighten, while the nonequatorial zonules relax. This has an effect similar to holding a balloon filled with water at its two poles and pulling it outward. The net result is a bulging in the center (ie, an increase in the anterior-posterior diameter). He postulates that the degenerative changes, which have been observed in the ciliary muscle of presbyopic eyes, may be related to disuse atrophy and not suggestive of age-related atrophy.

Both theories agree that during accommodation the lens bulges in the center. So when the lens starts hardening, as in cataract, there will be a loss of accommodation due to inability of the lens to bulge in the center. However, we are interested in the physiology of accommodation in the absence of lens hardening or cataract.

The concept of scleral expansion is under hot debate. Many studies have actually discounted Schachar's hypothesis. A. Glasser, MD[16] and S. Matthews, MD[17] demonstrated a decrease in the equatorial diameter of the crystalline lens as an effect of scleral expan-

sion. They also found no evidence of a dynamic change in power of presbyopic patients provided by Schachar.

Helmholtz stated that the ciliary muscle is relaxed when the eye is focused for distance. The relaxed ciliary muscle maintains the zonule under tension to flatten the crystalline lens for distance viewing. When the eye focuses on a near object, the ciliary muscle contracts and releases tension on the zonule. The release of zonular tension allows the crystalline lens to become more curved due to elastic forces in the lens. Fincham[18] added additional experimental support to the accommodative theory of Helmholtz and also offered evidence that presbyopia was caused by the inability of the lens capsule to mold the hardened lens substance into the accommodated form. Fisher and Pau[19] and Kranz[20] supported Fincham's theory of presbyopia by showing that the lens hardens with age.

In addition to the classical theories of accommodation and presbyopia that conflict with Schachar's ideas, there are additional reasons suggesting that further verification of the efficacy of scleral expansion surgery would be prudent. The reported evidence showing improvement in the human accommodative amplitude is based solely on subjective push-up measures.[21]

Matthews[17] found no evidence of a dynamic change in power of the eye, which is accommodation. Indeed, the methods employed are the best to objectively demonstrate whether accommodation is present.

Accommodation is not simply the ability to see clearly at near. By definition, accommodation is a change in the optical power of the eye. For example, a presbyope with a bifocal spectacle lens or a multifocal contact lens on the eye can see both at distance and at near, but this is by no means accommodation. Accommodation is a dynamic process.

Matthews suggested in *EyeWorld*[22] that some of the improved reading ability demonstrated with subjective push-up testing might be a result of inadequate testing procedures. It may be due to some kind of induced multifocality of the eye, either in the cornea or in the crystalline lens, as a consequence of these surgical procedures. Patients may be left with an aberration—either astigmatism or higher-order aberration of the eye—which allows them to have functional near and distance vision simultaneously. Matthews stated that it is difficult to find a physiological explanation for how a surgical procedure done on one eye should restore accommodation in the contralateral eye.

THE LIN-KADAMBI HYPOTHESIS

The Lin-Kadambi hypothesis attempts to explain the mechanism by which the LAPR procedure causes a positive effect on the range of accommodation. The immediate effect due to scleral thinning is an increase in the elasticity of the scleral "ring" as a whole. As shown in Figure 2, the ciliary muscle attached to the inner side of this more elastic scleral ring is now able to work more efficiently, as it works against less resistance. Myopic or hyperopic shift has not been reported after LAPR. Some studies seem to indicate a paradoxical increase in the scleral diameter. We are not convinced that there is any change in the scleral diameter, as there has been no reported change in the distance refractive status after LAPR. However, we do not rule out the possibility of this occurring in some cases. Perhaps full-thickness incisions and excisions may tend to produce this effect.

We do not totally discount the existence of the phenomenon of "posterior chamber crowding." We believe that this phenomenon may exist in many cases but may not be directly related to the physiology of accommodation in all cases. After our LAPR procedure, the ablated scleral groove is filled with subconjunctival tissue. Although this tissue forms a good barrier to infection and adds some amount of lateral strength to the wound, it is our contention that the tissue is still "softer" and more elastic. We also believe that the increased radial elasticity of the scleral ring is preserved as a whole and, hence, the positive effect on accommodation is retained. Under this scenario, it will not be surprising if some regression of effect is observed. Clinically, the regression has been reported as minimal over 2 years and more. We also believe that the "filling in effect" of the scleral grooves by the subconjunctival tissue plays a role in preventing regression. In acceptance of the Lin-Kadambi hypothesis, it naturally follows that there should be an immediate demonstrable improvement soon after the procedure or in the following days. This has been clinically observed (for a patient to see J3 even within 4 to 5 hours postoperatively). It takes a few days for the patient to subjectively demonstrate significant improvement.

ANALYSIS OF ACCOMMODATION

By scanning microscopic studies of the zonula in humans,[23] the ciliary body moves forward and inward when it is contracted, causing bulging and minor displacement of the lens toward the cornea. Accommodation of the lens is accomplished by changing the thickness and curvature of the elastic lens capsule. The elasticity is most likely in the lens capsule rather than in the interior portion of the lens. Due to the high water content, the lens is almost incompressible, and the hard nucleus, deeply buried in the soft cortex, is unlikely to contribute to the observed elasticity of the lens.

The equatorial diameter increases from an average of 5.8 mm in the newborn to around 9.0 mm in the adult. With the increase of lens cortex thickness (average of 1.0 mm), the radius of curvature of the anterior lens surfaces decreases with age, around 5 mm in average between age of 20 to 60, or about a 1.5-mm decrease every 10 years.

In addition to the change in size of the aged lens, aging is also associated with changes at the molecular level, especially involving the lens protein, which is the major constituent of its dry weight. Almost 95% of the lens structure protein is water soluble at birth and converted to a nonsoluble protein as aging proceeds. The changes in protein solubility result in a significant increase in light

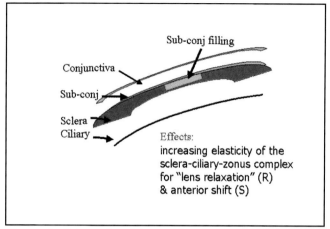

Figure 2. Schematic of laser-ablated sclera and the filling effect of subconjunctival tissue.

scattering and a decrease of its refractive index. The layers of the lens have a stepwise increase of refractive indices toward the interior. The refractive index for a young adult is about 1.37 in the cortex and rises to about 1.405 in the nucleus.[24] The lens nucleus refractive index increases with age from 1.405 (at birth) to 1.4125 (at age 60).

Koretz and Handelman[5] proposed a theory for presbyopia. They found that the older the individual, the more curved the lens becomes for a given accommodative demand because the refractive index of the lens decreases with aging, related to the known shift in its protein from soluble to insoluble form. The image is of a presbyopic eye hypershifted when the lens index decreases. They also found that the angle of zonular insertion should change with increasing lenticular size, weakening its effectiveness. As the lens increases in size with aging, the zonules come to exert a force that is tangential (or nearly so) to the surface of the lens so that zonular relaxation has less and less effect on the shape of the lens. In addition, the sclera tissue and ciliary body become more rigid in elderly people than in young people. The thickness of the lens capsule also increases with age but reduces its elasticity, in addition to increasing its curvatures.

The effectiveness of ciliary body contraction for lens relaxation (or accommodation) is therefore reduced by age due to the combined effects of the above-mentioned aging factors, including lens property changes (index, size, thickness, and curvature), tissue elastic changes (in sclera and ciliary), and the zonular tension change.

TENSION ANALYSIS

The stress patterns of the sclera, stroma, and limbus were studied by Maurice.[25] The cornea has a smaller tension than the sclera due to its smaller radius of curvature, where there is a discontinuity in the curvature of the globe. The tangential tension in the sclera (Ts) is not matched at the limbus by an equal tangential tension in the corneal stroma (Tc) and is balanced by another force (TL) toward the center of the eye. Maurice has compared TL to the force applied by a purse string drawn around a perfect sphere, forming the indentation at the limbus. TL is greater than either Ts or Tc, and the limbal region supports this extra tension by being thicker (and perhaps richer in circular collagen fibers) than either the central

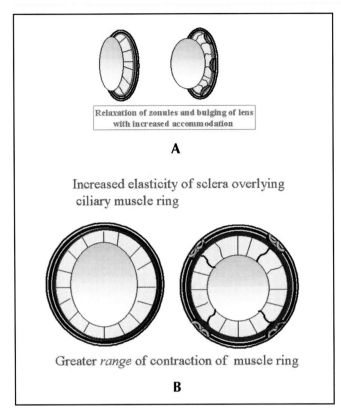

A

Increased elasticity of sclera overlying
ciliary muscle ring

Greater *range* of contraction of muscle ring

B

Figure 3. Mechanism of lens relaxation for accommodation after LAPR.

cornea or equatorial sclera. The sclera is reported to have an elastic modulus in circumferential tension about 100 times greater than for radial compressive stress, consistent with the concept that the collagen fibrils run in the circumferential direction.[26] Therefore, far less stress is needed in stretching the radial than the circumferential direction of the sclera.

Using a laser to ablate (remove) a portion of the sclera tissue in the radial directions decreases the radial tension of the sclera and causes it to expand or become more elastic. This expansion in turn increases the inward tension (TL) and causes the ciliary body to contract for lens relaxation, accommodating for near objects. In addition, the laser-ablated scleral groove is filled with subconjunctival tissue, which is more elastic than the original sclera tissue. As shown in Figure 3, this increased radial elasticity of the scleral ring is preserved as a whole, hence the positive effect on accommodation is retained. We also believe that the "filling in effect" of the scleral grooves by the subconjunctival tissue plays a major role in preventing regression.

Ciliary muscle contraction for forward and inward movement of the muscle causes stretch of the fiber system such that traction is taken up from the posterior zonular fiber, allowing the anterior zonules and lens to thicken. As shown in Figure 4, an inward movement of the ciliary body will generate two tension components (T1 and T2): T1 along the lens diameter to cause the lens anterior capsule to relax with decreased radius of curvature (or increased refractive power); T2 along the optical axis pushes the lens toward the anterior chamber, and the shorter chamber depth (S) will have increased power, about 1.25 D accommodation per millimeter of movement. Glasser and Campbell[27] reported a stretching experiment and showed that (for ages 31 to 39) the ciliary body move-

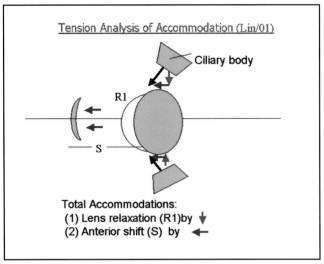

Figure 4. The tension analysis of lens accommodation and anterior shift.

ment (dC) is related to the accommodation power (D) by a slope of (0.8 – 2.6) D/mm depending on the range of C. For T2 only, we may calculate that accommodation is about (0.97 – 1.1) D/mm.

Total accommodation (TA) is proportional to the lens accommodation (LA) and is related to other components of the eye, as the following approximate analytic form illustrates:

$$TA = (1 - S/f_1)\ LA - 1336\ [dL/L_2 + dS/(f_1\ f_2) + dP/F_2]$$
(equation 3)

where S is the anterior chamber depth, f_1 is the corneal focal length, dL is the globe axial length change (with initial length of L), dS is the anterior chamber depth change, F is the effective focal length (governed by f_1, f_2, and S), and dP is the principle plane shift during lens accommodation.

Based on equation 3, we are able to predict some clinical outcomes of accommodation as follows:

1. Lens accommodation (LA) may be achieved by two components: the lens relaxation (due to ciliary body contraction) and lens anterior shift (dS, due to forwarding lens movement). Each millimeter lens anterior shift shall provide LA = (1.1 – 1.97) D depending on the values of lens radii (r_1, R_2).

2. Total accommodation (TA) is proportional to LA and reduced by a separation ratio factor (S/f_1) defined by the anterior chamber depth (S) and corneal focal length (f_1). This factor is about 0.6 (for S = 5.0 and f_1 = 31). Therefore, shallow chamber depth (smaller S) or "hyperopic" cornea (longer f_1) shall have larger overall accommodation (TA) for a given lens accommodation (LA). The TA value is calculated to be in an average of 0.66 x LA, and this reduction of 0.34 is caused by the principle plan shift (dP) of about 20% and the separation factor of about 16%.

3. Shorter initial globe length (L), anterior chamber depth (S), or smaller radii of curvatures of the lens (R_1, R_2) will have more total accommodation (TA) for a given lens accommodation (LA). However, our calculation also showed that LA is not sensitive to the initial value of f_1. The value of LA only changes about 2% for a wide range of f_1 = 28 to 35 mm (or cornea power changes from 38 D to 48 D).

In addition to the above optical parameters, the tissue elastic properties of the lens capsule, ciliary and sclera bodies as a whole, and the cumulative efforts or degree of need of accommodation of the lens relaxation may all influence total accommodation. For example, an older patient may have more accommodation than a young one because of a larger degree of need, and the young one may "reserve" some unneeded accommodation. The treated eye's accommodation may be affected by the untreated eye, which may be myopic or hyperopic. Patients with smaller pupil size will have "subjective" accommodation (about 1.5 to 2.0 D) due to depth of focus effects between ages 15 and 60.

SUMMARY

The effectiveness of ciliary body contraction for lens relaxation (or accommodation) may be influenced by combined aging factors, including lens property changes (index, size, thickness, and curvature), tissue elastic changes (in sclera and ciliary), and the zonular tension change. The scleral expansion techniques (SEB, SEP, ACS, SCI) suffer from major regression due to tissue healing, whereas LAPR showed a minimum regression even after 24 months follow-up. The fundamental difference between the mechanism behind LAPR and those of nonlaser methods is presented by the Lin-Kadambi hypothesis proposing that increasing elasticity of the sclera-ciliary units is achieved by subconjunctival tissue filling. This filling process also prevents scleral tissue healing, which closes the gap and leads to regression. We also present equations for mathematical modeling for the total accommodation affected by the optical and tissue conditions of the lens, cornea, and their relative position and globe length. In our analysis, we introduced two tension components that attribute to the lens accommodation and anterior movement accommodation.

To conclude, we believe that accommodation caused by laser or nonlaser techniques is a very complicated mechanism and can only be understood quantitatively by treating the eye as a "whole," where its refractive state is governed by many of the optical and tissue properties. Further studies, particularly the lenticular and aging aspects, must be measured before a complete and accurate picture of the cause and correction of presbyopia can be addressed.

REFERENCES

1. Brown N. The change in lens curvature with age. *Exp Eye Res.* 1974;19:175-183.
2. Farnsworth PN, Shyne SE. Anterior zonular shifts with age. *Exp Eye Res.* 1979;28:291-297.
3. Koretz JF, Kaufman PL, Neider MW, Goeckner PA. Accommodation and presbyopia in the human eye—aging of the anterior segment. *Vision Res.* 1989;29(12):1685-92.
4. Fisher RF. Elastic constants of the human lens capsule. *J Physiol (Lond).* 1969;201(1):1-19.
5. Koretz JE, Handelman GH. How the human eye focuses. *Sci Am.* 1988;259:92-99.
6. Weale R. Presbyopia toward the end of the 20th century. *Surv Ophthalmol.* 1989;34(1):15-30.
7. Pierscioneck B. Presbyopia: the riddle of the lens. The 6th Varilux Presbyopia Forum; June 2000; Portugal.
8. Pierscionek BK. Related articles, refractive index contours in the human lens. *Exp Eye Res.* 1997;64(6):887-93.
9. Slataper FJ. Age norms of refraction and vision. *Arch Ophthalmol.* 1950;43:3.
10. Saunders H. Age-dependence of human refractive errors. *Ophthalmology and Physiology Optics.* 1981;1:159-174.
11. Thornton S. Anterior ciliary sclerotomy (ACS): a procedure to reverse presbyopia. In: Sher NA, ed. *Surgery for Hyperopia and Presbyopia.* New York: Williams & Wilkins; 1997.
12. Schachar RA. Cause and treatment of presbyopia with a method for increasing the amplitude of accommodation. *Annals of Ophthalmology.* 1992;24(12):445-7,452.
13. Fukasaku H. Silicone expansion plug implant surgery for presbyopia. Presented at: American Society of Cataract and Refractive Surgery Symposium; 2000; Boston, Mass.
14. Baikoff G. Surgical correction of presbyopia: phakic refractive lenses or supraciliary segments? Presented at: ESCRS; Sept 1-5,2001; Amsterdam.
15. Helmholtz HV. *Helmholtz's Treatise on Physiological Optics.* Vol. 1. Southall JPC, trans. New York: Dover Publications; 1962:143.
16. Glasser A, Kaufman P. The mechanism of accommodation in primates. *Ophthalmology.* 1999;106(5):863-72.
17. Matthews S. Scleral expansion surgery does not restore accommodation in human presbyopia. *Ophththalmology.* 1999;106:873-877.
18. Fincham EF. The mechanism of accommodation. *Br J Ophthalmol.* 1937;8:5-80.
19. Fisher RF. Presbyopia and the changes with age in the human crystalline lens. *J Physiol (Lond).* 1973;228(3):765-79.
20. Pau H, Kranz J. The increasing sclerosis of the human lens with age and its relevance to accommodation and presbyopia. *Graefes Arch Clin Exp Ophthalmol.* 1991;229(3):294-6.
21. Yang GS, Yee RW, Cross WD, et al. Scleral expansion: a new surgical technique to correct presbyopia. *Invest Ophthalmol Vis Sci.* 1997;38(Suppl):S497.
22. Matthews S. Laser treatment designed to reverse presbyopia. *Eyeworld.* 2001;May:32.
23. Robert JW. Scanning electronic microscopic studies of the zonular apparatus in human and monkey eyes. *Invest Ophthalmol Vis Sci.* 1979;18:133-144.
24. Davson H, ed. *The Eye.* Vol 1. New York: Academic Press; 1969.
25. Maurice DM. The cornea and sclera. In: Davson H, ed. *The Eye.* Vol 1. New York: Academic Press; 1969.
26. Battaglioli JL, Kamm RD. Measurements of the compressive properties of scleral tissue. *Invest Ophthalmol Vis Sci.* 1984;25:59-65.
27. Glasser A, Campbell MC. On the potential causes of presbyopia. *Vision Res.* 1999;39(7):1267-1272.
28. Grosvenor T. Reduction in axial length with age: an emmetropizing mechanism for the adult eye? *Am J Opt Physiol Opt.* 1987;64:657-663.
29. Hemenger RP, Garner LF, Ooi CS. Change with age of the refractive index gradient of the human ocular lens. *Invest Ophthalmol Vis Sci.* 1995;36:703-707.
30. Dubbelman M, Van der Heijde GL. The shape of the aging human lens: curvature, equivalent refractive index and the lens paradox. *Vision Res.* 2001;41:1867-1877.
31. Koretz JF, Bertasso AM, Neider WM, True-Gabelt B, Kaufman PL. Slit-lamp studies of the rhesus monkey eye. II. Changes in crystalline lens shape, thickness and position during accommodation and aging. *Exp Eye Res.* 1987;45:317-326.
32. Kaufman PL. Accommodation and presbyopia: neuromuscular and biophysical aspects. In: Hart WM Jr, ed. *Adler's Physiology of the Eye, Clinical Application.* 9th ed. St. Louis, Mo: Mosby; 1992.
33. Pierscioneck B. Presbyopia: the riddle of the lens. Presented at: 6th Varilux Presbyopia Forum; June 2000; Portugal.
34. Lavinsky J. Synthesis of recent clinical studies. 5th Presbyopia Forum. International Symposium on Presbyopia; 1995.
35. Bullimore MA, Gilmartin B. Hyperopia and presbyopia: etiology and epidemiology. In: Sher NA, ed. *Surgery for Hyperopia and Presbyopia.* New York: Williams & Wilkins; 1997.
36. Miege C. Age-related changes in accommodation and refraction for presbyopes. The 6th Varilux Presbyopia Forum; June 2000; Portugal.
37. Lin JT. US Patent 5144630 and 5520679.
38. Lin JT. US Patent 6258082 B1 and 6263879 B1.

BIBLIOGRAPHY

Crawford KS, Kaufman PL, Bito LZ. The role of the iris in accommodation of rhesus monkeys. *Invest Ophthalmol Vis Sci.* 1990;31:2185-2190.

Fatt I, Weissman BA. *Physiology of the Eye.* Stoneham, Mass: Reed Publishing; 1992:9-11,85-90,209-211.

Garner LF, Smith G. Changes in equivalent and gradient refractive index of the crystalline with accommodation. *Optom Vis Sci.* 1997;74:114-9.

Garner LF, Yap MK. Changes in ocular dimensions and refraction with accommodation. *Ophthalmic Physiol Opt.* 1997;17:12-7.

Glasser A, Campbell MC. Presbyopia and the optical changes in the human crystalline lens with age. *Vis Res.* 1998;38:209-229.

Glasser A, Campbell MC. Biometric, optical and physical changes in the isolated human crystalline lens with age in relation to presbyopia. *Vision Res.* 1999;39:1991-2015.

Glasser A, Murphy CJ, Troilo D, Howland HC. The mechanism of lenticular accommodation in chicks. *Vision Res.*1995;35:1525-1540.

Koretz JF, Handelman GHA. A model for accommodation in the young human eye: the effects of lens elastic anisotrophy on the mechanism. *Vision Res.* 1983;23:1679-1686.

Koretz JF, Kaufman PL, Neider MW, Goeckner PA. Accommodation and presbyopia in the human eye-aging of the anterior segment. *Vision Res.* 1989;29:1685-1692.

Lin JT. Scanning laser technology for refractive surgery. In: Agarwal S, et al, eds. *Refractive Surgery.* New Delhi, India: Jaypee Brothers; 2000.

Lin JT, Mallo S, Hwang MY, et al. Abstract: Congress of the ESCRS, 2001;135,144.

Mutti DO, Zadnik K, Adams AJ. The equivalent refractive Index of the crystalline lens in childhood. *Vis Res.* 1995;35:1565-1573.

Schachar RA, Black TD, Kash RL, et al. The mechanism of accommodation and presbyopia in the primate. *Ann Ophthalmol.* 1995;27:58-67.

Schachar RA, Cudmore DP. The effect of gravity on the amplitude of accommodation. *Ann Ophthalmol.* 1993;25:404-9.

Schachar RA, Tello C, Cudmore DP, et al. In vivo increase of the human lens equatorial diameter during accommodation. *Am J Physiol.* 1996;271:R670-6.

Shump PJ, Ko LS, Ng CL, Lin SL. A biometric study of ocular changes during accommodation. *Am J Ophthalmol.* 1993;115(1):76-81.

Smith G, Atchison DA. Equivalent power of the crystalline lens of the human eye: comparison of methods of calculation. *J Opt Soc Am A.* 1997;12(10):2537-46.

Smith G, Pierscionek BK. The optical structure of the lens and its contribution to the refractive status of the eye. *Ophthalmic Physiol Opt.* 1998;18(1):21-9.

Stephen JR, Ginsberg SP, eds. *Ophthalmic Technology.* New York: Raven Press; 1987:137-142,277-286,324.

Strenk SA, Semmlow JL, Mezrich RS. Using magnetic resonance imaging to mathematically model the lens capsule. *Invest Ophthalmol Vis Sci.* 1994;35(Suppl):1948.

Winn B, Pugh JR, Gilmartin B, Owens H. The frequency characteristics of accommodative microfluctuations for central and peripheral zones of the crystalline lens. *Vision Res.* 1990;30:1093-1099.

Wyatt JH. Application of a simple mechanical model of accommodation to the aging eye. *Vision Res.* 1994;33:731-738.

Chapter 7

Contact Lens Alternatives for Presbyopia

Kenneth Daniels, OD, FAAO

INTRODUCTION

In the United States, there are approximately 70 million people with presbyopia and 4 million new cases of presbyopia each year (Figure 1).[1,2] Presbyopia is defined as the decrease in accommodative ability that occurs with aging (maturing). It is a deterioration of vision that identifies the onset of the psychological fact that the individual is no longer as youthful as he or she once was. It is a loss of the eye's muscular ability to supply the force to focus at near point objects, referred to as the "loss of accommodation." Plus (magnification) power is required to compensate for the inability to focus at the individual's customary near working distance. The cause of presbyopia is related to one or more aging events. These include lens sclerosis, ciliary muscle and zonular weakening with age, and amplitude of accommodation decreasing with age.

Presbyopic contact lenses are probably the most challenging method of correction and, if in the hands of a creative practitioner, will address the majority of patient needs with the least amount of visual compromise. However, as seen in Figure 2, there is an approximate 50% "drop-out rate" from contact lens use due to the perceived limitations of presbyopia and contact lenses. Many simply abandon contact lenses due to the lack of education regarding the alternatives or hesitation of the clinician to fit the patient (Figure 3).

Therefore, this chapter will discuss the vast array of options and fitting techniques for the patient with mature eyes. The real challenge of fitting the *mature eye* (a better phrase than presbyopia = older eyes), is not the actual fitting of the lenses, but understanding the needs of the patient. To properly fit the patient is to simply ask the right questions:

1. What are the needs of the presbyopic patient?
2. What are the options for the presbyopic patient?
3. What are the expectations and motivation of the patient?
4. How is the patient's ocular health and will it support a contact lens?
5. How does the fitter address the variety of visual needs of the presbyopic patient?
6. How does one address the contact lens alternatives for an astigmatic presbyopic patient?
7. How does the fitter introduce contact lens options to a new emmetropic-presbyopic patient?

PATIENT SELECTION

The presbyopic patient is unique due to the variety of visual demands for distance, intermediate, and near. The variety of demands on their eyes will create new factors that will influence their contact lens wear. It is the complexity of the visual demand that makes the contact lens fit even more complex. Patients no longer complain of difficulty with reading a book or newspaper, but they will also present with complaints while using the computer, during sports activities (golf, archery, shooting, tennis, and so forth), while at the same time demanding clarity of vision at distance. The clinician must properly educate the patient on the possibilities and limitations of a presbyopic fit. This is the real challenge. Once the patient demonstrates a reasonable understanding of the limitations, the rest is somewhat easy.

The success of presbyopic contact lens fitting depends upon many factors. The primary factor is motivation. A patient's motivation is hinged upon discouraging preconceptions of contact lenses and presbyopia and re-educating the patient about the variety of contact lens options. Contact lenses for presbyopia must not be presented as a "cure all," but as an alternative with known compromises to overall level of visual quality. The fitter should explain that a visual compromise is not negative but a subtle change to the quality of vision that the patient may presently appreciate. Realistic expectations must be developed or failure will most definitely occur.

In order to establish realistic expectations, it is a useful technique to demonstrate a subtle monovision effect when refracting the patient in the phoropter or trial frame. Simply add plus power to the near dominant eye and allow the patient to visualize distance and near. The examiner will receive positive or negative feedback instantaneously. If positive, an introductory technique is to fit the patient with daily disposable soft lenses in a subtle monovision scenario. Once again, the examiner will have an instantaneous positive or negative feedback of acceptance by the patient. "Open the door and they will enter" is my philosophy.

Prior to proceeding with a contact lens fit, an informed consent process is beneficial. The informed consent should define presby-

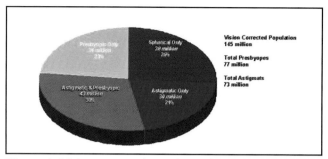

Figure 1. Vision-corrected population by type of correction (courtesy of Dwight Akerman, OD, Ciba Vision).

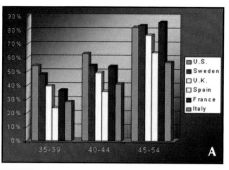

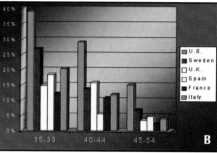

Figure 2. Demographics of the presbyopic market. A: Patients requiring vision correction; B: percent of individuals wearing contact lenses is diminished by 50% after age 45 (courtesy of Dwight Akerman, OD, Ciba Vision; HPR Reports, 2000).

opia, discuss the various methods of lens correction, the advantages and disadvantages of contact lenses, and the potential for visual compromise.[3]

> Presbyopic correction with contact lenses may create a compromise that may reduce visual acuity and depth perception for distance and near tasks. You understand that this compromise can create an increased risk when operating a motor vehicle, dangerous machinery, or performing other potentially hazardous activities…[4]

> It is the goal of the fit to establish adequate and acceptable vision for the multitude of tasks that you are presented with on an everyday basis. However, due to the complexity of the optics of contact lenses, you must realize that perfect 20/20 is not always achievable. It is our goal to establish comfortable visual function at distance, intermediate, and near biased to your individual demands. In order to do so, ancillary spectacles may be required for sun protection, safety, and/or enhancement for near or distance when you feel it is required.

A questionnaire or proper, repeatable format to a clinical interview is vital in the success of a presbyopic contact lens fit. The interview should be specific to the patient's motivation, needs, occupation, avocation, in addition to the standard medical-ocular history. Table 1 lists the major components of the interview.

CLINICAL CONSIDERATIONS

As one matures so does his or her anatomy. Ocular anatomy and function will have a more defined role in presbyopia, varying dramatically from the more youthful patient. The clinical examination will assist in determining not only the design of the required lens but also the potential for success. A complete examination needs to define the functionality of the eyelids, tear film, cornea, clarity of ocular media, retinal integrity, and finally the assessment of visual function inclusive of acuity and contrast sensitivity.[5]

OCULAR ADNEXA AND MUSCLES

A reduction in the tonus of the adnexa is proportional to the age of the patient. The younger presbyopic patient will demonstrate a more taut eyelid musculature versus the more senior patient. A reduction in the tonus, an increase in the orbital fat, and loss of dermal elasticity will directly influence the positioning of the contact lens on the eye. Apposition of the lid and puncta toward the globe will define the tear film distribution and support the lens on the ocular surfaces. Additionally, variance in lid structure and glandular

support may also induce a misdirection of lashes, known as trichasis or loss of lashes. For example, a rigid gas permeable translating lens is dependent upon the tautness of the lids to allow for proper movement. If the lids are flaccid, the lens will malposition and not translate. In contrast, an extremely taut lid will impede the translation of the lens. Additionally, lid laxity, as well as the dexterity of the patient, will affect the patient's ability to properly insert and remove lenses.

Ptosis, entropion, ectropion, and lagophthalmos will adversely affect the outcome of the lens fit. Ptosis will cause a malposition of the lens as well as obscure the optics. An upper lid entropion will enhance a superior positioning of a lens and decrease proper translation and movement. A lower lid entropion will prevent a proper translation of a lens and increase lens awareness. In contrast, an upper lid ectropion will decrease the ability of the lid to properly move, increasing lens-lid attachment, while an inferior ectropic lid will not allow the lens to maintain centralization on the cornea. Lagophthalmos will simple impede proper lens movement, thus decreasing tear film exchange and inhibit proper translation over the corneal surface (Figure 4).

TEAR FILM

Secretory functions decrease with aging, thus decreasing the ability to properly support a contact lens on the eye with sustained comfort. Dry eye symptoms tend to become more predominant as an individual matures. A variety of environmental insults and the adverse effects of medications on tear film production and supportive glands exacerbate symptoms (Figure 5).

The lipid layer of the tear film is approximately 0.1 µm thick and produced by various glands, such as the meibomian, Zeis, and Molls.

TABLE 1	INTERVIEW QUESTIONS FOR PATIENTS WITH PRESBYOPIA

Motivation to wear contact lenses with realistic expectations	Occupation: requirements for distance, intermediate, and near vision
Previous refractive correction (eg, spectacles or contact lenses)	Avocation: requirements for distance, intermediate, and near vision
Environmental factors (eg, safety requirements)	Travel requirements: frequency (defines the level of convenience required)
Previous ocular and/or blepharoplastic surgeries	

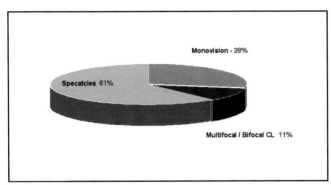

Figure 3. Contact lens versus spectacle correction for presbyopia (courtesy of Al Vaske, Lens Dynamics).

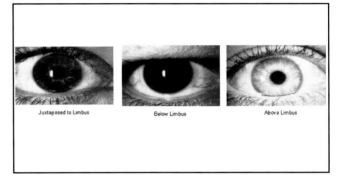

Figure 4. Lid position in relation to the cornea.

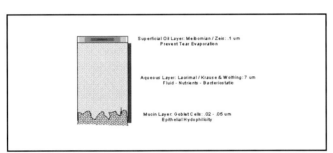

Figure 5. The tear film.

Over time, the number of functioning glands decreases in efficiency, leading to an increase in tear evaporation and less support for a contact lens on the eye. The aqueous layer, which approximates a thickness of 0.7 µm, is produced by the various lacrimal, Wolfring, and Klaus glands and is vitally important in producing lactoferrin, lysozyme, and B-lysin. All of these constituents are essential in the defense mechanism and wound healing process of the cornea. A depletion in aqueous production due to age or the introduction of medications such as diuretics, antiovulation agents, hormone replacements, antipsychotic agents, and antihistamines will lead to symptomatic keratoconjunctivitis sicca and make it difficult to support contact lenses on the eye.

Finally, the oil layer produced by the goblet cells of the conjunctiva is approximately 0.05 µm thick and acts as the mechanical protective layer against frictional insult. Once this layer starts to diminish, increased irritation occurs from any exogenous matter or biomaterial on the eye. Symptomatically, the patient will complain of decreased wear times with contacts as well as an increase in ocular redness. Clinically, this is observed as an early yellow or keratinization of the conjunctiva, paralimbal chemosis, conjunctival

drag with lenses, and persistent level of ocular injection. Many ascribe the "newer" onset of symptoms as an allergy and treat it as such. In reality, they do not have an allergy and in fact many medicinals, particularly over-the-counter remedies, will exacerbate the condition.

If the oil, mucus, and aqueous layers of the tear film are insufficient, the lens cannot be supported on the corneal surface comfortably and there will be poor lens surface wetting. If the lens surface poorly wets, the patient will have a persistent complaint of variable to "filmy" vision. Additionally, the lack of an adequate aqueous layer decreases the available enzymatic support to reduce the proteinaceous insult of the eye on the lens, leading to increased deposition. Finally, if the mucus layer is deficient, then the conjunctival and corneal surfaces will suffer from mechanical irritative frictional forces on the ocular surface manifested as increased ocular injection, superficial punctate epithelialopathy, photosensitivity, and a decreased tolerance for the lenses. Therefore, the clinician must consider supportive therapy to enhance contact lens wear. These therapies would include supplemental drops and nocturnal ointments, antioxidant therapy (topical or oral), and punctal occlusion.

CORNEA

The regenerative ability of epithelial cells will also slow with maturity (Figure 6). The average cell regenerative cycle is 5 to 7 days, but with the persistent microtrauma of a contact lens, the cell regeneration may be slightly retarded. Squamous cell loss occurs at a greater rate, while maturation of the wing and columnar cells are slowed. Additionally, the basement membrane attachments to the columnar cells are weakened, allowing for a higher rate of contact lens-related–age-related EBM (epithelial basement membrane) difficulties (Figure 7). Add ultraviolet light insult to the contact lens insult on the cornea; and lens-induced trauma to the cornea increases.

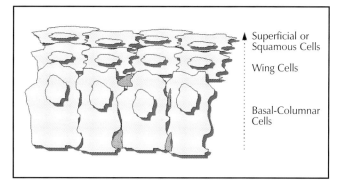

Figure 6. Regenerative cells of the corneal epithelium.

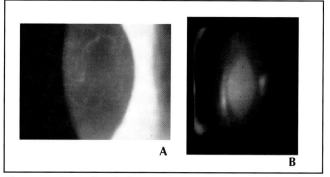

Figure 7. Age-related changes. A: EBMD; B: nuclear sclerosis.

The contact lens acts as a mechanical barrier to oxygen transport to the cornea. Thus, if the dK (diffusion coefficient) of the lens is not sufficient, the cornea suffers from edema. Microcystic edema, more commonly found in extended-wear patients, may also become a more pronounced issue with the presbyopic cornea. As edema occurs to the cornea, the stromal fibrils are adversely affected by an osmotic draw through the endothelium. If edema to the cornea occurs, the balancing mechanism is an increase in the endothelial pump, thus increasing the intumescence of aqueous into the stroma.

Upon examination, the observer will note an increased polymegathism (change in cell size) and pleomorphism (change in cell shape) of the endothelium associated with age, which is amplified by the constant use of contact lenses and the change to the endothelial pump. It is a natural course to lose the regenerative endothelial cells during one's lifetime, however the contact lenses will expedite a loss of cells associated the induced hypoxia (lack of oxygen) and hypercapnia (increase of carbon dioxide). If the edema persists, the stromal fiber bundles will lose their integrity and start to demonstrate a level of haze, yielding diminished vision.

One can intervene and prevent many of these changes by selecting a lens design with high dK levels, high water content lenses, low dehydration rates, and lenses that allow for a freedom of movement on the cornea. Supportive therapy is also required to maintain proper lens hydration and support of the cornea metabolism. Therefore, it is highly recommended to encourage the patient to utilize tear supplements, in particular electrolyte balanced and/or antioxidant drops, approximately three to four times per day (with meals). Encourage the patient to use a cushion drop in the bowl of the lens prior to insertion (prevents microtrauma and yields immediate comfort), and always use a wetting drop prior to lens removal. This will make the lens buoyant on the eye and reduce the forcefulness of aggressive lens removal techniques.

IRIS AND PUPIL

Fortunately, as the patient matures, the pupil size becomes more consistently miotic, as does the near triad (slow oscillatory scans of the eye, reduced convergence and accommodation, and decreased pupil response to light). The fitter can exploit consistency of the triad that allows for an increased depth of focus and field, decrease in paraxial aberrations, and reduction in the retinal blur circle. The drawback is the potential atopic position of the pupil and lack of rapid reaction to variant levels of illumination.

The pupil size becomes the key defining factor in fitting presbyopic contact lenses. Pupil size limits the ability to fully utilize a concentric or translating design. Small, slowly reactive pupils of 2 to 3

mm limit the ability to utilize pupil-dependent lenses such as aspheric, diffractive optics, or concentric designs. Patients with small pupils may be better fit with monovision due to the depth of focus and field, while avoiding the inability to center complex optics of bifocal or multifocal lenses. Conversely, large pupils may make these designs less effective by not allowing the patient to appreciate the defined optics of the lens.

Photopic and scotopic conditions will have a direct effect on the pupil and proper lens selection. In younger patients, the average pupil size in photopic conditions is approximately 5 mm, and 8 mm in scotopic conditions. As one matures into the 40s, the pupils approximate 4 mm and 6 mm, respectively. In more senior years, the pupils vary approximately 1 mm in either condition. Therefore, where at one time a patient may have been successful in a translating, aspheric, or concentric design, he or she may literally "grow out" of the design. Paradoxically, in the younger presbyopic patient where monovision works well, translating, aspheric, and concentric designs may not be accepted based on the low add requirements. The most optimal scenario for a bifocal or multifocal design is one that requires a defined add power and has sufficiently large (4 to 6 mm) reactive pupils. These fitting issues will be discussed at greater length later in the chapter.

CRYSTALLINE LENS

The lens of the eye can be the most limiting factor outside the pupil influence. It is common knowledge that the lens develops additional membrane layers as one ages. These layers are compressed on one another and after time become sclerotic and less malleable (see Figure 7). This, in turn, restrains the ease of lens flexure required in proper accommodation. At the same time, the lens develops a brunescence (yellowing), which is a subsequence to the absorption of ultraviolet light, causing a reduction in the visibility of the blue wavelengths, and leading to a loss of contrast sensitivity, decrease in retinal illumination, and potential dispersion of incident light. The lens capsule also thickens, causing a subsequent lack of elasticity consistent with the loss of accommodative function.

Supportive therapy consists of selecting polymers with ultraviolet (UV) protective chemistry or inhibitors. UV-protecting sunglasses should be encouraged at all times. Additionally, antioxidant therapy has been demonstrated to enhance the metabolic capabilities of the lens by getting rid of free radicals, thereby protecting the lens and decreasing the sclerosing process.

VITREORETINAL INFLUENCES

An example that can be given to the patient is the retina is

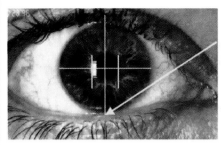

Lid position/tightness
Corneal/iris diameter
Pupil size/dynamics
Fissure width

Lower lid to pupil edge

Location/amount of astigmatism
Ocular health

Figure 8. Ocular examination—required measures prior to lens fitting.

equivalent to the film of a camera. If the film ages, it may not be as capable of accepting the light to process an image. Any type of vitreoretinal anomaly will deleteriously affect the quality of light emerging through the media to be processed. Many factors in retinal health occur over time. Preservation of retinal function has been the core of much research in past years. The research is based upon several factors such as preservation of photoreceptor function, preservation of the supportive retinal pigment epithelium, and vasculature integrity changes of the choriocapillaris. Once again, supportive therapy is protective in nature. UV protection and antioxidants; specific extracts such as bilberry, grape seed, ginkgo bililoa; and xanophylls are important nutrient sources in cell chemistry and protection.

Contact Lens Designs and Techniques

There are a multitude of lens designs that are available for the presbyopic patient. The ultimate question is, "Which one will work?" This question is not so easily answered in one quick response (Figure 8). The answer is highly dependent on three factors:

1. It is important to determine the visual, occupational, and avocational requirements of the patient.

2. The health of the patient's eyes and ability to physiologically accept a contact lens on the eye.

3. The experience of the fitter and availability of the various designs.

Advise to the fitter and an explanation of the complexity of the fit to the patient follows:

> There is a recipe that we need to define, and sometimes to make the recipe work, we will need several modifications. We hope that the first choice is the best, but it is not unusual to require several modifications. If you are willing to work with me, I am more than glad to work with you.

It is important to be honest and define the negatives of a presbyopic fit so that the patient does not assume high expectations. There are compromises that will be induced—they will be minimized—but they will exist. Reality and motivation of the patient are essentially. Without these, frustration will pursue.

When developing an approach for a presbyopic contact lens fit, explain to the patient that there will be an appreciable level of blur or decrease in the overall quality of vision. A phrase called "a balanced blur or equality of blur at distance and near" is appropriate. The achievable goal for acuity should be a level of visual equality at distance and near of approximately 20/25. In contrast, if the patient is able to see a crisp 20/20 at distance but only 20/30 at near, he or

she will consistently notice a blur at near and be uncomfortable and frustrated with visual correction. The fitter will hear: "I can see well when I read, but street signs are blurred." If the patient is fit with an "equal balance of blur," you will not hear this complaint.

The second part of developing a concept for a presbyopic fit is the question of the patient's acceptance for a "presbyopic contact lens correction." Understanding the advantages and disadvantages of contact lens and spectacles is important. Glasses and contact lenses do not and will not deliver the same quality of perceptual acuity. Contact lenses will afford different benefits versus spectacles. It is important that the patient have a realistic expectation of contact lens correction by understanding the variances between the two corrective modalities, as seen in Table 2.

Patient selection is premised by age and refraction when developing a concept for presbyopic contact lens correction. The younger presbyope will adapt to a presbyopic contact lens correction more easily than an older patient. Likewise, a patient requiring a lower add power will also be more accepting of a presbyopic contact lens correction than a patient requiring a higher add power. Finally, hyperopes tend to be better candidates than myopes, while emmetropes or purely astigmatic patients are generally the least accepting of a visual compromise induced by presbyopic corrections.

Determination Of Ocular Dominance

There are several techniques to determine ocular dominance for distance and near. These include the "hole in the hand" method, plus lens test, alternate occlusion test, and the "camera to the eye" or "targeting eye" method. In all forms of presbyopic fitting, a dominant eye will need to be selected in order to bias one eye for distance and the other for near refractive error (Table 3).

To determine the patient's ability to tolerate a reduction in visual quality, the fitter should perform the following procedure: The fitter should "push plus at distance" in the manifest refraction in order to reduce the need for a strong add power at near—"maximum plus maximum visual acuity (MPMVA)" (Table 4).

Lens Design Options

There are many lens designs available, each having a different level of complexity in fitting and ability to satisfy the visual and environmental needs of the patient. The designs include monovision, modified monovision, translating bifocals, simultaneous view bifocals, modified bivision, and diffractive bifocals.

The lens design selection is premised by accounting for many of the previously mentioned factors. It would be advantageous for the fitter to utilize a standardized method to present the designs (Table 5.

Monovision

Monovision is a method that allows for a quick and efficient way of introducing a "presbyopic correction" to an individual. The method simply utilizes the patient's present contact lens design, spherical and/or astigmatic, with a subtle power adjustment to bias one eye to near and the other to distance. In the early stages of presbyopia when the add power is low (ie, +.75 to +1.00), this might be referred to as a "near bias" technique.

The most difficult part of this technique is first convincing the patient that "one eye near–one eye distance" will not be detrimental to his or her vision. It is best to explain that by the time the patient reaches 40, the visual mechanism is well-cemented neurologically and that monovision will not affect the mechanics and

TABLE 2	*ADVANTAGES/DISADVANTAGES OF PRESBYOPIC CONTACT LENS CORRECTION*

Advantages	*Disadvantages*
Lessened limitations of vision at distance, intermediate, and near	Compromise to the quality of perceivable vision
Broadened and full field of view with enhanced peripheral vision	Decreased visual abilities in dim illumination
Versatility in visual correction at distance, intermediate, and near	Decreased contrast detail
Cosmetically enhancing	Requires additional spectacles to enhance distance or near vision and/or sunglasses
Allows for freedom of body motion (eg, sports) from restrictive eyewear	Adverse complications associated with contact lenses
Constant level of visual correction without the requirement of carrying an optical appliance (spectacles)	May require an ancillary pair of spectacles for visual enhancement
Enhanced transition of vision from distance to intermediate and near	Variance to vision based on climate and environmental factors
	Difficulty driving at night
	Increase in glare or hazing of vision

abilities of the eyes to work together and recognize visual cues. The younger patient will have a higher success rate in being fit with monovision due to a lesser add power requirement, leading to a lesser visual compromise.

Patient selection is premised by the need for a near point correction. If monovision or near biasing is introduced too soon, the patient will not be able to visually adapt. The patient must have a near point visual complaint and/or accept a minimum of a +1.00 add. A +1.00 spectacle add will translate to a +.75 contact lens add, leaving the patient with a subtle blur of approximately 20/25 or 20/30 at distance and near. A lesser add is used with monovision in order to minimize near and distance disparity.

Where once binocularity assisted the patient, the fitter has induced an interruption or disparity to the patient's binocular acuity. There is a level of aniseikonia that is insignificant with monovision.[8] The patient must learn to suppress or accept the slightly blurred image. He or she will develop a subtle level of suppression for the blurred image.[9] Patients will tend to adapt very quickly to monovision, generally within a few minutes or days of the initial trial. Distance cues and binocular precepts will remain in place. These are "learned" cues that cannot be broken or significantly disturbed once neurologically cemented. However, this does not imply the visual quality will remain as good as it was with full binocularity. Stereopsis and contrast sensitivity will be decreased by the monovision modality but can be limited to an acceptable level as perceived by the patient.[10]

When refining a monovision correction, the near eye should be able to achieve a distance visual acuity of approximately 20/40 to 20/50 vision, as seen in Figure 9. This level is critical in operating a motor vehicle. Documentation of distance and near visual acuity should always be noted. It is important to note that stereopic vision is reduced proportionally with the degree of monovision and the induced disparity between eyes. Even though stereopsis is reduced, the individual has learned three-dimensional cues and, therefore, is generally not greatly affected by the subtle decrease in stereopsis. However, if this becomes an issue, the patient can be given ancillary spectacles to assist at visually discriminating times or can consider modified monovision or bifocal contact lens options.

Refinement of monovision should start with the addition of plus in the distant eye. If the patient is capable of accepting additional plus in the distant eye without affecting distance acuity, it will only enhance near and intermediate ranges. After the addition of plus to the distant eye, try additional plus in the near eye while the patient views distance. Again, if distance vision is not diminished, this will be a benefit for close-range work. If additional power, plus or minus, does not improve the quality of vision, the fitter can suggest a spectacle overcorrection for distance or near, modified monovision, or a bifocal contact lens fit (Figures 10 and 11).

The limitations of monovision occur particularly in dim or low-contrast lighting situations (eg, driving at night) or during sport activity. The patient should be given an option to utilize the "third lens" method or an ancillary pair of spectacles. The third lens method is to simply supply the patient with a spare distance lens to be used when the patient will knowingly be in a "distant only" environment (eg, sports activity). This is inexpensively accomplished with the use of disposable hydrogel lenses, preferably a daily disposable secondary to ease of tracking and affordability.

A second alternative for visual enhancement with monovision is a spectacle overcorrection. A near point overcorrection should have a suitable add power to assist the near point biased eye. The power should be trial framed rather than prescribed based upon the spectacle add. The fitter will find that the required add over the distance-corrected eye will be approximately 20% less than the manifest add power for spectacles. If the spectacle overcorrection is required for distance, the lens should be prescribed as a photosensitive (photochromatic) or "clip-on" sunglass lens to enable the patient the versatility in day and evening situations at a less expensive cost and minimal inconvenience.

Contraindications for monovision encompass existing binocular problems and individuals who have critical distance vision demands. If the patient has critical distance demands but desires contact lenses, one should consider modified monovision or bifocal contact lenses. If a patient has a refractive or strabismic amblyopia, it would not be appropriate to induce any further decrement to vision. However, if the patient has an alternating tropia, relatively good acuity in each eye, and is capable of active suppression, this could work in the favor of a monovision fit.

TABLE 3	SELECTION OF THE DISTANCE DOMINANT EYE[6,7]

Method	Technique
Hole in the Hand Demonstrates visual dominance and alignment	1. The patient is asked to fully extend the arms and place the hands together, making an opening the approximate size of a quarter. 2. The patient is asked to view an isolated letter on the acuity chart. 3. The fitter then covers one eye and then the other. 4. The eye that sees the target through the "hole" is the dominant eye.
Plus Lens Test Demonstrates ocular dominance and level of "blur toleration"	1. Place the best distance refraction into a trial frame. 2. Place a +1.50 lens in front of each eye in an alternating fashion as the patient views the distance acuity chart. 3. Ask the patient: "When the lens is held over your eye, which eye is least disturbed or appreciates the least amount of blur?" 4. The eye that appreciates the least amount of blur is the eye that should be selected for distance dominance. 5. Note: The test should be performed with an add power +.25 D to +.50 D less than the patient's spectacle add. 6. Less add power is required due to the vertex effect. Closer to the corneal plane adds plus to the overall power.
Alternate Occlusion Demonstrates the dominant eye for distant visual quality	1. This method uses the cover test method to determine the distant-dominant eye. 2. Simply have the patient view the acuity chart while occluding the eyes in an alternating format. 3. Ask the patient which eye appreciates the sharpest quality of vision while alternating the occluder. 4. After determining the distant-dominant eye in this method, proceed to the "plus lens" method to determine the level of "blur tolerance" at distance and near.
Camera to the Eye or Targeting Eye method Defines the distant-dominant eye	1. Place the final distance correction into a trial frame. 2. Have the patient take a camera and place it to the eye that he or she would normally use when taking pictures. This is the distance-dominant eye. 3. If a patient is active in sports that require firearms, archery, and so forth, ask the patient which eye he or she would usually use for targeting. Again, this would be the distance-dominant eye. 4. After the dominant eye is determined, proceed with the introduction of plus lenses over the near eye to determine the tolerance for blur.
Refractive Variance	Generally, the more myopic or less hyperopic eye will accept less plus at the near point. Therefore, the more myopic eye should be biased for the distance correction.

TABLE 4	DETERMINING POWER TOLERANCES FOR MONOVISION AND MULTIFOCAL FIT

1. Place subjective refraction into a trial frame.
2. Occlude the near-dominant eye. Add plus power in +0.25 D increments in front of the distant-dominant eye until there is a "just noticeable" decrease in visual quality when viewing distance. Place the power into the trial frame.
3. Occlude the distant-dominant eye. Place the subjective add power into the trial frame. Reduce plus power in +0.25 D increments until there is a "just noticeable" decrease in visual quality when viewing near. Place the power into the trial frame. The reading distance should be recessed to 16 to 18 inches.
4. When the fitter completes this evaluation, the distant-dominant eye should have an additional +0.25 to +0.50 D as compared to the spectacle prescription, while the near-dominant eye should have -0.25 to -0.50 D.
5. The overall add power should be reduced approximately +0.25 to +0.50 D as compared to the spectacle prescription.

TABLE 5	SATISFACTION OF VISUAL DEMAND WITH VARIOUS PRESBYOPIC CONTACT LENS OPTIONS				
Factor	Monovision	Modified Monovision	Translating Bifocal	Simultaneous Design	Modified Bivision
Visual demand at distance	✓✓	✓✓✓	✓✓✓	✓✓	✓✓✓
Visual demand at intermediate	✓	✓✓	✓	✓✓✓	✓✓✓
Visual demand at near	✓✓	✓✓	✓✓✓	✓✓	✓✓✓
Add power	<+1.75	<+2.50	<+2.50	<+1.75	<+2.50
Pupil dependency	None	Minimal	Variable	Variable	Variable
Pupil size limitations (mm)	No limitation	>3 mm	3 to 4	3 to 4	3 to 4
Available lens designs	Rigid and soft	Rigid and soft	Rigid only	Rigid and soft	Rigid and soft

✓ = below average; ✓✓ = average; ✓✓✓ = above average

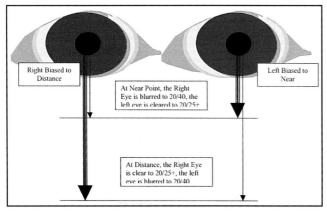

Figure 9. Balancing monovision.

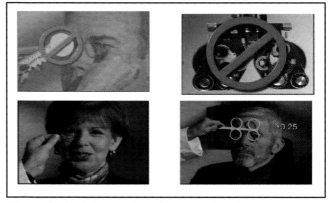

Figure 10. Refining presbyopic contact lens fits. Do not use a phoropter. Always refine binocularly, never monocularly. Always utilize a trial lens or flippers: ±0.25 or ±0.50.

Simultaneous View Annular Bifocals

Multifocal contact lenses can be described as "simultaneous view designs" due to their position over the pupil utilizing an annular, aspheric, or diffractive design. Multifocal lens designs can also be referred to as "pupil dependent or pupil sharing." This phrase implies that the lens has to be properly centered over the pupil and visual axis to yield the optimal visual effect. Any decentration of a "pupil dependent" lens design will degrade the visual quality and yield an image jump or "ghost/shadow" image adjacent to the primary image due to its axis eccentricity, causing an image awareness similar to that of an old-style black and white television set.

The annular or concentric design multifocal lens utilizes two distinct optical zones. These lenses are either designed as a near center-distance peripheral or distance center-near peripheral. These lenses require various annular widths that should complement the patient's pupil size in mid-dilation. This implies that the central optic should be visible to the examiner in red reflex at mid-dilation or should cover 50% of the entrance pupil.[11] Concentric designs will have either discrete junctures between the distance and near portions or can be designed with an aspheric interphase. The lenses can be constructed with either front or back surface optics (Figure 12).

Concentric bifocal contact lenses will have a distinct and measurable central and peripheral power. The most prevalent disadvantage of concentric-designed lenses is the induced blur circle created by the lens optics at the juncture of the distant and near annulus.

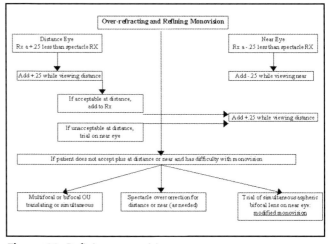

Figure 11. Refining monovision.

This can be minimized if the juncture is blended or the manufacturer utilizes an aspheric progression throughout the juncture. Optically, these lenses will produce relatively bright blur circles. These circles will tend to compete with well-focused images, leading to image confusion. Suppression and/or adaptation of the "out of focus" image is difficult due to its intensity.

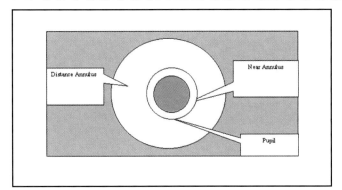

Figure 12. Annular-concentric lens design.

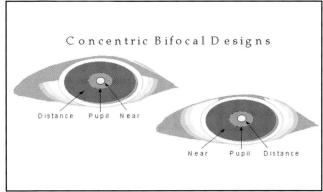

Figure 13. Annular-concentric bifocal designs.

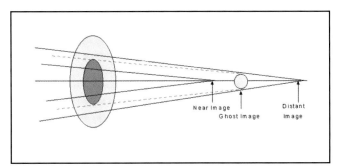

Figure 14. Annular-concentric bifocal optics/ghost-prismatic image.

With simultaneous vision lenses, 50% of the available light is designated for distance and 50% for near imaging. The retinal photoreceptors have an ability to utilize a summation of receptive fields in order to suppress certain portions of the image while amplifying the remaining light. This has been described as Airy's circle. It is a process of utilizing adjacent photoreceptors to intensify light.[12]

Annular designs can be fabricated from rigid or hydrophilic materials. The optics can be ground onto the front or back surface of the lens via lathe or cast molding technologies. In many designs, the manufacturer will make various segment or annulus diameters and add powers available. This allows the fitter to bias the segment or annulus and add on one or both eyes based upon the individual's pupil size and visual requirements. Noting that the lens must position over the visual and pupillary axis implies that the lens must be fit in alignment to the corner or slightly steeper in order to avoid excessive translation. Increased translation of a concentric design lens would only induce variable blur and increased appreciation of a ghosting image (Figure 13).

Lens decentration will decrease the image and increase ghosting ("image jump") due to the misalignment of the lens to the visual axis (Figure 14). Lens centration can be improved by utilizing a steeper base curve as long as it maintains the proper ocular physiological balance. Image jump can be reduced by splitting the segment size and bifocal power between the two eyes. This acts as an "image blending" technique, allowing for a modified bifocal effect. For example, the right eye may have a segment width of 2.5 mm with a +2.00 add, while the left eye may utilize a 4.0 mm segment width and a +1.00 add. The right would act as an intermediate and near eye, while the left eye would act as an intermediate and distance eye.

Center-near designs are used to maximize vision in variable lighting conditions optimized when the pupil is mid-dilated. The dilation of the pupil permits more light to enter through the distant peripheral portion of the lens while in bright light the pupil constricts, limiting the optics to the near annular. In contrast, center-distance designs are used to maximize the optics in better lighting conditions. This design limits the light entry through the distance portion of the lens when the pupil is constricted.

An astigmatism is not a contraindication to monovision. The astigmatic patient would be fit with the same method as the purely myopic or hyperopic patient. The only limitation that exists is the limited parameters in certain lens series for astigmatism. Hydrophilic disposable lens are now readily available in a wide range of parameters. However, if a patient starts to approach a greater level of astigmatism (greater than 2.00 D of cylinder), a rigid gas permeable—possibly a bitoric design—may be more appropriate.

The major limitation to the distance-centered design is that in normal working conditions, room lighting will limit the functional near point ability of the lens. In order to combat this problem, one could utilize different segment sizes on each eye or use inverse designs. For example, the right eye could be fit with a near-centered designed and the left fit with a distance-centered design. The power would be biased such that the right eye would facilitate near and intermediate while the left eye would be biased to intermediate and distance.

An aside to annular or concentric designs is the Pinhole lens. The Pinhole bifocal (Breger-Mueller-Welt contact lenses, Chicago, Ill) is a single-vision distance lens combined with a concentric near add that has a pinhole effect. The pinhole, as does a near annular, acts as an aperture stop before the entrance pupil, collimating light into amplified bundles that decrease the longitudinal and spherical aberrations while increasing the depth of focus and depth of field. In actuality, this is the oldest form of bifocal correction, dating back to the 16th century, and was later developed into the first still photographic techniques.

Modified Monovision, Modified Bivision

When patients do not accept monovision as well as a simultaneous or multifocal lens fit on both eyes, one can compromise. A technique that allows for a compromise and merger of fitting techniques tends to be one of the more successful overall methods of fitting a presbyope. Modified monovision is a method that encompasses the use of the distance-dominant eye to be fit with a single-vision distance lens. Contralaterally, the opposite eye will be fit with a bifocal or multifocal simultaneous view lens.

To optimize the effect, the distance-dominant eye is fit with a slight near bias by the method of MPMVA. The near-dominant eye

TABLE 6	TECHNIQUES FOR SUCCESSFUL MODIFIED MONOVISION AND MODIFIED BIVISION FITTING	

Distance Eye	Near Eye
Modified Monovision	
Single vision for distance	Bifocal with distance and near
Single vision distance	Bifocal with intermediate and near
Bifocal distance and intermediate	Single vision for near
Toric distance lens	Single or toric lens for near
Modified Bivision or Trivision	
Bifocal distance and intermediate	Bifocal for intermediate near
Concentric bifocal, small optical zone distance and near	Concentric bifocal, large optical zone for intermediate and near
Aspheric distance-centered design	Aspheric near-centered design
Translating bifocal distance near	Translating bifocal intermediate near
Concentric design, distance centered	Concentric design, near centered
Toric-concentric bifocal, distance centered	Toric-concentric bifocal, near centered

is then fit with a simultaneous view lens that is biased to an intermediate and near lens power range. This will afford the patient maximum range of vision without a dramatic compromise at distance or near. This technique should allow the intermediate/near eye to visualize distance to at least 20/40 to 20/50 level. In contrast, pure monovision would decrease the distance acuity of the near eye to 20/80 or worse. For near point enhancement, a simple ancillary pair of reading glasses could be prescribed but is usually unnecessary.

As a note, if a patient requires an astigmatic lens in one eye, that eye should be biased to a full distance correction. If the patient requires a toric lens in both eyes, a rigid gas permeable lens is preferred. However, several companies are now manufacturing toric multifocals. These are limited due to higher complexity of design, compounding visual variables, and increased cost of lenses.

This same technique can be accomplished with multifocals or bifocals on each eye, called "modified bivision" or "modified trivision." In this scenario, the multifocal or bifocal fit is pure distance and near, and tends to yield adequate vision but is not subjectively acceptable. In a modified technique, the distance-dominant eye is fit with a lens that has the full distance annulus correction but only a partial near annulus correction biased toward the intermediate range. Contralaterally, the opposite eye is fit with a lens that biases the distance annulus to intermediate and the near annulus to the full near add. This technique works remarkably well for patients with a vast array of visual demands.

In either technique, a combination of lenses have been utilized to imply that the patient may be wearing different materials on each eye as well as each lens having different base curves and fitting relationships (Table 6). In the majority of cases, it is best to start with a manufacturer that offers single vision, toric, and bifocal lenses.

Simultaneous View Aspheric and Multizonal Multifocals

Aspheric multifocal designs utilize a pseudoannular design that is generally referred to as progressive aspheric power design. Aspheric multifocal lenses are designed with a front or back surface that allows for enhanced fitting characteristics with an enhanced multifocal effect. The lenses will either have a central distance portion with the progressive peripheral flattening yielding less minus, an increase in plus power, or a central portion biased to near with a

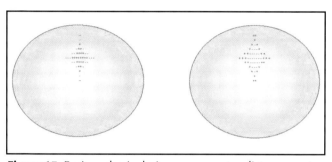

Figure 15. Basic aspheric designs: near center-distance center.

progression to distance power in the periphery. The major limiting factor of these lenses is the amount of affordable add power due to the eccentricity, or "e" value. At best, an aspheric lens delivers an approximate add power of +1.50 to +1.75. Therefore, a biasing technique of modified monovision or modified bivision must be applied when higher add powers are required (Figures 15 and 16).

Simultaneous view aspheric multifocals (Figure 17) have the advantage of allowing for a wide range of correctable vision at near, intermediate, and distance without adjusting the head or eye position. The designs allow for the fitter to be creative in addressing the variety of visual needs of the patient. Aspheric lens designs will require the fitter to bias one eye to distance (infinity) and a far intermediate (25 to 35 inches), while the contralateral eye is biased to approximately intermediate (18 to 24 inches) and near (14 to 18 inches).[13-16]

There are various aspheric lens designs (Figures 18 to 23) that enable one to meet the visual and physiological needs of the patient. Restriction to a single lens design can limit the fitter's success rate. In turn, the success rate can be enhanced by abiding to the key principles of the lens design that mandate pupil and visual axis centration, adjusting powers to meet the patient's needs, and selecting the appropriate material to meet the ocular physiological requirements.

Aspheric lenses are pupil- and visual-axis dependent—the same as annular designs. The fitter needs to explain to the patient that there will be some compromise to the quality of vision by this design; however, the patient will appreciate an enhanced level of

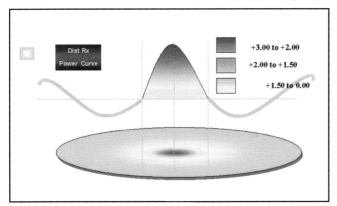

Figure 16. Focus-progressive power curve of a near-centered aspheric lens (courtesy of Dwight Akerman, OD, Ciba Vision).

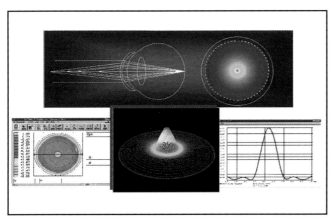

Figure 18. Focus progressive design by Ciba Vision. Lens optic surface topography (courtesy of Dwight Akerman, OD, Ciba Vision).

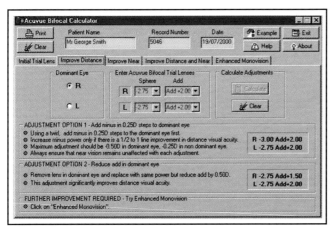

Figure 20. AcuVue bifocal online calculator.

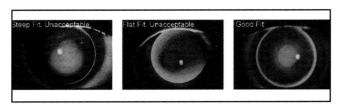

Figure 22. Rigid gas permeable back surface aspheric: VFL3 (courtesy of Randy Campbell, Conforma Labs, Norfolk, Va).

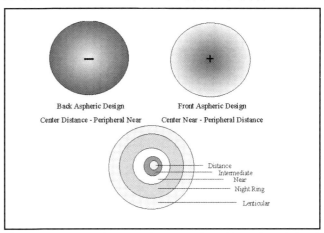

Figure 17. Front, back aspheric, and multizonal multifocal designs.[21,22]

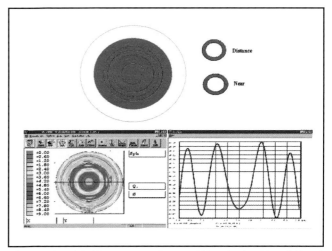

Figure 19. Multizone annular multifocal: AcuVue bifocal (Johnson and Johnson, Jacksonville, Fla).

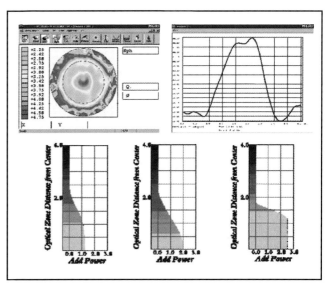

Figure 21. Sunsoft aspheric near center design: three aspheric profiles.

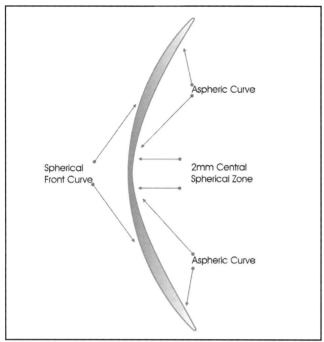

Figure 23. Back surface aspheric rigid gas permeable: Metro aspheric progressive (courtesy of Metro Optics, Dallas, Tex).

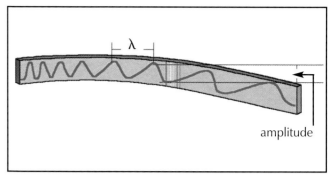

Figure 24. Sine wave: lambda (λ) and amplitude.

Diffractive Multifocals

Diffractive multifocal designs create simultaneous vision that will deliver light from distance, intermediate, and near through a centralized optical system. Diffractive optics utilize a variation of Fresnel prisms. This creates a deviation of the light based upon the apical angles of a series of circular prismatic rings.

A diffractive lens, sometimes referred to as a holographic lens, utilizes a combination of refraction and diffraction. Refraction is defined as the change in the velocity of light and emergence of light through a media due to the variance in the index of refraction based upon Snell's law. Diffraction is defined as the interaction of light waves with an obstacle(s), which will control the functionality and characteristics of the light wavefront (Figure 24).

The diffractive optic multifocal uses a front surface refraction and a back surface diffractive phase plate that adds or subtracts portions of the incoming light. A phase plate is a clear optical medium that will split incoming light between near and distance foci. The phase plate alters the light by amplifying, either additively or subtractively. The phase plate is referred to as an echelon with "echelettes." Amplification of light will vary on base curve, index of refraction, and spacing and depth of the echelettes (Figure 25). This demonstrates the amplification of entering light onto a specific focal point via refraction and diffraction. The echelettes are cast molded onto the back surface of the lens at a 3-micron depth. The depth determines the intensity of the wave amplification or additive effect. The spacing between the echelettes, viewed as concentric circles, will determine the add power. More numerous echelettes will deliver a higher add power but will require tighter spacing.

Unwanted visual side effects of diffractive optics include ghosting, halos, and contrast reduction. If the diffractive lens is significantly decentered away from the visual axis, the patient will appreciate a ghost image. This will appear as a sharp, intense image surrounded by a second out-of-focus or hazed image. Due to lens decentration and the prismatic effect of the echelettes, the patient may perceive "halos" or color infringement patterns. Additionally, since the lens is separating incoming light, the patient may appreciate reduced contrast sensitivity particularly in low illumination. The patient should always be instructed to read in good light. If the patient finds that it is difficult to read fine detail, it is suggested that a +1.00 enhancement spectacle be worn over the contact lenses as needed.

Diffractive lenses are not pupil-dependent but should be fit steep enough to maintain a centralized optic at all times. There are no rotational factors that would diminish the image quality. The lens utilizes a full aperture optic that allows for a complete capture of

vision at various ranges. If the lens displaces significantly upon gaze or blink, the patient will appreciate a variability in the quality of vision and/or experience a ghosting image. Therefore, aspheric as well as concentric annular designs must be fit with a slightly steeper base curve to allow for the minimization of lens translation. This creates a fine balance of a good fit for optimal vision while maintaining adequate criteria for proper physiological maintenance. Therefore, high dK rigid gas-permeable (RGP) lenses or high water content hydrophilic lenses are encouraged.

There is no one design that will suffice the total visual needs of the patient; therefore, combinations of powers and designs must be tried. For instance, a fitter may need to utilize front or back aspheric on both eyes or may want to use a front aspheric for the near eye and a back aspheric for the distant-dominant eye. The bottom line is to follow the specific guidelines developed by each manufacturer for the initial trial fitting and then apply creativity and clinical experience to determine the appropriate refinement.

Aspheric multifocals are designed based upon an eccentricity value (e value). The degree of flattening is directly proportional to the increase in the eccentricity. Front surface aspheres are generally used for presbyopic correction. The amount of add required for an aspheric lenses will require an e value of 1 to 1.3, where a value of 1 would be analogous to a low add such as +1.00. In contrast, an e value of 1.3 would be equivalent to a +2.50 add. e values of 0.4 to 0.6 are usually prescribed for nonpresbyopic patients and used to enhance fitting characteristics of the lens.[17,18]

$$ESR = s/2 + d^2/8s$$
(ESR = equivalent sagitta radius, s = sagitta, d = chord)
ESR for the determination of aspheric back surface

$$e = (1-b^2/a^2)^{1/2}$$
(e = eccentricity value, b = prolate chord, a = oblate chord)
(equation 1: eccentricity value)[19]

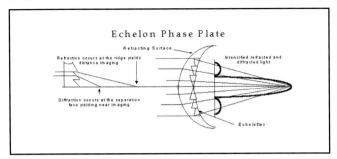

Figure 25. Echelon diffractive optic bifocal.[22-24]

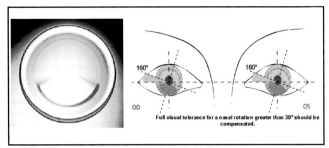

Figure 26. Presbylite translating inversed crescent bifocal.

entering light while enhancing the critical resolution of the image. Finally, it allows for enhanced binocular vision and intermediate visual ranges. The optimal diffractive effect is accomplished with a near biasing of the near-dominant eye or the use of a combination of the diffractive optic bifocal on the near-dominant eye with an back surface aspheric on the distance-dominant eye.

Translating or Alternating Bifocal Lens Designs

Translating or alternating bifocal lens designs differ significantly from other multifocal designs. These lenses are essentially "miniature" executive, flat top, or crescent-style pupil-dependent bifocals. All light will pass through the distance or near zone based upon the eye and lens position.

Hydrophilic translating designs have not proven to be effective due to the lack of significant alternation between distance and near. Hydrophilic lenses will conform to the corneal topography, thus restricting an ease of translation. Rigid translating bifocals can be fabricated in front, back, and bitoric designs, addressing the needs of the presbyopic astigmatic patient. Translating bifocal lenses, particularly single-piece lenses, are 30% to 40% thicker than standard rigid spherical lenses.

Pupil size in bright, moderate, and dim light must be measured. Large pupil diameters will limit the success of a crescent or segmented bifocal. Palpebral aperture width and lid tension will also have a significant effect on lens fitting. Tight lids will not allow the lens to translate properly as well as possibly displacing the bifocal segment superiorly into the midpoint of the pupil. Flaccid lid anatomy will allow the lens to displace below the inferior lid, thus making it difficult to properly place the bifocal segment into the appropriate position.

Finally, the patient should have experience with rigid lenses prior to fitting a rigid translating bifocal. Inexperienced patients will have tightened lid posture upon the introduction of the lens, thus erroneously dislocating the lens. The introduction of anesthetic to the eye will facilitate a patient's initial comfort and lens measures.

The lens will assume an inferior position on primary distance gaze. Therefore, the lens design requires stabilization, ballasting, and truncation similar to that of toric lenses. The prism ballast acts as a "brake" to prevent the lens from migrating behind and below the inferior lid margin upon downward near point gaze. In other words, as the patient switches gaze from distance to near, the lens will be forced to translate, vertically aligning the add segment with the visual axis. Thus, the lower lid, in conjunction with the ballast of the lens, acts as a buttress to inhibit excessive downward translation of the lens and allow the lens bifocal segment to center over the pupil zone.

Rigid translating bifocals can be designed in a variety of ways,

including one piece, such as the Presbylite (Figure 26) or MetroSeg, executive style such as the Tangent Streak, crescent shaped (Figure 27), and fused straight-top design such as the Paragon ST (Paragon Vision Sciences, Mesa, Ariz) bifocal. Basic fitting of these lenses does not vary significantly from standard gas permeable techniques. These lenses require a palpebral aperture or inferior aperture position. An experienced rigid lens patient who is to be refit with a translating design should be forewarned that the lens position will be low in comparison to his or her present lens.

A low-riding lens may yield a slight lens awareness due to its interaction with the inferior lid margin. The difficulty in these lens designs is their increased weight. A low-riding lens may not be due to the base curve but to the lens weight. Therefore, excessive inferior positioning of the lens may not be easily rectified by changing the base curve.

The optimal fitting scenario for a translating bifocal is to position the segment line below the pupillary fringe at mid-dilation. Any impingement within the pupil while viewing distance will disrupt vision. This would be most apparent in dim illumination.

It is important to pay attention to the tautness of the lower lid. As mentioned before, the lower lid acts as a "buttress" to assist in the proper translation and positioning of the bifocal segment. If the lid is excessively taut, it may force the lens to rest high, causing the segment to impinge within the pupil. If the lid is flaccid, the lens must translate behind the lid margin, not allowing the segment to translate vertically into the region of the pupil during reading. The only remedies for an excessive lid tightness is to design a low segment with an "on K" or slight steep base curve to limit the amount of translation. To remedy a poor translation due to a flaccid lid is to flatten the base curve to encourage a greater lid interaction. In this scenario, do not increase the prism ballast of the lens because it will only cause the lens to decenter inferiorly and cause an increased lens awareness.

Another method of measuring the segment height is to simply place the trial lens on the eye and adjust the room lighting while the patient views the distance acuity chart. If the patient appreciates a blur or image jump after dimming the room light, the segment is too high. An additional method to determine an optimal position of the segment is to have the patient look at a near point card positioned directly in front of him or her. Have the patient lower the reading card slowly into his or her customary near point reading position. The patient should take note of at what point the vision clears for near. Is this a comfortable position, too high, or too low?

To measure the segment height, observe the segment position in primary gaze and then have the patient look slightly down and inward, and observe the translation of the segment. This is best accomplished by using a cobalt blue filter with the slit lamp rheostat set to moderate to low illumination. The segment should never position itself within the pupil upon distance gaze but should have a complete coverage of the pupil upon near gaze.

The segment height will vary based upon the lens design. One-piece designs, such as the Tangent Streak or Paragon ST bifocal segment will encompass approximately 33% to 50% of the total lens surface. This is equivalent to a segment height of approximately 3 to 4.5 mm high. A fused bifocal design such as the Paragon ST has segment heights available from 3 to 5 mm, with the average order between 3.4 and 3.6 mm.

Translating lenses should be fit with slightly steeper alignment than flat keratometric fit. To compensate for excessive steepness, an optic zone equal to or slightly smaller than the base curve should be used. This will facilitate proper translation without resistance. Additionally, the fitter should incorporate the appropriate prism ballast to allow the lens to settle evenly on the inferior lid margin. The prism ballast for a minus lens will be 2 to 2.5 D, while a plus lens will require a 1.5 to 2 D. To enhance the prism ballast and reduce overall lens thickness, a truncation can be added. Truncation should range from 0 to 0.4 mm, noting that 0.2 mm is usually sufficient.

Rotation of a translating lens is considered problematic if the segment encroaches into part of the pupil or is excessively nasal or temporal. Lens rotation can be corrected by specifying the base apex line. This is done in the same manner as adjusting for a toric rotation using the LARS (left add, right subtract) principle.

For example, a right eye lens that is observed to rotate 10 degrees to the examiner's right should order the base apex line of the prism ballast at axis 80 degrees. This would shift the prism ballast weight of the lens to the lower left edge of the truncation, forcing the rotation toward the left. Another method is to taper and polish the inferior right aspect of the truncation to reduce its weight and shift the ballast to the left aspect of the truncation.

A further adjustment for excessive rotation can be accomplished by base curve and/or optic zone diameter adjustments. A steeper base curve of approximately 0.05 mm may straighten the lens as long as it does not restrict translation. Additionally, the optic zone diameter can be increased, which will also yield a subtle steepening effect.

To avoid superior lid attachment, the peripheral curve system can be designed steeper than the fitter would normally do. For example, if the fitter's traditional rigid lens secondary curve is 1.2 mm flatter than the base curve and the peripheral curve is 2.8 flatter than the base curve, the fitter may want to design the lens 0.8 mm and 2.0 to 2.4 mm flatter than the base curve. Additionally, a superior CN bevel (anterior surface edge thinning) or superior tapering of the front surface will limit superior lid grab or interaction.

If the patient requires intermediate vision correction, the contact lens power should be adjusted to a modified bivision design. This requires the fitter to prescribe the full distance and near power to the distant-dominant eye while the near-dominant eye is fit to intermediate and near. The intermediate power should be equivalent to less than 50% of the add power, while the add power for that eye is adjusted to maintain the same total add as the opposite eye.

For example, if the binocular subjective refraction is -2.00 D with a +2.00 add, then the distant dominant eye would be fit with a -2.00 with a +2.00 add. The near dominant eye would be -1.00 with a +1.00 add. This will maintain a +2.00 add binocularly. This is referred to as a modified bivision design. Modified bivision bifocal fitting will yield a high success rate, particularly for patients

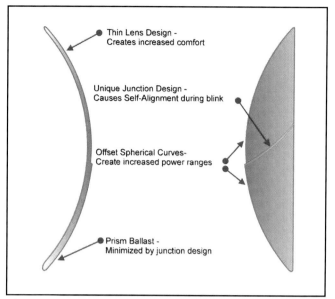

Figure 27. Crescent segment translating bifocal (courtesy of Metro Optics, Inc, Dallas, Tex).

using computers, making presentations, or those with a large amount of intermediate vision requirements.

Finally, as with segmented spectacle bifocals, image jump at the intersection of the segment and carrier lens can be disruptive to vision. Translating bifocal contact lenses are diminished by displacing the segment's optical center at the upper edge of the segment or, as with executive-style translating lenses, the lens is monocentric. These are called "no jump" designs due to the rapid translation into the segment and displaced optics.

Translating bifocal lenses are best designed from RGP materials. Hydrophilic materials lack adequate ability to properly translate and are, therefore, limited to aspheric and annular designs. Translating designs give the greatest level of freedom in design, inclusive of astigmatic options. Additionally, there is more freedom in developing modified monovision and/or bivision options.

NEW MONTHLY REPLACEMENT LENS

Frequency 55 multifocal is the new monthly replacement multifocal lens from CooperVision, Inc, Irvine, Calif. It is an "inverse geometry lens system," resulting in a modification and enhancement to monovision utilizing a multifocal design. The system requires a D lens (distance) for the dominant eye and an N lens (near) for the nondominant eye. The lenses have a spherical central zone surrounded by an aspheric annular zone, followed by a spherical peripheral annular zone (Figure 28). The central zone diameters vary between the D lens (2.3 mm) and N lens (1.7 mm) so as to maximize both the visual performance at various focal points of distance, intermediate, and near. The inverse geometry lens system results in optimizing binocular visual acuity at both distance and near.

The fitting process is straightforward and best shown below:
Acuity Expectations
Binocularly: Distance 20/20, near 20/20
D lens: Distance 20/20, near 20/40 or better
N lens: Near 20/20, distance 20/40 or better

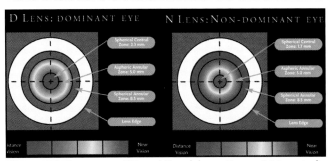

Figure 28. Frequency 55 multifocal from CooperVision. Left: D lens. Right: N lens

CONCLUSION

It is a disservice to a patient not to discuss the contact lens options for presbyopia. Not being involved with the fitting of contact lenses for presbyopia is the most devastating mistake in practice management. The population of present contact lens patients is getting older, and they will not surrender their contact lenses. Therefore, it is mandatory that the clinician address the presbyopic needs of the patient via the variety of contact lens modalities discussed in this chapter. Explore the triad of modalities—monovision, alternating, and simultaneous deigns—and the combinations and modified modalities. Experience with the various modalities will define ultimate success.

Success in fitting presbyopic contact lenses starts with listening to the patient. The second step is designing a system that will address the needs of the patient. This may not occur on the first dispensing visit but will arise on subsequent aftercare visits. Presbyopic contact lens fitting is not perfect; it has limitations that can be minimized with the proper lens design and, more importantly, proper patient education, development of realistic expectations, and motivations.

REFERENCES

1. White P, Watanabe R. Presbyopic contact lens care. *Contact Lens Spectrum.* 1996;8;34-40.
2. Karp A. Presbyopes hit critical mass. *Vision Monday.* 1996;June 10:23.
3. Harris MG, Classe JG. Clinicolegal considerations of monovision. *J Am Optom Assoc.* 1988;59(6):491-494.
4. Harris MG. Keep presbyopic contact lens wearers informed. *Contact Lens Spectrum.* 1993;8.
5. Jurkus JM, Nichols SL. Contact lenses and the aging eye. *Optometry Today.* 1999;April(Suppl):53-60.
6. Wood WW. Five ideas for improving your success with monovision. *Contact Lens Spectrum.* 1992.
7. Wood WW. Six more ideas for improving your success with monovision. *Contact Lens Spectrum.* 1992;Aug.
8. Lebow KA, Goldberg JB. Characteristics of binocular vision found for presbyopic patients wearing single vision contact lenses. *J Am Optom Assoc.* 1975;46:1116-1123.
9. Collins MJ, Brown B, Verney SJ. Peripheral visual acuity with monovision and other contact lens corrections for presbyopia. *Optom Vis Sci.* 1989;66:370-374.
10. Schor C, et al. Effects of interocular blur suppression on the ability of monovision task performance. *J Am Optom Assoc.* 1989;60(3):188-192.
11. Erickson P, et al. Performance characteristics of concentric hydrogel bifocal contact lenses. *AJOPO.* 1985;62(10):702-708.
12. Benjamin WJ, Borish IM. Presbyopia and the influence of aging on prescription of contact lenses. In: Rueben M, Guillion M, eds. *Contact Lens Practice.* London: Chapman & Hall; 1994:785-786.
13. Lapierre M, et al. Success rate evaluation of simultaneous center add soft contact lenses. *ICLC.* 1991;19(3):157-161.
14. Shapiro MB, et al. A prospective evaluation of Unilens soft multifocal contact lens in 100 patients. *CLAO.* 1994;20(3):189-191.
15. Key JE, et al. Perspective clinical evaluation of the Sunsoft multifocal contact lens. *CLAO.* 1996;22(3):179-184.
16. Maltzman BA, et al. Experience with soft bifocal contact lenses. *CLAO.* 1985;2(11):73-77.
17. Baude D, Meige C. Presbyopia with contact lenses: a new aspherical progressive lens. *British Contact Lens Association.* 1992;15(1):7-15.
18. Goldberg JB. Basic principles of aspheric contact lenses. *Contact Lens Forum.* 1998;May:35-38.
19. Ruben M, Guillion M. Contact lens practice. In: Ruben M, Guillion M, eds. *The Verification of Soft Lenses in Clinical Practice.* London: Chapman & Hall; 1994:176-177.
20. Lifestyle Frequency Progressive (Specialty Progressive) Fitting Guideline; 1996.
21. Unilens Fitting and Technical Guidelines for Unilens, Simulvue, Unilens RGP, System 250; 1996.
22. Gailmard NB. Clinical investigation of the Hydron echelon bifocal hydrophilic contact lens. *Contact Lens Spectrum.* 1989;Oct:51-56.
23. Cohen AL. Bifocal contact lens optics. *Contact Lens Spectrum.* 1989;June:43-52.
24. Cohen AL, Cohen HA. Diffractive bifocal designs vs. simultaneous vision. *Contact Lens Spectrum.* 1989;Mar:49-51.

SECTION II

Scleral Modifications to Correct Presbyopia

Chapter 8

Scleral Expansion Band Instrumentation and Anesthesia

Gene W. Zdenek, MD; Gregg Feinerman, MD;
and Nora Emmons, RN

INTRODUCTION

Three decades ago an ophthalmic revolution began, lead by the vast technology acquired from both the private and government sectors. The first decade was that of the intraocular lens. This era brought many new surgical approaches supported by many new instruments. Phacoemulsification was one of many technologies to help advance this era. The second decade was that of laser-assisted in situ keratomileusis (LASIK). Technology led our quest for refractive perfection. An interesting perspective on these two decades is the first was lead by surgical skills and supported by technology, whereas in contrast the second decade was just the reverse. With LASIK, technology leads the way, albeit surgical skills are a requirement.

In the present decade, the key word is presbyopia. Like the first decade, the current emphasis is surgical skill; however, technology is meeting the challenge to improve, simplify, and refine the procedure.

The surgical reversal of presbyopia (SRP) using scleral expansion band (SEB) segments is a great example of how important the synergy is between surgical skills and technology. SRP can be divided into eight basic steps:

1. Oblique quadrant marking at the limbus
2. Conjunctival opening and exposure
3. Hemostasis
4. Scleral marking
5. Sclerotomy
6. Belt loop formation
7. Segment insertion
8. Conjunctival closure

Of these basic steps, the new automated device called the PresbyDrive (Presby Corp, Dallas, Tex) is capable of eliminating half of the steps (#3 to 6) (Table 1).

The relationship of the PresbyDrive to SRP is analogous to the microkeratome advancing photorefractive keratectomy (PRK) to the current LASIK procedure. In contrast to the microkeratome, the PresbyDrive has only one moving part and is much more dependable. Unlike LASIK, where the microkeratome is an integral and necessary component, SRP can be successfully completed without the PresbyDrive.

EYELID SPECULUM (PRESBY PY ES 5)

This speculum contains solid blades for retraction of the lashes and drapes. The convenient "setscrew" assembly allows for maximum exposure along with patient comfort.

WIRE SPECULUM (PRESBY PY ES 12)

This basic wire speculum offers surgeons another option for lid retraction.

AXIS QUADRANT MARKER (PRESBY PY AM 3)

Proper placement of the SEB segments is of fundamental importance in SRP surgery. The surgical result will be suboptimal if the SEB segments are not properly positioned. Additionally, improper placement of the segments can lead to anterior segment ischemia. The quadrant marker is used to mark the *axis location* of the SEB segments. Prior to the procedure, it is important to mark the 12 o'clock position at the slit lamp with the patient in the upright position. At the beginning of the surgery, the surgeon lines up the handle of the axis quadrant marker at the 12 o'clock position. Twelve marks are created near the limbus. The marks represent the axis orientation for proper placement of the SEB segments but do not always define the anatomical location of the limbus. Each quadrant has a 1.0 mm radial central mark that represents the oblique (45 degree) meridians relative to the 12 o'clock mark. There are two pointed marks on each quadrant that are 4.0 mm apart. At the completion of the procedure, the SEB segments should be centered over the oblique axis 45-degree mark, and the ends of each SEB segment should be in line with the pointed marks.

Ink should be applied sparingly with a sterile surgical marking pen. Applying the ink a few minutes prior to use may give better, longer-lasting results. The surgeon will need to refer back to these

	PRESBYCORP INSTRUMENTATION KIT	

Part Number	Description	Used in Step
Presby PY ES 5	Eyelid speculum	1 to 8
Presby PY ES 12	Wire speculum	1 to 8
Presby PY AM 3	Axis marker	1
Presby PY WB 10	Conjunctival scissors, blunt	2
Presby PY WS 11	Conjunctival scissors, sharp	2
Presby PY BF 1	Scleral forceps	2
Presby PY CF 7	Tissue forceps	2, 7
Presby PY SM 4	Four-prong marker	4
Presby PY PD 1	PresbyDrive (optional addition)	4 to 6
Presby PY BL 2-4	Scleral belt loop marker	4, 6
Presby PY P 15	Incisional diamond blade	5
Presby PY P 9	Lamella diamond blade	6
Presby PY SF 2R	Scleral fixator-right	6, 7
Presby PY SF 2L	Scleral fixator-left	6, 7
Presby PY SP 1-4	Double-ended spatula	6, 7
Presby PY IN 6	Segment injector	7
Presby SH 1	Insertion forceps	7
Presby PY NH 30	Segment holder, needle holder	7
Presby EB 4	Scleral expansion band segments	7
Presby PY TF 26	Tying forceps	8

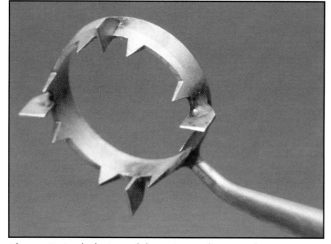

Figure 1. Angled view of the axis quadrant marker.

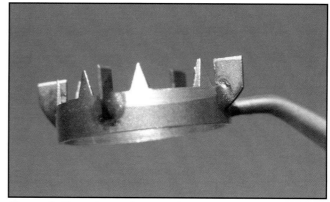

Figure 2. The axis quadrant marker.

marks throughout the procedure. If the marks fade, they can be remarked directly with a surgical pen (Figures 1 and 2).

CONJUNCTIVAL SCISSORS AND TISSUE FORCEPS (PRESBY PY WB 10, WS 11, CF 7)

A peritomy is created with .12 forceps and Wescott scissors (both blunt and sharp are provided, either or both may be used). The conjunctival peritomy is extended to 1 to 2 mm beyond the pointed 4 mm mark to assure adequate exposure. Care should be taken not to damage the underlying sclera during Tenon's dissection (Figure 3).

PRESBYDRIVE AUTOMATED BELT LOOP MAKER (PRESBY PY PD 1)

The PresbyDrive is an automated device consisting of a rotating arcuate blade that passes through a foot plate designed with an entrance and exit slot. This allows the PresbyDrive to make a precise belt loop 400 microns deep and 4.0 mm long (Figures 4 to 7).

The disposable blade (Figure 8) advances to form the belt loop with the foot pedal control (Figures 9 and 10). The control unit has a convenient abort button if progression of the blade needs to be stopped.

After completion of the belt loop, the PresbyDrive automatically senses the completed belt loop and retracts to the original position in preparation for the next belt loop.

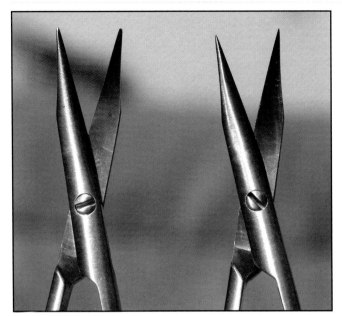

Figure 3. Blunt and pointed scissors side by side.

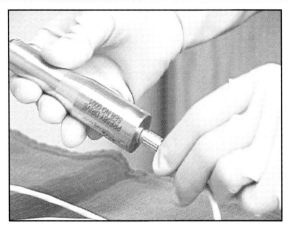

Figure 4. The hand piece.

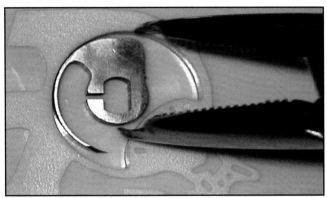

Figure 5. Forceps removing the PresbyDrive blade.

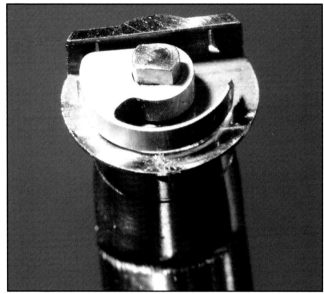

Figure 6. PresbyDrive head, front view.

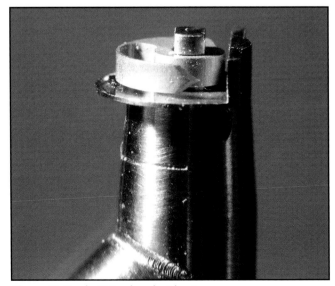

Figure 7. PresbyDrive head, side view.

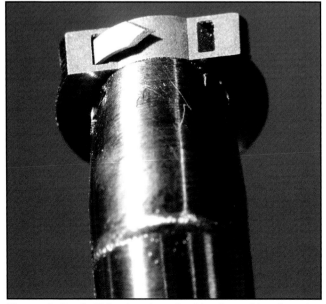

Figure 8. PresbyDrive head, underside view with advancing blade.

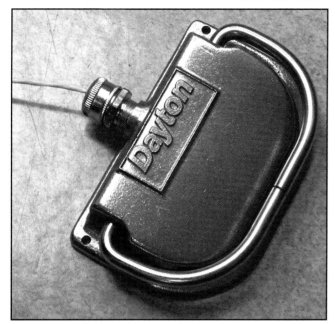

Figure 9. PresbyDrive foot switch.

As mentioned earlier, the PresbyDrive will eliminate four major steps in the SRP procedure. The surgical time can be shortened even more if all four belt loops are made at once. This avoids passing the PresbyDrive back and forth to the scrub technician. Following are the steps necessary for manual belt loop formation.

Scleral Belt Loop Marker (Presby PY BL 2-4)

The scleral belt loop marker is used to mark the position of the scleral belt loop. The pointed prongs are 4.0 mm apart. The parallel rectangular prongs are 1.5 mm long and 3.5 mm posterior to the pointed prongs. The parallel posterior marks define the location for the sclerotomy (Figure 11).

Four-Prong ("Two-by-Four") Marker (Presby PY SM 4)

This instrument is included in the Presby kit to double-check the proper location of the scleral belt loop marks. One pair of prongs is 4.0 mm apart for determining the distance between the sclerotomies. The other end of the instrument has prongs that are 3.5 mm apart and used to verify that the sclerotomies are 3.5 mm posterior to the limbus. In the past, the sclerotomies were made 2 mm posterior to the limbus, which gave the instrument the name "two-by-four." An improved accommodative effect occurs with the sclerotomies located 3.5 mm posterior to the limbus. The ends are labeled with rubber identification sleeves (Figures 12 and 13).

Incisional (Scleral Punch) Diamond Blade (Presby PY P 15)

This is a square diamond blade that is used to make the 300 µm

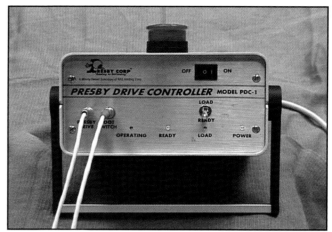

Figure 10. PresbyDrive control panel.

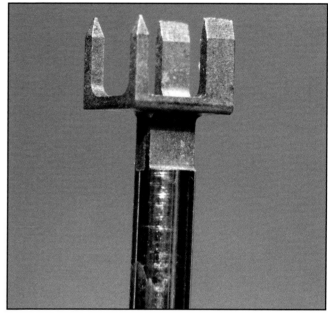

Figure 11. Scleral belt loop.

deep sclerotomy. It is retractable and guarded, and is 150 µm thick and 1500 µm wide to create the 1.5 mm-wide scleral belt loops. Before making the scleral punch, it is important to make sure that there is no Tenon's capsule present at the site of the parallel marks. Otherwise, if Tenon's capsule is present, the sclerotomies will be shallower than 300 µm (Figure 14).

Scleral Fixator, Right and Left Twist Picks (Presby PY SF 2R and 2L)

A scleral fixator is used to provide control over the globe. It allows the surgeon to move the eye in the x, y, or z-axis. In SRP with SEB segments, the scleral fixator provides countertraction and prevents rotation of the globe during creation of the belt loop, and later for insertion of the SEB segments.

Presby Corp has supplied two types of scleral twist pick fixators. The scleral twist pick is designed for fixation to the eye by either clockwise or counterclockwise rotation depending on surgeon preference. It has a pair of sharp-tipped spiral prongs that only penetrate

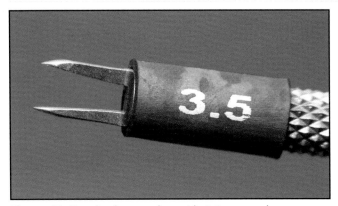

Figure 12. Two-by-four marker with 3.5 mm end.

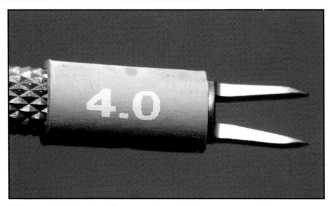

Figure 13. Two-by-four marker with 4.0 mm end.

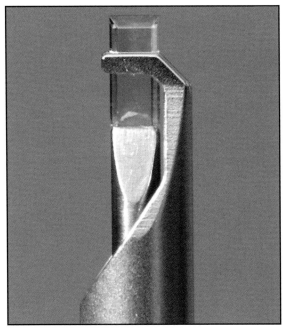

Figure 14. Sclerotomy diamond blade.

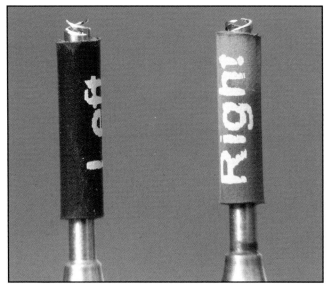

Figure 15. Left and right twist pick fixators.

the sclera 300 to 400 µm. It is important to clear away Tenon's capsule at the site of intended scleral fixation so that the surgeon maintains good fixation. The ends of the twist pick have rubber identification sleeves that identify their intended direction of use. They also protect the lamellar diamond blade from damage if the blade touches the twist pick (Figure 15).

Bores dual fixation forceps (Storz #1671, Gmbh, Germany) can also be used for scleral fixation. They have two 0.12 mm forceps that are spaced 3.0 mm apart. The Bores dual fixation forceps grasp the sclera at two points parallel to and behind the sclerotomy site. The lamellar diamond blade can easily pass between the fixation points. It is important to grasp the sclera firmly for good control during creation of the belt loop and for insertion of the SEB segments.

LAMELLA DIAMOND BLADE (PRESBY PY P 9)

The lamella diamond blade is used to make the scleral belt loop. The blade is 1.5 mm wide, 150 µm deep, 5 mm long, and is set at an angle. The extra millimeter in length of the blade assures it will exit the sclerotomy. Only the rounded tip of the blade is sharp. It is of

excellent quality, which allows for easy passage through the sclera during formation of the belt loop. The blade retracts into the handle when not in use (Figure 16).

After a successful belt loop has been completed, the following instruments are used to finish the SRP procedure.

SEGMENT INJECTOR (PRESBY PY IN 6)

Insertion of the segment is performed after creation of the scleral belt loop. The SEB injector is a spring-loaded plunger system. The surgeon applies pressure to the plunger, which pushes out the SEB segment. The segment can be loaded either flat side up or flat side down. If injected flat side up, the SEB segment must be rotated within the scleral belt loop after completion of the pass. After loading the injector, approximately one-third of the segment will protrude from the tip. Before injecting the SEB segment, it is important to use a scleral twist pick on the opposite end of the belt loop. The scleral fixator should be placed about 2 mm from the exit side of the belt loop. The tip of the SEB segment is inserted into the belt loop, and the surgeon gently applies pressure to the plunger so that the SEB segment is advanced slowly. Pressure is applied on the scleral twist pick to ensure that the tip of the SEB segment points slightly upward. It is important to keep the injector in line with the belt

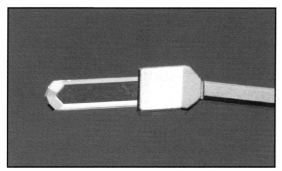

Figure 16. Lamella diamond blade.

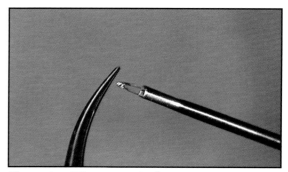

Figure 17. SEB segment in the injector.

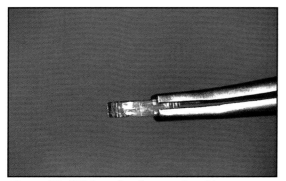

Figure 18. SEB insertion forceps tip with segment.

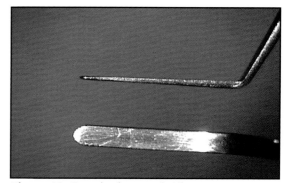

Figure 19. Spatula, front and side views.

loop as the SEB segment is advanced. Force is applied with the scleral twist pick in the opposite direction of the segment insertion. This injector is also designed to allow leading edge lift of the advancing segment during injection. This steep angle eases segment insertion in difficult cases (Figure 17).

SEB INSERTION FORCEPS (PRESBY SH 1)

The SEB insertion forceps are two square-tipped, channeled forceps that snugly hold the SEB segment. This aids insertion of and allows direct visualization of the SEB segment. The surgeon can regrasp the SEB segment and apply different torsional movements. One significant advantage of the SEB insertion forceps is that they provide the ability to pull the SEB segment out of the belt loop. The injector can only push the segment forward but cannot pull it back out if necessary. Another advantage is the ability to rotate the SEB segment using the same instrument. The only disadvantage is a limitation of the steep angle often necessary during difficult SEB segment insertions (Figure 18).

DOUBLE-ENDED SPATULA (PRESBY PY SP 1-4)

This 1.4-mm-wide spatula is used to check continuity of the belt loop from entrance to exit. It is also used to assist exiting of the SEB segment from the belt loop and for repositioning the sclera under the ends of the SEB segment (Figure 19).

COLIBRI-STYLED FORCEPS FOR SEB ROTATION

The Colibri-styled forceps (my personal preference) have 0.12 mm teeth and 2.0 mm angled platforms. They are used to rotate SEB segments that are inserted upside down (flat side up). The advantage of using this instrument for SEB segment rotation is that it is smaller and will cause less stretching of the belt loop during rotation. These forceps are also used for the routine surgical steps concerning the conjunctiva (Figure 20).

SCLERAL EXPANSION BAND SEGMENTS (PRESBY EB 4)

The four polymethylmethacrylate (PMMA) SEB segments are supplied in a gas-sterilized pouch. They are 5 mm in length and 1.22 mm wide. There are two notches at each end of the base to help prevent segment extrusion. Additionally, the segments are wider than they are tall to prevent them from rotating postoperatively (Figures 21 and 22).

CONJUNCTIVA CLOSURE

After properly placing the SEB segments, it is important to reposition the conjunctiva and Tenon's capsule. It is important to cover the SEB segments with the conjunctiva and Tenon's capsule to pre-

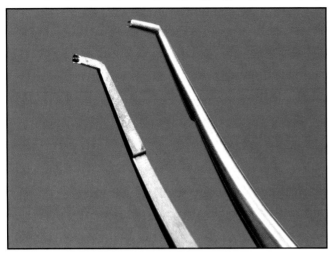

Figure 20. .12 forceps for SEB segment rotation.

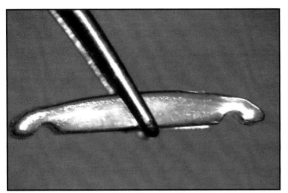

Figure 22. SEB segment held by forceps, high magnification.

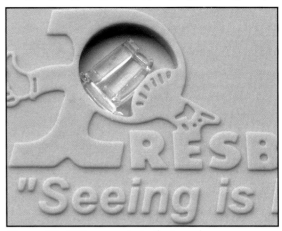

Figure 21. SEB segments in their package.

vent extrusion. A single suture at the 6 or 12 o'clock position is all that is needed for closure. A small needle holder can be used to pass 10-0 sutures through the conjunctiva, and the knot is buried under the conjunctiva and tied with assistance from .12 forceps if additional traction is necessary.

ANESTHESIA

Nora Emmons, RN

INTRODUCTION

Patients today have the capability of doing extensive research when it comes to issues related to their health and medical treatment. Individuals who fall into the presbyopia category are for the most part very computer savvy and frequently utilize the Internet as a source of information. Many times, when a patient comes into the office to be seen, he or she has already checked a variety of websites and feels that he or she has a pretty good understanding of what is going on with and what can be done about his or her eyes. It is still very important to offer the patient as much information as possible to ascertain if his or her research is correct and comprehension is accurate.

A well-educated patient is going to tolerate any procedure more easily. For this reason, it is believed that there is more to anesthesia than just the medication. Patients should know that they will be awake for the procedure and that they will feel touch while the eye is being operated on. When the segment is placed, they may experience quite a lot of pressure, which should be relayed to them beforehand. If they know that they are able to communicate their feelings with their doctor, who will give them more anesthetic, they will be more at ease and willing to help out. The patients should be given reasons for choosing local anesthesia over general. These should include the fact that recovery will be much shorter, and compromise to their cardiovascular and pulmonary status through the induction of a full general anesthetic is not warranted. During the SRP using SEBs, it is very helpful to have patients look in different directions while making the belt loops and inserting the segments. If they are able to look in the opposite direction from the quadrant in which the surgeon is working, it makes the approach much easier. Letting patients know about their ability to help out during the procedure (and therefore make it progress smoother and faster) adds to their understanding of the need to be awake.

PREPARATION

Although many physicians perform the SRP using SEBs under local and topical anesthesia, some surgeons prefer to have an anesthesiologist or nurse anesthetist present. Taking a brief history and physical preoperatively will alert the medical personnel to any potential medical problems that may arise. Since patients often have a habit of mentioning only medications that are prescribed by their medical doctor, it is a good idea to specifically question them about taking aspirin or aspirin-containing medications. Due to the inhibition of platelet aggregation that aspirin-containing medicines cause, they should be asked to discontinue use for 2 to 3 weeks prior to their surgery.

Since the patient is not given a general anesthetic, there is no need for a 6- to 8-hour NPO (nothing by mouth) status; but for safety and comfort, a 4-hour NPO status is often recommended. This is a sufficient amount of time to have an empty stomach but not enough time to cause hypoglycemia and the associated discomforts that a patient may experience by not eating for an extended period of time. Mannitol (Abbott Labs, Abbott Park, Ill) 20%, 250 cc is infused immediately postoperatively. The purpose of this is prophylactic treatment to avoid the incidence of malignant glaucoma (see Chapter 9 for rationale and explanation). The diuresis produced by the Mannitol combined with NPO status is another good reason to address the patient's history. Assuring that their cardiac status is stable will help to thwart any probability of congestive heart failure. Since this is an elective procedure and the patients who are having it performed are generally young and healthy, chances are very slim that there would be any major medical problems. However, as the age range for the success of the procedure is widening, one is better to err on the side of safety. Additionally, with the success that SRP is gaining in the treatment of primary open-angle glaucoma, individuals presenting for this surgery will become a bit more varied.

PREOPERATIVELY

For surgeons performing this procedure without the assistance of an anesthesiologist, Ativan (orazipam) 1 to 2 mg or Valium (diazepam) 10 to 20 mg given 1 hour preoperatively provides light sedation. Since the mannitol needs to be infused intravenously postoperatively, it is beneficial to start on intravenous (IV) lactated ringers or dextrose preoperatively. This access will make it possible to inject Versed (midozolam) 1 to 4 mg, along with a narcotic if necessary throughout the procedure. Whether this procedure is performed with the assistance of an anesthetist or not, it is still imperative that that patient be appropriately monitored. The use of Ativan, Valium, and Versed are commonly used benzodiazepines and are classified as agents used during conscious sedation, which warrants monitoring of blood pressure, electrocardiogram (ECG), respiratory rates, and oxygen saturation. If no anesthetist is present, a registered nurse may monitor the patient, give oxygen, and give IV sedation at the direction of the surgeon. These guidelines are recommended practices suggested by the Association of Operating Room Nurses.

Prior to taking the patient into the operating room, 0.5% proparacaine is instilled into the eyes. Although it is not as long-acting as tetracaine, it is kinder to the epithelium and the duration of action is sufficient. Due to the possibility of rotation of the eye occurring, the limbus is marked at the 12 o'clock position while the patient is in an upright position. Instillation of proparacaine is done at this time, which will also be sufficient for anesthesia prior to preparation of the first eye to be operated on.

INTRAOPERATIVELY

Xylocaine 4% or lidocaine is available in 50 mL bottles, which come in a sterile solution for topical anesthesia. A small quantity (5 cc) on the sterile field may be used to saturate a Merocel sponge (3M, St. Paul, Minn). It is applied only to the part of the eye that is being operated on. It should be used initially to anesthetize the conjunctiva prior to dissecting it from the sclera. The lidocaine is then used on the quadrant on which the surgeon is operating. The

saturated sponge is held in place for about 3 to 5 seconds to provide sufficient anesthesia. If subsequent anesthesia is necessary, the same technique can be used on the surface of the sclera after the conjunctiva is dissected away. Avoid injecting xylocaine or xylocaine with epinephrine due to the additional trauma it causes to the conjunctiva. Retrobulbar or peribulbar injection should also be avoided. These modes of anesthesia cause additional and unwanted edema of the conjunctiva. They also take away the ability of the patient to help out by looking in the direction opposite from which the surgeon is working.

POSTOPERATIVELY

When the SRP using SEBs is performed bilaterally, the dominant eye is operated on first. By the time the surgery is completed on the second eye, the patient may be starting to experience some aching or pain in the first eye. Oral administration of acetaminophen may be all that is necessary. Many patients need something stronger, such as hydrocodone. Most likely this is only needed for the first 24 to 48 hours. Immediately postoperatively, a cold compress across the eyes and forehead for 15 minutes at a time makes the patient more comfortable.

Many surgeons instill pilocarpine 1% at the end of the case. This is to ensure that the pupil will constrict concentrically. The unlikely development of anterior segment ischemia should be avoided by noting the occurrence of miosis. Unfortunately, significant brow ache that accompanies the instillation of pilocarpine can be quite upsetting for patients. Letting them know in advance that they may experience this sensation will make it a little easier to tolerate and manage.

CONCLUSION

As described above, SRP lends itself nicely to the locally anesthetized patient. Due to the straightforwardness of the procedure, the need to change or amend the approach is not really necessary. As with many other surgical procedures, as the surgeon becomes more proficient, the time taken to perform the surgery will shorten, the amount of anesthetic will diminish, and the recovery and healing time will decrease. Surgeons who initially use the assistance of an anesthetist may find that as their comfort level and expertise rise, the desire to use straight local anesthesia will be greater.

The information presented in this chapter is intended to offer the reader a brief comprehensive picture of the needs of the patient undergoing SRP using SEBs. Incorporated in this chapter are the applications of anesthesia as they relate to the specifics of the procedure.

Chapter 9

Scleral Expansion Bands

Patient Selection, Preoperative Evaluation, Technique, and Prevention of Complications

Gene W. Zdenek, MD and Nora Emmons, RN

INTRODUCTION

With the growing popularity of LASIK, one must remember the contrasting differences between operating in a "clean" case and maintaining aseptic technique during an actual surgical procedure. The surgical reversal of presbyopia (SRP) is truly a surgical procedure and should be treated as such. Care should be taken to adhere to aseptic technique throughout the procedure. During the first few cases, the time taken to perform the procedure may be a little lengthy and there is a direct correlation between the time the sterile field is established and the length of exposure to airborne contaminants. Personnel should don full surgical attire and the patient should be prepped and draped according to the policy of the facility at which one is working.

The prevention of complications as they relate to this procedure are incorporated into this chapter so that the reader will understand the reasoning for many of the steps taken while performing the surgery. A detailed explanation of the complications that could arise are thoroughly detailed in this chapter. The complications outlined here are related to the technical components utilized while performing the procedure and are actually discussed so as to avoid problems that could potentially decrease the effect of the procedure. Confirmation of measurements and the ability to offer a variety of ways to address segment insertion will make the surgeon's course much more successful.

PATIENT SELECTION AND PRE- AND POSTOPERATIVE EVALUATION

The ideal SRP patient may fall anywhere in the age range of 40 to 70 years old. Obviously, the patient must be aware of difficulties while performing near vision tasks. Patients with the highest level of motivation appear to be individuals whose jobs or lifestyles require considerable near vision activities.

The patients on the upper limit of the age range should have thorough informed consent due to the fact that by age 70, there may be some atrophy of the ciliary muscle. This atrophy could cause ineffective results.

Emmetropes who are now facing presbyopia are the most ideal candidates. With possibly never having experienced a trip to an eye doctor's office in the past, the idea of imperfect vision is usually upsetting to these patients. They may be reluctant to accept the idea of wearing reading glasses or creating monovision with contact lens or laser-assisted in situ keratomileusis (LASIK). These patients would be receptive to a discussion on the merits of reversing the effects through surgery. Additionally, patients already wearing glasses or contacts to correct their distant vision may be good candidates after having LASIK or photorefractive keratectomy (PRK) to perfect their distance vision. Surgical results will be optimal with distance vision corrected. SRP with scleral expansion band (SEB) segments may be performed safely approximately 4 to 6 weeks post LASIK or PRK. However, should SRP be performed first, refractive correction can still be accomplished safely.

SRP may be considered an optional cosmetic procedure with the same inherent issues. Therefore, it may not be for everyone. Patients need to be aware of the need to exercise and work at strengthening the muscle for several months after the procedure to gain optimum effects. The SRP patient's eyes will be quite red for a few weeks following the surgery. Postoperative expectations given prior to the procedure are extremely important.

When taking the patient's history, the physician should note the following contraindications:

+ Insulin-dependent diabetes mellitus
+ Severe hypertension
+ Blood dyscrasias
+ Chronic or recurrent uveitis, iritis, scleritis, herpes simplex
+ Previous eye surgery (including cataract, corneal transplant, glaucoma filtering surgeries, retinal detachment repair)
+ Patients on Heparin or Coumadin
+ Sjögren's syndrome
+ Chronic systemic disease (ie, systemic lupus erythematosus, Crohn's disease, collagen vascular disease, rheumatoid arthritis)

In the preoperative evaluation of the patient, include the following:

+ Distance visual acuity with correction in place
+ Visual acuity at 40 cm, 30 cm, and 20 cm
+ Visual acuity starting at 70 cm and bringing the eye chart

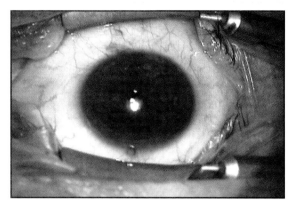

Figure 1. Twelve o'clock mark made upright at the slit lamp.

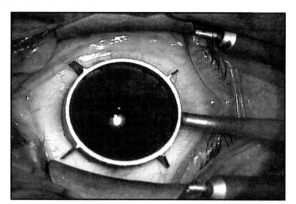

Figure 2. Quadrant marker.

closer until the smallest line read starts to blur (this test gives you the diopters of accommodation that the patient has. The formula to measure this is 1/distance in centimeters x 100 (ie, if the patient is able to read the line clearly up to 50 cm, the formula applied would be 1/50 x 100 = 2 diopters [D] of accommodation)

✦ Axial length measurement and corneal topography

Step 3 above is also important in the postoperative evaluation to measure the amount of accommodation gained. When repeating this step postoperatively, it is important that the patient use the same line that he or she was able to see preoperatively (even if it was only 20/200). Bring the eye chart in toward the patient as before to find the gain in accommodation. To illustrate (continuing from the example in step 3): if the patient is able to clearly see the same line on the eye chart when brought up as close as 20 cm, this would result in 5 D of accommodation.

Axial length results should not be affected as a result of the surgery. Corneal topography may show induced astigmatism immediately postoperatively. In all cases, this astigmatism disappears within 3 months. At the time of this writing, SRP with SEB segments has completed US Food and Drug Administration (FDA) Phase I trials. Included in the trial data were the corneal topography and axial length readings. Upon FDA acceptance of the SRP procedure, these tests will not be necessary.

THE PREOPERATIVE COURSE

As mentioned in Chapter 8, this procedure may be safely performed under local and topical anesthesia. The addition of light sedatives is beneficial to the comfort and well-being of the patient. If the surgeon feels more secure with the assistance of an anesthetist, he or she should remember the benefits of minimal sedation so as to incorporate the patient's assistance by looking in various directions during the case. This will allow exposure of the quadrant of the eye being operated on.

After the instillation of 0.5% proparacaine, the patient should have the eyes marked with a skin scribe or marking pen at the 12 o'clock position. It is documented that up to 10 to 15 degrees of torsion or eye movement can occur when the patient is in a supine position as compared to the upright position. If this mark is not placed accurately, the segments may be off by as much as 20 degrees. This inaccuracy in positioning may be sufficient to compromise the anterior circulation of the eye. As will be discussed later, anterior

segment ischemia is a complication that could arise if segment placement is not accurate. The design and placement of the SEB segments have been modified in order to address and therefore curtail this unwanted situation (Figure 1).

A relatively new addition to the preoperative regime has been the instillation of brimonidine tartrate or Alphagan (Allergan, Irvine, Calif). The alpha adrenergic properties of Alphagan have been beneficial for hemostasis. It may be instilled 30 and 15 minutes prior to the start of surgery.

THE INTRAOPERATIVE COURSE

Once the patient has been prepped and draped, the lid speculum is positioned. Without the use of retrobulbar anesthetic, the patient may be a little uncomfortable between the light of the microscope and the insertion of the speculum. Open the speculum only part way until the anesthetic has been applied to make the patient more comfortable.

If the eye was just prepped and proparacaine was instilled, the quadrant marker is ready to be used. If not, topical anesthetic should be applied prior to using the quadrant marker. The anesthetic may be applied by using a Merocel sponge or dropped directly onto the eye. When marking the sclera with the quadrant marker or axis marker, one must realize that these marks do not delineate the limbus but rather the position in which the SEB segment will be placed in its oblique quadrant (Figures 2 and 3). It is important to note that during the case if fading of these marks is observed, the surgeon should re-mark directly on the limbus with the sterile marking pen to avoid any confusion when relying on these marks as guides for future segment insertions (Figure 4).

Now a corneal cover may be placed on the eye with either a thick artificial tear or a small amount of viscoelastic beneath it to hold it in place and keep the cornea moistened. A corneal shield may be positioned to keep the light out and prevent corneal drying or abrasion, but it is best to wait until after the quadrant marker has been used (Figure 5). Now the patient is a little more comfortable and the speculum may be fully opened.

At this point the application of topical 4% xylocaine or lidocaine may be instilled. Instead of dropping it onto the entire surface of the eye, it is preferred to use a Merocel sponge saturated in the anesthetic. This way it may be directly applied only to the area on which the surgeon is working.

The conjunctival opening and exposed surgical field should be

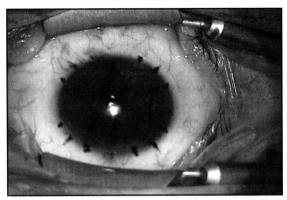

Figure 3. Quadrant marks.

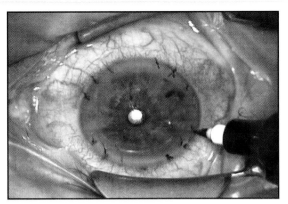

Figure 4. Pen used to enhance quadrant marks.

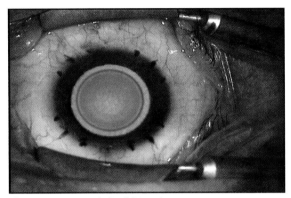

Figure 5. Corneal shield in place.

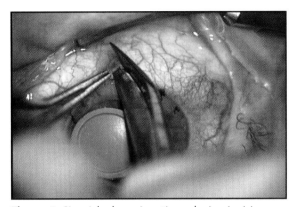

Figure 6. Six o'clock conjunctiva relaxing incision.

large enough so that the surgeon does not have to fight the conjunctiva when making the marks and inserting each segment. Different surgeons have different approaches to the order in which they like to insert the segments. Many surgeons like to insert the inferior segments first and then finish with the superior segments. The reasoning behind this is due to the fact that the anesthesia often pools into the inferior fornix if the superior segments are inserted first. By the time these are completed and the surgeon starts with the inferior quadrant, the area has already completed one or two stages of anesthesia and is beginning to wear off. This not only produces some hyperemia and conjunctival edema, but can also cause postanesthesia dysthesia or hyperesethesia.

Using either blunt or sharp Wescott scissors (whichever is preferred for dissection) and a Colibri or .12 forceps, start the conjunctival opening in the inferior quadrant at the 6 o'clock position (Figure 6). Open the conjunctiva at the limbus and dissect it free of the sclera going about 6 mm back from the limbus.

Complete the incision by starting at the 12 o'clock position and extending it to make a complete peritomy, which will allow for the best exposure. It is important to carefully dissect Tenon's capsule away from the sclera to assure proper belt loop formation. Do not use any cautery at this time. Instead, wait for natural hemostasis to occur. Extensive use of cautery can thin the sclera and potentially decrease the effect of the procedure. Too much cautery may also cause a thicker (deeper) than normal belt loop. If cautery is necessary, it should be a pencil or eraser type of bipolar coagulation.

Starting with the inferior portion of the globe, one should approach the quadrant that is bleeding the least and cauterize only as necessary for good visualization. Many surgeons will only cauter-

ize in two different areas. Some vessels that will interfere with visualization posterior to where the segment will lie may be cauterized if necessary. The area where the actual incisions are to be made may be lightly cauterized. This will be about 3.5 mm back from the limbus and lined up with the marks made with the quadrant marker. This cautery is used very lightly so that no darkening, discoloration, or shrinkage of the sclera occurs (Figure 7).

Performing the procedure in this manner helps to avoid conjunctival complications. When the second quadrant is to be approached, natural hemostasis will have occurred. Once the conjunctiva is dissected free and the surgeon is ready to start working on the sclera, it is a good idea to apply the topical anesthetic to the quadrant of the sclera that is going to be addressed next (Figure 8).

PRESBYDRIVE AUTOMATED BELT LOOP MAKER

Numerous surgeons have been performing the SRP surgery worldwide and have found a variation of accommodation. Since these variations are consistent with the FDA Phase I trials, further investigation was warranted. The findings revealed variability in the depth of the belt loop. A surgeon's natural instinct is to create a shallow belt loop. A lack of depth will result in a decrease in the gain of accommodation. This variable is eliminated through the development of the automatic belt loop maker called the PresbyDrive (Figures 9 and 10).

The PresbyDrive device has a rotating arcuate blade that passes through a slotted foot plate to make a belt loop 400 microns deep. The disposable blade advances to form the belt loop with foot pedal control. The control unit has a convenient abort button if progression of the blade needs to be stopped (Figures 11 to 13).

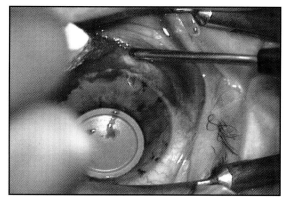

Figure 7. Cauterizing only where necessary.

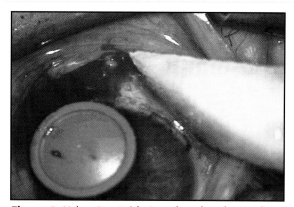

Figure 8. Xylocaine 4% being placed on bare sclera.

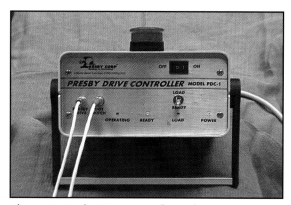

Figure 9. PresbyDrive control panel.

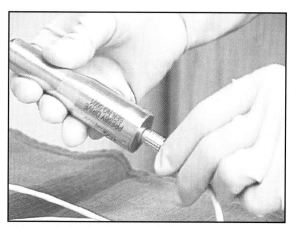

Figure 10. PresbyDrive hand piece.

After completion of the belt loop, the PresbyDrive automatically senses the completed belt loop and retracts to the original position in preparation for the next belt loop. The speed and precision of belt loop formation with the PresbyDrive enables the surgeon to form all four belt loops consecutively.

It is apparent that the PresbyDrive will eliminate the need for the sclerotomy diamond blade and lamellar diamond blade in formation of the belt loop. Additionally, the PresbyDrive has a limbal mark on its neck, and the base plate is sized for a perfect belt loop length. These features eliminate the four-prong marking step necessary during manual belt loop formation. Because scleral marks and visualization of the lamellar blade as it passes through the belt loop are not required, cautery is not necessary. Eliminating cautery saves time and decreases postoperative inflammation. Early clinical experience has demonstrated a marked improvement in postoperative recovery time using the PresbyDrive.

After the conjunctiva and Tenon's layer have been dissected, the PresbyDrive is placed on the sclera in the appropriate quadrant. The twist pick provides countertraction for stable and precise positioning while activating the PresbyDrive on the surface of the eye (Figure 14).

When ready, the surgeon simply steps on the pedal to activate the PresbyDrive (Figure 15). The ease of operation and handling of the PresbyDrive makes it an invaluable adjunct to SRP. The PresbyDrive replaces nearly half of the steps in the SRP procedure, reducing operating time by as much as 50%. The surgical time can be shortened even more if all four belt loops are made at once (avoiding passing the PresbyDrive back and forth to the scrub technician).

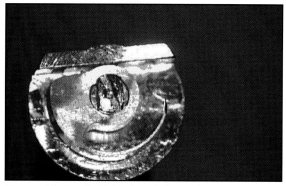

Figure 11. PresbyDrive head, front view.

Manual Technique—Belt Loop Formation

When using the scleral four-prong marker, note the difference between the two sets of prongs. Two of them are pointed and are 4.0 mm apart from each other. The other two prongs are also 4.0 mm apart from each other are 1.5 mm long. The distance between the pointed prong and the 1.5 mm prong is 3.5 mm. These prongs should be inked prior to their use. Using a Merocel sponge to dry the sclera and push the conjunctiva back out of the way, hold the four-prong marker with the pointed prongs on the surgical limbus at the location of the corresponding marks made by the quadrant marker. Keeping them in place on the limbus, tilt the marker back so that all four prongs are in contact with the sclera. Some pressure should be exerted so that a slight indentation is made into the scle-

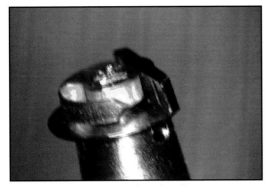

Figure 12. PresbyDrive head, side view.

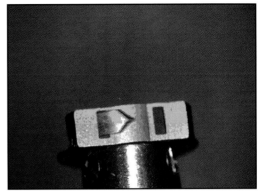

Figure 13. PresbyDrive head, underside view with advancing blade.

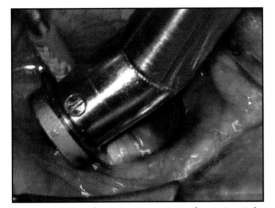

Figure 14. PresbyDrive in position by twist pick.

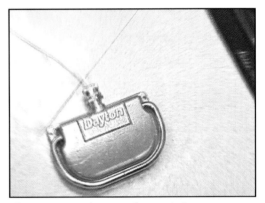

Figure 15. PresbyDrive foot switch.

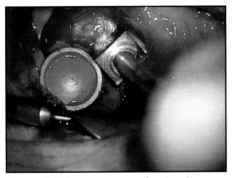

Figure 16. Four-prong marker in place.

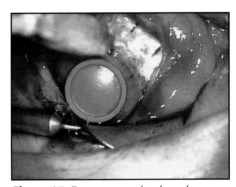

Figure 17. Four-prong scleral marks.

ra. These marks will be used for location of the sclerotomy. Remember that the initial marks placed by the quadrant marker are to be used for clock hour positioning and may not lie directly on the surgical limbus. For this reason it is important to make sure that the four-prong marker is placed on the limbus and not necessarily on top of the marks created by the quadrant marker (Figures 16 and 17).

When performing the sclerotomy, only mild fixation is necessary. More importantly, ensure that all of the conjunctiva and Tenon's layer have been dissected free from the sclera. The diamond sclerotomy blade is guarded and set to achieve a depth of 300 microns. If Tenon's layer were in the way, the incision may not attain the desired depth and a shallow belt loop would result. When making the sclerotomy, the blade should be left in place long enough to cause an indentation of the sclera by the guard of the diamond blade. Placing the blade directly on top of the inked marks should result in perfect placement of the belt loop (Figure 18).

If there is any question as to the proper placement of the sclerotomy incisions, they can easily be checked with an instrument created for this purpose. A double-ended measuring device that has a set caliper of 4.0 mm on one end and 3.5 mm on the other may be utilized. The 3.5 mm end is used to confirm that the anterior end of the sclerotomy incision is placed 3.5 mm from the surgical limbus. The opposite end is used to confirm that the two sclerotomy incisions are parallel to each other at a distance of 4.0 mm. If it is noted that the incisions have been placed too far apart (or too close together), measurements should be reconfirmed and a new sclerotomy should be carried out. If the incisions are too far apart (resulting

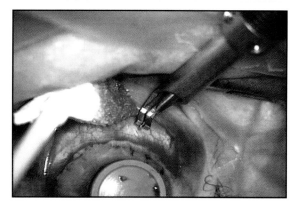

Figure 18. Sclerotomy diamond blade in use.

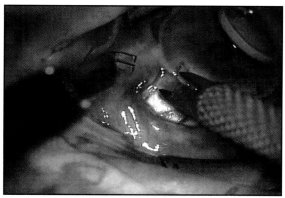

Figure 19. 3.5 mm marker checking distance from the limbus.

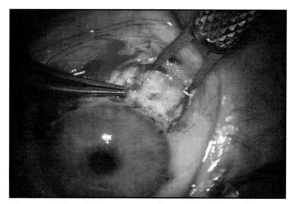

Figure 20. 4.0 mm marker checking distance between sclerotomies.

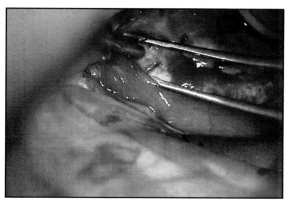

Figure 21. Twist pick fixator in relation to the exit sclerotomy.

in a longer belt loop), the SEB segment will not be protruding from both ends of the belt loop. This positioning is imperative to create optimum effects. Since the notches are placed on the bottom side of the segment 4.0 mm apart from each other, a long or short belt loop will negate the ability of the notches to aid in stabilization of the segment (Figures 19 and 20).

Creation of the belt loop with the diamond lamellar blade requires good fixation of the globe. This is best achieved by utilizing a scleral fixator or twist pick. When placed properly before making the belt loop, it may be left in place while moving onto the next step—insertion of the SEB segment. The fixator should be placed about 2 mm out from the sclerotomy that is going to be the exit end of the belt loop. This will allow for adequate fixation as well as protection so that the end of the diamond lamellar blade does not run into the fixator when it is completing the belt loop (Figure 21).

Once fixation has been achieved, the diamond lamellar blade is used at the entrance sclerotomy. Good visualization is imperative so as to see that adequate blade depth is being maintained. The diamond blade should approach the sclerotomy entrance at about a 45-degree angle. As it enters the sclerotomy, it is then leveled so that it is crossing the sclera in a fashion parallel to the surface. Since the sclerotomy is 300 microns deep, this should be the depth of the entire belt loop. Again, visualization of the sclera over the belt loop will help to achieve this. If the blade is actually visualized through the sclera, then the belt loop is too shallow. A shallow belt loop allows the sclera to be more elastic, stretch more, and have a decreased scleral expansion effect. The blade may be retracted and advanced again, but deeper. If no blade and no effect is seen, then

that blade is too deep in the sclera. If the belt loop is too deep, the segment can easily tear the floor of the sclera within the belt loop and have a tendency to enter the suprachoroidal space. Also, a deep belt loop makes it very difficult to insert the SEB segment. One should actually be able to see the effect of the blade as it crosses through the sclera. It will create a slight rise or "hill" across the sclera. Since the end of the diamond blade is beveled, just before the rise or "hill" reaches the second or exiting sclerotomy, the fixator should be slightly depressed. This will create a slight opening in the sclerotomy as well as help to allow for the diamond lamellar blade to make its exit. Due to the curved tip of the blade, one needs to make sure that the blade exits completely so that the width of the exit incision is as wide as the entrance. This is necessary to accommodate insertion and positioning of the SEB segment. Due to the quality of the diamond lamellar blade, formation of the belt loop should easily be accomplished. Movement through the belt loop should be straight with as little side-to-side movement as possible. This will make for a tight fit of the SEB segment, which has been shown to create a better effect and not allow for migration of the segment out of the belt loop (Figures 22 to 24).

Segment insertion is the most difficult step of the surgery. The surgeon must know whether he or she is working with a deep or shallow belt loop. A shallow belt loop allows the SEB segment to be inserted very easily and in the correct position. However, there appears to be less of an effect in reference to the range of accommodation that is achieved. With a deep belt loop, the range of accommodation may in fact be greater, but the difficulty of inserting the segment is also greater. The belt loop is tighter, and more

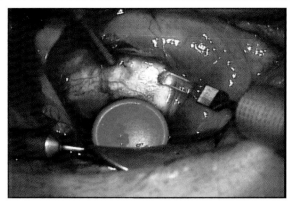

Figure 22. Lamellar diamond blade starting the belt loop.

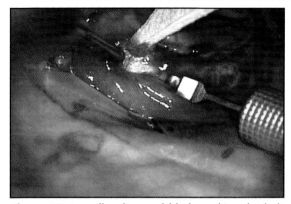

Figure 23. Lamellar diamond blade making the belt loop.

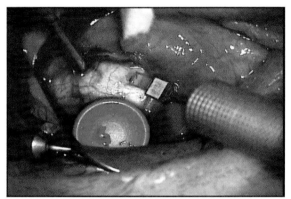

Figure 24. Lamellar diamond blade making the belt loop.

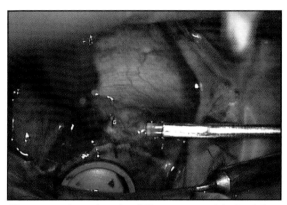

Figure 25. Inserting the SEB segment with the injector.

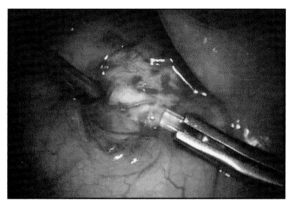

Figure 26. Inserting the SEB segment with channeled forceps.

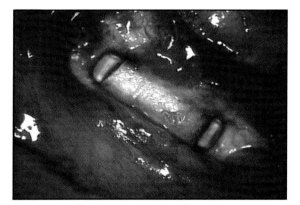

Figure 27. The SEB segment in place.

force has to be applied to the SEB segment as it is inserted. Inserting the segment upside down and then rotating it to the proper position is the preferred technique when dealing with a deep belt loop.

Surgeons have a variety of methods that may be employed to insert the SEB segment. It may be held with a large needle holder, an injector (Figure 25), or with the newest instrument—an insertion forceps that holds the segment (Figure 26). While maintaining fixation with the scleral twist pick, the SEB segment is inserted into the entrance of the belt loop. Pressure must be maintained on the inserter to keep the segment parallel across the belt loop. Due to the curve of the top side of it, the segment has a tendency to "dive"

down into the sclera. Keeping the insertion forceps in a position where it is actually angling the segment upward will help to get the segment into the belt loop. The fixator does not need to be depressed as the segment is exiting. It is important to make sure that no conjunctiva is caught under the segment. If the belt loop is correctly made, equal amounts of the segment will be sticking out from the ends of the belt loop. The SEB segment is designed with a notch at each end (4.0 mm apart) on the underside that corresponds with the end of the belt loop. This will allow the edge of the sclerotomy and its scleral tissue to wedge up into the notch and help hold the segment in place (Figure 27).

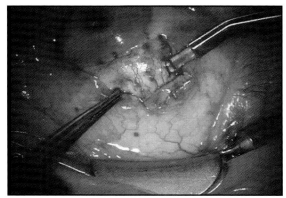

Figure 28. Inserting the SEB segment upside-down with channeled forceps.

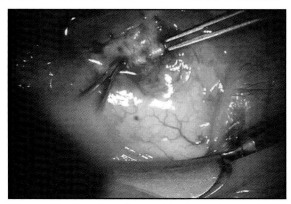

Figure 29. Rotating the upside-down–inserted SEB segment.

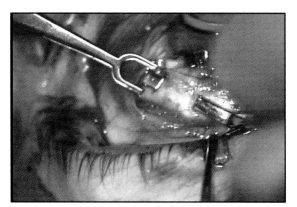

Figure 30. Spatula in the belt loop.

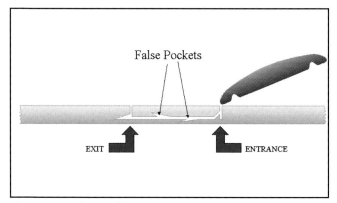

Figure 31. False pockets.

If too much resistance is met when inserting the segment, there is a variety of different approaches to try. As mentioned earlier, the SEB segment may be inserted upside down. The upside down approach is good if the belt loop is deep (Figure 28). Some surgeons routinely insert them in this manner, but others feel this approach may slightly stretch out the belt loop. The disadvantage to this method with its inherent stretching of the belt loop would be a looser fit of the segment that could possibly lead to movement. Additionally, as mentioned previously, a looser belt loop may create a lessened effect (Figure 29).

If the segment is unable to be inserted all the way through the belt loop, the spatula may be inserted into the belt loop to ensure a patent opening. The spatula may also be used to slightly depress the floor of the belt loop. This too may aid in segment insertion (Figure 30).

Another approach to segment insertion may be achieved by removing the fixator, placing it at the entrance end, and inserting the segment through the exit end of the belt loop. When creating the belt loop, if one starts to go too deep or too shallow, pull the diamond blade back and start to advance it again in a slightly different plane. This will create small false pockets (Figure 31). They really are not a problem if they are approached from the opposite side. This way, the segment cannot get caught in the pocket (Figure 32). Again, it is important to make sure that there is no Tenon's layer or conjunctiva caught under the segment and that both ends of the segment are equally out of the belt loop.

If the segment is inserted upside down, make sure that both ends are equally extending out of the belt loop. Using Colibri or .12 forceps, position the wrist and hand in such a fashion so as to antici-

pate the 180-degree rotation required. Often, due to poor exposure or other difficulties this cannot be achieved. Utilizing a second forceps, grasp the other end of the segment. Once the segment is rotated halfway, the other forceps are used to grab the opposite end of the segment and rotate it the remaining 90 degrees. If the segment is not extended evenly on either side of the belt loop, the edge of the segment that is least prominent should be the one that is grasped by the forceps and rotated. The reason for this is that as one rotates with the forceps, the segment has a tendency to pull out, and if one were to grab the edge of the segment that is projecting the most, the other end may fall back into the belt loop. Because it is believed that the accommodative effect may be proportional to the depth of the segment, the tendency for experienced surgeons is to place the segment deeper. The deeper the segment, the more likely it will have to be put in upside down.

A very important part of this procedure is the closure of the conjunctiva after all four segments have been inserted and checked for proper positioning. Prior to closing, it is a good idea to reapply the topical anesthetic to the operative site. Conjunctiva along with Tenon's layer should be pulled over the segment as close to the original insertion as possible. Only a single suture at the 6 or 12 o'clock positions should be necessary, and a small bite of sclera should be included in the suturing (Figure 33). If the conjunctiva has been stretched or torn, a larger bite of conjunctiva will need to be taken and puckered at that clock hour position. This suture securely pulls the conjunctiva tightly over the segment and achieves complete coverage. If there is up to a 1.0 mm recession of the conjunctiva from its original insertion, this would still be acceptable. However,

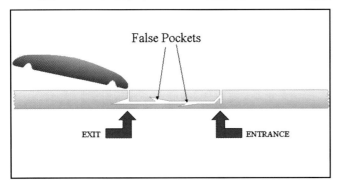

Figure 32. False pocket—inserted from the exit end.

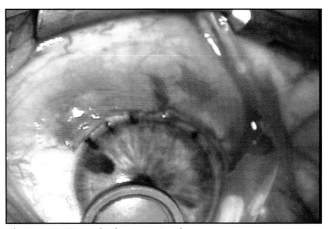

Figure 33. Six o'clock suture in place.

if this becomes a 2- to 3-mm recession of the conjunctiva, it will need to be sutured. The suture may be inserted at the location of the recession, or at the 6 or 12 o'clock position, so as to pull the conjunctiva tighter and closer to its original insertion site.

Many surgeons prefer to use 10-0 nylon suture and bury the knot. Most of the time these sutures do not need to be removed. If at a later date suture irritation occurs, they can be easily removed at the slit lamp using topical anesthesia. Another suture used by surgeons is 9-0 or 10-0 Biosorb by Alcon (Fort Worth, Tex). This is a coated absorbable suture. If this suture is used, the surgeon should be sure to cut the ends of the knots as short as possible. As edema of the conjunctiva subsides, the suture becomes more prominent in relation to the tissue around it and can create an incredible foreign body sensation to the patient. Sutures should be removed no sooner that 7 to 10 days postoperatively to ensure complete coverage of the segment.

As mentioned in the beginning of the chapter, anterior segment ischemia is a potential complication that has been documented and addressed. One method that can be utilized to ascertain that SEB segments are accurately positioned is the instillation of 1% pilocarpine. The surgeon should observe a rather dramatic and immediate constriction of the pupil in a very concentric manner. The observation of an elliptical or tear-shaped pupil could mean a compromise in circulation. The surgeon should be able to slightly shift a segment that is located in the direction of the drawn-up pupil. Return to a round shape should then be observed. Many patients respond quite dramatically to the constrictive effect of the pilocarpine. Making the patients aware of this in advance may make it more tolerable. Many surgeons will omit the routine instillation of pilocarpine if they are able to see normal pupillary constriction at the end of the case. Routine postoperative medications, including antibiotic and anti-inflammatory eye drops, should be continued by the patient.

THE POSTOPERATIVE COURSE

The patient undergoing SRP is often quite motivated and anxious to "see what I can read." Many patients are able to gain some lines on the reading chart immediately after surgery. Many just want to lie down. Postoperatively, patients may need analgesics or narcotics for the discomfort they experience. These may be needed for the first 24 to 48 hours after surgery. Intravenous (IV) administration of 250 cc of 20% mannitol should be infused within half an hour. A cold compress across the eyes and forehead often provides comfort, especially if the pilocarpine is bothering them. For those patients who are anxious to read, it is best to remind them that as the swelling begins within the first 24 hours, they may find that their tear film is not as it should be and is interfering with their progress. This may be the case for the next few days.

Patients should continue their use of antibiotic and anti-inflammatory eye drops for 2 to 3 weeks. Artificial tears are very beneficial to the patient's comfort as well as visual rehabilitation and should be used frequently in the first few weeks postoperatively.

CONCLUSION

SRP using SEBs has been performed long enough for surgeons to have researched and decided on a uniform procedure to gain optimum results. Although each surgeon has his or her own techniques and approaches, the one described were outlined for new surgeon success. In the years that this procedure has been around, many have tried personal approaches to various steps in the surgery. It is for this reason that potential changes should be first discussed with a surgeon who routinely performs the surgery.

SRP using SEBs is a surgeon-friendly procedure with a quick learning curve. With adherence to technique, one should feel confident performing the procedure.

Chapter 10

Scleral Expansion Band Surgical Technique

Christopher J. Engelman, MD and Edward E. Manche, MD

INTRODUCTION

Given the dramatic advances in our ability to treat myopia, hyperopia, and astigmatism, the concept of surgically reversing presbyopia has been aptly referred to as the "last frontier" in the efforts to correct refractive disorders.[1] In distinct contradiction to the long-accepted Helmholtz's theory of accommodation,[2] Ronald Schachar has proposed that aging is accompanied by a predictable increase in equatorial crystalline lens growth.[3] This growth reduces the ability of the ciliary body, via equatorial zonular fibers, to induce peripheral lens flattening and increase central lens curvature, which normally provides the optical power necessary for focusing at near.[3] Although this novel theory has been the subject of considerable criticism,[4,5] it has served as the basis for several innovative surgical procedures developed to correct presbyopia, including anterior ciliary sclerotomy[6] and anterior ciliary sclerotomy with silicone expansion plug insertion.[7] The most extensively studied method and the subject of this chapter is scleral expansion band (SEB) surgery, which has been reported to allow recovery of on average 3.25 diopters (D) of accommodation.[8] This procedure, which is designed to restore the pre-presbyopic working distance between the ciliary muscle and equatorial lens (Figure 1), has undergone several important modifications since it was introduced by Jose de la Garza Viejo, Antonio Garza, and Ronald Schachar in 1992. The procedure involves four basic steps including conjunctival peritomy, scleral belt loop placement, expansion band insertion, and conjunctival closure, all shown in Figure 2.

PREOPERATIVE CONSIDERATIONS

Surgical reversal of presbyopia with SEBs can be considered in patients between 40 and 70 years of age who maintain less than 1.00 D of distance refractive error and have normal binocular vision for which other measures to correct presbyopia are not satisfactory. The procedure is contraindicated in patients with advancing cataracts requiring imminent removal, prior intraocular surgery (cataract extraction, trabeculectomy, scleral buckle, pars plana vitrectomy, etc), evidence of scleromalacia, collagen-vascular disease, or coagulopathy. Patients who are older than 70 years of age, monocular, suffer from severe dry eyes, or have poorly controlled diabetes are likewise not ideal candidates. As with any surgical procedure, the patient must demonstrate an adequate understanding of not only the potential risks and benefits but also the requirements for postoperative near vision exercises, which are reported to be essential to the procedure's eventual success.

PATIENT PREPARATION

Topical antibiotics as well as anti-inflammatories can be given preoperatively. Topical anesthesia with proparacaine 0.5% usually provides adequate anesthesia for marking. Tetracaine is less desirable given the associated toxicity to the corneal epithelium. An intravenous (IV) line should be placed to facilitate sedation, although this can be done orally as well with diazepam. If IV sedation is used, the equipment necessary to monitor vital signs as well as resuscitate cardiorespiratory complications should be available according to each institution's standards of patient safety. While the procedure can be performed in a minor procedure room, we prefer the more controlled environment of the operating room, as it provides the accessibility of nursing, anesthesia, and equipment resources that would be difficult to achieve otherwise.

SURGICAL TECHNIQUE

INSTRUMENTS

All necessary surgical instruments are included in the Presby Corp kit (see Table 1 in Chapter 8).

SURGICAL MARKING

All of the necessary instruments for marking are provided in the Presby Corp kit, as shown in Figure 3. With the patient sitting upright, a mark is placed on the cornea at the 12 o'clock position to aid in the proper placement of the four SEBs in each quadrant. Incorrect positioning of the SEBs near the 12 to 6 o'clock or the 3 to 9 o'clock meridians increases the risk of damage to the anterior ciliary circulation and consequences of anterior segment ischemia. Marking can be performed at the slit lamp or using loupe magnification. The surgical field is then cleaned and draped in a sterile manner.

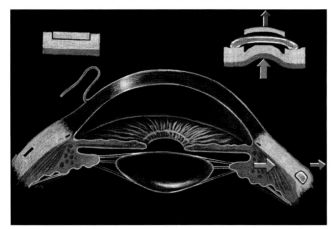

Figure 1. Restoration of pre-presbyopic working distance between the ciliary body and equatorial crystalline lens by expanding the space between the lens and sclera with a scleral expansion band (courtesy of Presby Corp).

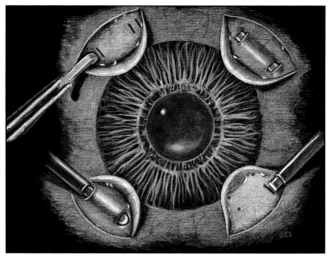

Figure 2. Clockwise from lower right, scleral belt loop incision, scleral tunnel creation, scleral expansion band implant insertion. Conjunctival peritomy shown for illustration only (courtesy of Presby Corp).

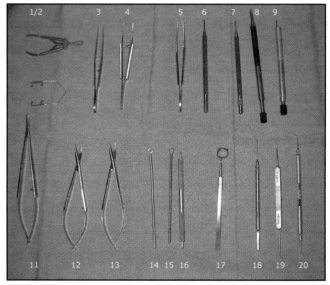

Figure 3. Presby Corp surgical instrument kit.

An eyelid speculum is then placed to attain adequate exposure. After gently drying the cornea with Weckcell sponges, the quadrant axis marker is used with the handle directed in the 12 o'clock position to identify the 45-degree meridians where the SEB segments are to be placed.

CONJUNCTIVAL PERITOMY

Supplemental anesthesia with subconjunctival 2% lidocaine should be injected into each of the oblique quadrants from the 12 o'clock and 6 o'clock positions. Limbal conjunctival incisions are then placed perpendicular to the limbus again at the 12 o'clock and 6 o'clock positions. A fornix-based conjunctival peritomy is then performed using tissue forceps and blunt conjunctival scissors from 10:30 to 1:30 superiorly and from 4:30 to 7:30 inferiorly. Vertical relaxing incisions at the 12 o'clock and 6 o'clock positions improve the exposure necessary for dissection to bare sclera extending approximately 5 mm posterior to the surgical limbus. The corners of each incision can be tagged with 10-0 Biosorb to facilitate proper alignment of conjunctival closure at the end of the procedure. Eraser tip cautery is conservatively applied to achieve hemostasis. It is important to avoid excessive cauterization, especially in the planned regions of the SEBs, in order to prevent any compromise in tissue integrity.

SCLERAL BELT LOOP

The locations of each planned scleral belt loop are first marked using the four-prong marker, which provides two parallel lines designating the location, length, and orientation of the incisions. Measurements should be made based upon the most posterior aspect of the limbus where the gray limbal tissue meets white sclera. The marker should be placed 2.75 mm posterior to this landmark and aligned to straddle the previously placed 45-degree quadrant marker lines. This placement is critical, as the most anterior portion of the scleral belt loop should be between 2.75 and 3.25 mm from the posterior limbus corresponding to the area overlying the ciliary body. Any further posterior and the subsequent effect on accommodation will be diminished.

Using the incisional diamond blade, a 5.0 mm long and 1.5 mm wide scleral tunnel is then created, connecting each previously placed SM4 mark. First make 0.3 mm deep incisions perpendicular to the surface plane of the eye along each of the parallel marks. To assist in globe fixation, the scleral fixator can be used to provide more stability than forceps fixation. For optimal control, it should be placed approximately 2 mm away from the planned exit incision. The blade is then placed in one of the groove incisions to the full 0.3 mm depth and then angled in a tangential plane while it is advanced toward the paired exit incision. The appropriate tunnel depth can be maintained by ensuring that the tip of the blade is not easily visible through the sclera while the remaining portion is seen during advancement. To facilitate the blade's exit at the full depth of the second vertical incision, slight pressure can be applied at this site with the scleral fixator or tissue forceps while simultaneously angling the lamellar blade up just before completing the tunnel. Because the length of the blade is 5.0 mm and the beveled tip 1.0 mm, the entire tip should be visualized beyond the tunnel to ensure a complete 4.0 mm length. The 1.4 mm double-ended spatula should then be placed through the tunnel to better evaluate the wound's completeness and integrity.

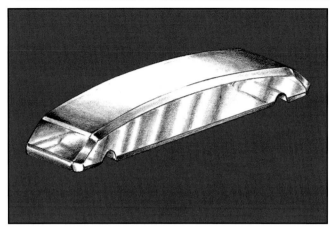

Figure 4. PMMA scleral expansion band segment. Length: 5.5 mm; width: 1.38 mm; height 925 microns (courtesy of Presby Corp).

Scleral Expansion Band Insertion

After completion of each of the four scleral belt loops, the SEB segments can be placed into each tunnel using the segment inserter. Each segment, made of polymethylmethacrylate (PMMA), is 5.5 mm in length, 1.38 mm wide, and 925 microns in height (Figure 4). The segment to be placed is positioned into the tip of the SEB injector such that the grooves are facing upward (ie, upside down). At this point, approximately one-third the length of the SEB will be exposed and is inserted into the tunnel lumen. Moderate downward pressure should be applied at the entrance wound to help ensure movement of the segment through the belt loop rather than toward the interior of the eye. Using small, controlled, push-and-release or pumping movements, the SEB segment is advanced through the scleral belt loop while providing moderate downward pressure on the exit wound with the scleral fixator as the segment approaches the terminal end of the tunnel. Alternatively, the segment inserter forceps can be used to complete SEB insertion. After implantation, the SEB segments are carefully rotated such that the grooves face the sclera and are centered in the scleral tunnel. The above steps are completed in each of the four quadrants.

Conjunctival Closure

After inspection to ensure the proper positioning of each SEB, identify the previously placed tagged corners of conjunctiva to aid in closure. Using a small episcleral fixation bite, the 10-0 Biosorb knot is buried at the 12 o'clock and 6 o'clock positions.

IMMEDIATE POSTOPERATIVE CONSIDERATIONS

Prior to completing the procedure, pupillary size and response to light is assessed to ensure adequate anterior circulation to the iris. One drop of topical 2% pilocarpine should result in prompt constriction to provide assessment or occasionally iris fluorescein angiography can be obtained to provide additional assurance that the anterior circulation has not been compromised. Mannitol 20%, 500 cc, is given to all patients intravenously over 30 minutes unless otherwise contraindicated. A combination antibiotic-steroid is then placed in the operated eye. No patching is necessary unless regional anesthesia was used (ie, peribulbar or retrobulbar blockade), which generally is not necessary.

Postoperative Care

Routine postoperative visits should be scheduled for 1 day, 1 week, 2 weeks, and 1 month following surgery. The antibiotic-steroid combination can be continued four times daily for 1 to 2 weeks assuming an unremarkable period of healing. Additionally, lubricants can be used as needed to alleviate minor irritation related to exposed sutures and/or conjunctival healing. Accommodative exercises including changing focus from near to far are said to be an integral component of the procedure and should be performed as frequently as possible for optimal results. Instruct patients to hold the eye chart at a length of 10 cm, focusing on the smallest line of print until the next smallest line comes into focus. Focus should be maintained while slowly moving the eye chart further away to arm's length and then back again to 10 cm. Exercises should be repeated as frequently as possible at least four times per day with six repetitions per session. For patients not compliant with these exercises, pilocarpine 0.5% twice every other day should be prescribed. While mild brow ache, tearing, photosensitivity, and conjunctival hyperemia are fairly common during the initial postoperative period, one should always be alert to the more serious potential complications described in subsequent chapters.

SUMMARY

Preliminary results using the current technique of SEB surgery described in this chapter are promising and currently undergoing prospective, multicenter FDA clinical trials in the United States. If proven successful, this alternative approach to the treatment of presbyopia has the potential to overcome many of the limitations encountered by our present treatment options, which include reading spectacles, monovision (ie, inducing myopia in the nondominant eye with contact lenses, corneal refractive surgery, phakic intraocular lenses, or following cataract surgery), and multifocal contact or intraocular lenses. However, before widespread clinical application, we must await the results of further studies to determine both the safety and long-term efficacy of this potentially universally applicable surgical procedure.

REFERENCES

1. Marmer M. The surgical reversal of presbyopia: a new procedure to restore accommodation. *Int Ophthalmol Clin.* 2001;41(2):123-132.
2. Southall JPC, trans. *Helmholtz's Treatise on Physiologic Optics.* Vol 1. New York: Dover Publications; 1962:143.
3. Schachar RA, Black TD, Kash RL, et al. The mechanism of accommodation and presbyopia in the primate. *Annals of Ophthalmology.* 1995;27:58-67.
4. Glasser A, Kaufman P. The mechanism of accommodation in primates. *Ophthalmology.* 1999;106:863-872.
5. Matthews S. Scleral expansion surgery does not restore accommodation in human presbyopia. *Ophthalmology.* 1999;106:873-877.
6. Thornton SP, Shear NA. *Surgery for Hyperopia and Presbyopia.* Baltimore, Md: Williams & Wilkins; 1997:33-36.
7. Fukasaku H, Marron, J. Anterior ciliary sclerotomy with silicone expansion plug implantation: effect on presbyopia and intraocular pressure. *Int Ophthalmol Clin.* 2001;41(2):133-141.
8. Schachar RA. The correction of presbyopia. *Int Ophthalmol Clin.* 2001;41(2):53-70.

Ultrasound Biomicroscopy After Scleral Expansion Band Surgery and Postoperative Exercises

Barrie D. Soloway, MD, FACS

Scleral expansion band (SEB) implantation has been developed as a strategy for rehabilitating the human eye's decreasing ability to accommodate with age based on Schachar's theory.

In the US trials that were performed at the New York Eye and Ear Infirmary on March 29, 2000, SEB segments manufactured by Presby Corp (Dallas, Tex) were implanted as described in earlier chapters. During these trials, ultrasonic biomicroscopy (UBM) was used postoperatively to evaluate the space created and attempt to correlate this with the results. It was found that an increase in space between the ciliary muscle origin and the lens capsule is required in order for the patient to have the anatomic ability to accommodate for near objects. Further investigation has demonstrated that after this additional space is created, efforts at increasing the muscle tone of the ciliary muscles can further improve the patient's ability to resolve near objects. This should come as no surprise to anyone familiar with the need for physical therapy after prolonged disuse of any striate muscle system in the body, as ciliary muscles are of a striate nature. This chapter will provide UBM data to show the importance of the position of the implants in providing this additional space, as well as exercises used for patients after SEB implant surgery.

ULTRASOUND BIOMICROSCOPY AND SCLERAL EXPANSION BANDS

Ultrasound biomicroscopy was performed 6 months after SEB implant surgery in each of five eyes operated on during Phase I of the US Food and Drug Administration (FDA)-monitored clinical trials at the Ocular Imaging Laboratory of the New York Eye and Ear Infirmary in 2000. The model P-40 Ultrasonic Biomicroscope (Paradigm Medical Industries, Salt Lake City, Utah) (Figure 1) with a 50-MHz probe, 50-micron resolution, 5-mm tissue penetration was used. A 5 x 5 mm field of view was obtained.

The patients were examined in the supine position with a 22-mm saline-filled eye cup for immersion (Figure 2).

The ultrasound probe was oriented perpendicularly to the surface of the eye and the SEB segment. All four segments were visualized in each of the five eyes examined. The scleral spur was used as a reproducible landmark to measure the position of the implants.

During this study, the average position of the SEB was found to be 2.8 mm with a standard deviation of ±0.18 microns from the scleral spur, as shown in Figure 3.

We were unable to determine the depth of the SEB in the sclera due to variable conjunctival thickness and echoing of the ultrasound from the polymethylmethacrylate material of the SEBs.

No alteration of the anterior segment structures or anterior chamber angle was found. The ciliary body showed no anatomic change, effusion, or detachment. An elevation of the ciliary body was recognizable along the anterior edge of the implant (Figures 4 and 5).

The average distance of the four implants in each patient was calculated and plotted against the increase in accommodative amplitude found for that patient. Despite the small number of patients examined, a positive correlation was found relating the distance from the scleral spur and the increase in accommodative amplitude (Figure 6).

As more patients undergo SEB implant surgery for presbyopia reversal surgery, UBM will continue to provide information on the importance of the positioning of segments to improve the results of surgery.

EXERCISE AFTER SCLERAL EXPANSION SURGERY TO REVERSE PRESBYOPIA

Exercise of the accommodative muscle complex is proving to be effective in improving the abilities of patients to accommodate near objects after SEB implant surgery. According to Schachar's theory, the crowding of the ciliary muscles by the progressive growth of the ectodermal lens causes them to have a resting flexure and decreases their ability to flex further to reshape the lens. This leads to a cycle of reduced resistance to flexure and a reduction in the muscles' ability to be effective in focus. Compounded by the use of external optical magnifier lenses to continue to see clearly at near, the muscles weaken further from disuse. As with any muscle complex in the body, it is presumed that the disuse of these muscles leads to their atrophy. We are frequently asked if the use of the eyes for focusing close after SEB implantation surgery is adequate for restoring accommodation. We have found that the exercises are helpful in returning patients to the best of their abilities because they work the

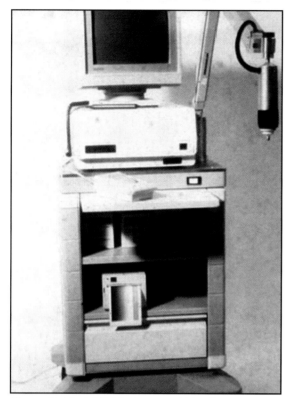

Figure 1. Model P-40 ultrasound biomicroscope.

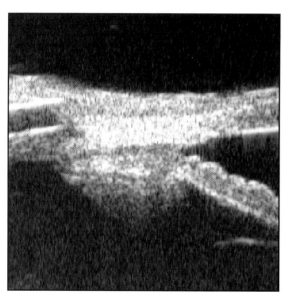

Figure 4. Ultrasound biomicroscopy photo of an implant.

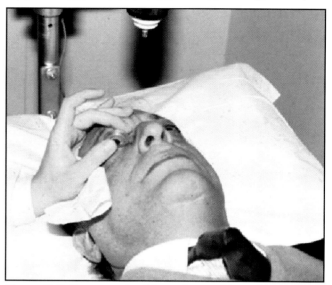

Figure 2. Patient examined in supine position with a 22-mm saline-filled eye cup.

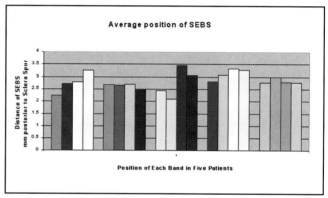

Figure 3. Average position of SEBs in five patients.

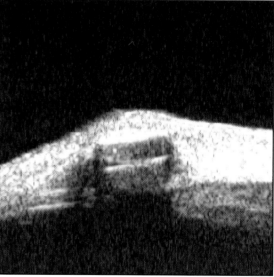

Figure 5. Ultrasound biomicroscopy photo of an implant.

muscles to their extreme levels instead of simply allowing them to work at a minimal level. Although patients who have undergone SEB implant surgery have been able to return to excellent accommodative amplitudes on their own, the specific exercises designed to increase the strength of the muscles of accommodation can help to improve the time it takes to restore accommodation, as well as yield greater levels of accommodative amplitude and faster reading speeds. This is accomplished by the exercises producing an alternating tension and relaxation in the accommodative musculature to enhance its ability to focus.

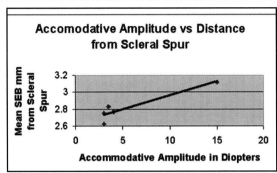

Figure 6. Accommodative amplitude versus distance from the scleral spur.

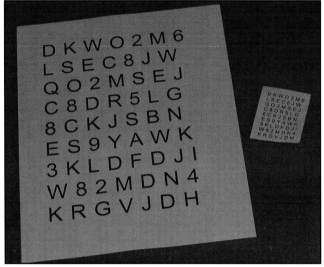

Figure 7. Hart chart.

Although more time is demanded of a patient's typically busy schedule, it is preferable to exercise each of the eyes individually in order to obtain the maximum accommodative effect and to remove the problem of headaches, diplopia, or suppression due to diminished accommodative convergence found in presbyopic patients. We have found that the problem of diminished accommodative convergence is easier to improve later, after the patient is seeing a clearer image up close and is therefore better able to binocularly fuse the images. During the early stages of accommodative exercise, an eye patch is used to occlude the eye that is not being exercised, then switched in order to allow the patient to work with each eye individually.

One of the most important aspects of the postoperative care of patients who have had SEB surgery to reverse the effects of presbyopia is preoperative education. Patients must be made aware of a number of aspects of the recovery process. One fact that cannot be overemphasized is that unlike other refractive procedures such as excimer laser reshaping of the cornea for distance refractive problems, these patients will need to play an active role in the rehabilitation of their near vision with exercise. By informing patients of these facts before they agree to undergo surgery, patients who might have been unwilling to comply with the exercises or who were unaware of the need for them postoperatively will be able to reassess their goals and better determine if they want to undergo the surgery. Another important fact to stress with the patient preoperatively is that this rehabilitative process will not be painless. As the postoperative SEB patients start to use and strengthen their ciliary muscles for reading, many of them feel a degree of pain that is best described as brow ache. This pain is believed to be directly related to soreness in the relatively atrophied ciliary muscles and has been termed *accommodative scleromyalgia* by scleral implant surgeon Dr. Gene Zdenek. This pain is very similar to the type that glaucoma patients feel when they are started on pilocarpine drops. Fortunately, just as this pain passes in patients after using pilocarpine for some time, the accommodative scleromyalgia diminishes as their muscle tone improves. We have found that by informing patients of this pain before they have surgery, they are better able to work through the pain. Their level of concern about it is lessened, as they know in advance that it will be present and will ultimately disappear.

HART DISTANCE AND NEAR CHARTS

A Hart chart is used to help increase the flexibility and tone of the ciliary muscles. As is seen in Figure 7, the Hart chart has two parts. The content of the two charts is identical, however one is printed in a substantially larger point type than the other.

The instructions given to the patient are as follows:
1. The larger point-sized Hart chart is affixed to a wall that is at least 2 m from the patient at eye level. This distance allows the chart to be clearly visible to the patient without having to use any accommodative effort.
2. The smaller point-sized chart is then held in good light at the patient's preferred reading distance. In order to read this chart, the patient will need to invoke accommodative effort to resolve the letters.
3. The patient is instructed to look at the far wall chart and read out loud each letter of the first line individually.
4. The patient is then instructed to look at the near chart and read the same line letter by letter.
5. After finishing the first line, the patient resumes distance focus on the far chart and reads the second line letter by letter.
6. On return to the next line on the near chart, the chart should be held slightly closer than it was for the earlier line.
7. This is repeated line by line until the patient has completed each line of the two charts. The eye patch is then placed on the other eye, and the process is repeated from the start.

Patients are encouraged to read the letters as quickly as possible while slowly decreasing the distance from the eye to the near chart while maintaining clear focus. For those patients who have difficulty reading the near chart at any distance, an alternative near chart, again with identical letters to the wall chart but printed with a slightly larger font size, is supplied to start. As the patient has more and more success with this larger near chart being held closer and closer, he or she can then progress to the smaller font near chart.

After performing these exercises for the first few weeks, patients typically find that it becomes easier and easier to jump their focus to the near chart, and the exercise can be done faster and faster. At this time, we ask them to start alternating from the far chart to the near chart on a letter by letter basis instead of line by line to further develop their ability to focus up close.

ACCOMMODATIVE ROCK EXERCISES

The use of low power plus/minus flipper lenses is another

method that is used to exercise the ciliary muscles and improve patients' ability to accommodate for near focus. Once again, the important aspect of alternating the need for near and distance focus is accomplished with these exercises. Patients are again advised to perform these exercises monocularly at first in order to avoid the potential interference of diplopia and discomfort of a relative convergence insufficiency. As they become more adept at maintaining near focus, once again the problem of binocular fusion diminishes with the sharper image seen.

The postoperative scleral expansion band patient is initially supplied with flipper lenses (Bernell, Mishawaka, Ind, www.bernell.com) (Figure 8). These are composed of a pair of +0.75 diopter (D) lenses on one side, and -0.75 D lenses on the other side. With these exercises, the patient is instructed to read something of his or her choice, such as a newspaper or novel. The reading material should be held at the standard reading distance of 30 to 40 cm with good lighting.

The instructions given to the patient for these accommodative rock exercises are as follows:

1. The patient should hold the flipper lens holder such that the +0.75 D side is in front of the eye.

2. The patient should clear the print and read the first line.

3. The flipper lens holder is then reversed to use the -0.75 D side over the eyes, maintaining the same distance with the reading material.

4. The patient should then try to clear the print and reread the same line word by word as quickly as possible.

5. The patient then reverses the flipper lenses to the plus lens side again and goes on to the next line.

6. Here again, the patient should continue the exercise line by line, slowly decreasing the distance from the eye, if possible, until the end of the material is reached.

While performing the accommodative rock exercises, there are two things that the patient must remember: the first is to hold the lens close to the eye to avoid magnification and minification. The second is that the flip from one side to the other must be accomplished as quickly as possible.

After a few weeks of exercise, the patient can begin to perform the accommodative rock exercises binocularly. During this time, the patient must be aware that he or she might start suppressing the vision from one eye if he or she cannot fuse the images of the two eyes individually. When performing these exercises with flippers binocularly, it is advisable for them to hold an object such as a pencil halfway between the flipper and the reading material. The patient is instructed that he or she should see two pencils at all times regardless of which side of the flipper lens is being used. This is an indication that both eyes are working together. If the patient finds that he or she sees only one pencil at any time, he or she needs to stop and blink a few times to try to resume seeing the pencil again with both eyes. As a last resort, the patient can position the reading material a little further away, allowing for less need for convergence.

Recording sheets are provided to the patient so that he or she can chart progress with the exercises. These are dated by the patient with the distance that he or she was able to hold the Hart chart, which eye was easier to see, the level of pain experienced, and any episodes of binocular suppression are recorded. These provide the patient with the positive reinforcement needed to continue the exercise process. These log sheets also give the surgeon a view as to the amount of effort and success that the patient is having and

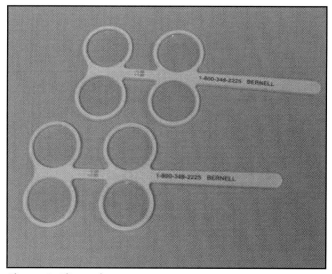

Figure 8. Flipper lenses.

allows the surgeon to individually tailor the exercises for the patient.

MEDICAL EXERCISE

At times, it can be difficult for patients to begin these exercises, as they are frustrated with their inability to see close letters clearly. In the early postoperative period, medication can be used sparingly to help strengthen the ciliary muscles. We have found the use of pilocarpine 1% drops used on alternate days to be an effective way to help patients clear near print. Prior to prescribing pilocarpine, a complete eye examination is performed to avoid the known complications of this medication. Although we have had patients using pilocarpine for up to 1 year after SEB implant surgery, long-term use of pilocarpine is not advised, as it can become a crutch for the patient.

OVERCOMING PATIENT PROBLEMS WITH EXERCISE

There are a number of common obstacles to exercise that patients can have after SEB implant surgery. One of the most common problems encountered during the first months after surgery is dryness on the corneal surface, causing a degradation of image quality. This has the effect of decreasing acuity in distance as well as up close. This is similar to the dryness seen in all patients who have had extensive conjunctival surgery, such as postoperative scleral encircling band surgery for retinal detachment and limbal approach strabismus surgery. The location of the implants and their elevation can worsen this problem and in extreme cases might cause localized dryness from poor lid flushing of the tear film. Here again, patients are advised about this preoperatively, and they are placed on frequent use of artificial tear lubricating drops during the day and a gel or ointment for long-term lubrication overnight. Preservative-free artificial tears are prescribed to avoid the medicamentosa effects seen from the frequent use of preserved tear solutions. In severe cases, silicone punctal plugs can be used to slow the drainage of their tears.

Investigational studies with the use of cyclosporin solution drops show promise toward improvement in the surface epithelial vitality and smoothness. Cyclosporin drops are prescribed to be used four times daily for the first month and twice daily thereafter. Resolution of dry eye symptoms can occur in the first month or two, however patients continue to use cyclosporin solution for 3 to 4 months before they will be able to discontinue its use fully. Typically, patients will still require the use of artificial tear lubrication supplements while they use the cyclosporin drops.

Frustration is another obstacle to patients' performance of the exercises needed to obtain the best possible results from SEB surgery and improve their accommodation to its highest level. It is important to spend time during the postoperative visits reviewing the exercise log sheets, having the patient perform the exercises to monitor that he or she is performing them properly, and providing positive reinforcement that is essential to their continuance.

We are frequently asked if the exercise process can be used to restore accommodation without surgery. This led us to attempt a study to see if this was possible. Unfortunately, the greatest obstacle to success and even continued use of the exercise in presbyopic patients was their inability to clear near print without aid. With all the exercises described in this chapter, the patient must have some ability to clear the near print for the exercises to work. Further long-term study is required to determine if these exercises can be effective in staving off the effects of presbyopia when started in the pre-presbyopic patient. These studies, however, are beyond the scope of this chapter.

Scleral expansion implant surgery appears to be a safe and effective method for restoring accommodation in presbyopic patients when the implants are properly positioned. This absolute requirement is undergoing refinement with the use of better localization methods such as high-definition ultrasonic biomicroscopy. Control of the depth of the implants with advances, such as the automated PresbyDrive, will continue to improve the results of the surgery. The use of accommodative exercise has been shown to help augment the effects of this surgery. Proper patient selection, cooperation, and level of expectation remain important facets in the surgery as well. The goal of the surgeon should be to use every method available in his or her armamentarium to help patients perform as well as they possibly can.

Chapter 12

Supraciliary Segments

Georges F. Baikoff, MD

INTRODUCTION

Surgical treatment of presbyopia is the next objective in refractive surgery. Correcting myopia, hypermetropia, or astigmatism has become routine due to the excimer laser (photorefractive keratectomy [PRK] and laser-assisted in situ keratomileusis [LASIK]) and refractive implants on phakic eyes. All human beings suffer from presbyopia during the second half of their lives, and today research is engaged in that direction.

Several directions of research are proposed:
+ Corneal (LASIK, different lasers, conductive keratoplasty, intracorneal inlay)
+ Crystalline (multifocal pseudophakic implants, accommodative pseudophakic implants, and multifocal phakic implants)
+ Scleral (incisions, implants, scleral ablation with laser)

We have decided to carry out research in two different areas:
+ Supraciliary segments
+ Anterior chamber foldable phakic intraocular lenses (IOLs)

The common denominator of these two techniques is their reversibility (ie, if the result is not up to expectations, it is possible to remove either the intrascleral segments or the phakic implant and more or less return the patient to his or her initial state). It is also possible to theorize that these two techniques are adjustable and the implant or segment can be exchanged. Both of these methods have their advantages and disadvantages.

SUPRACILIARY SEGMENTS

EVOLUTION OF THE CONCEPT

Between 1990 and 1995, the development of intrascleral implants was initiated by Schachar. He believed that it was possible to restore accommodation by pulling on or stretching the large diameter of the crystalline lens. This led him to believe that the observations made on balloons could be applied to the eye. If one pulls on a balloon, which can be compared to the crystalline lens, the periphery will be flattened and the center of the balloon will bulge. From there, and in complete contradiction with the theory

described by Helmholtz over a century ago, a new theory was born. According to Schachar, during the process of accommodation, certain parts of the zonula would appear to have a pulling effect on the crystalline lens, flattening its periphery and consequently creating a central steepening effect, increasing the refractive power of the lens itself. This argument is purely inductive, and scientific evidence leads one to think that Helmholtz's theory is perfectly valid and that any other theory is just hypothetical.

However, it is strange to observe that a certain number of patients operated on with Schachar's scleral expansion segments showed an improvement in their near vision. Therefore, an effect is produced when a segment or foreign body is inserted into the sclera. Thus, it is important to understand this mechanism in order to reproduce and quantify it.

I was fortunate to come across a case of congenital aniridia and artificially apply pulling or compression movements to the sclera of this eye. Effectively, if one pulls on the sclera facing the ciliary body, distortion of the periphery of the crystalline lens can be observed due to zonular tension, and this zone appears to be flattened. A Schachar effect can be observed—by pulling on the sclera, the periphery is flattened and steepening occurs in the center (Figure 1). On the other hand, if one has a minimum amount of clinical or surgical experience, in particular in retinal detachment surgery, it is impossible to believe that a scleral lift could be permanent. Any sort of foreign body resting on and exerting a centrifugal force on the sclera will create a cheese wiring effect, and this pressure toward the exterior will cause wearing and perforation of the superficial sclera; eventually the segment itself will be rejected.

During examination of this same patient, the sclera facing the ciliary body was depressed (centripetal force) and a contrary effect was noted. It is possible to relax the zonular tension (this brings us close to physiological accommodation), and it is clear to see that the diameter of the crystalline lens decreases, causing the whole crystalline lens to bulge. With this indentation procedure, it is then possible to imagine a "restoration" or assistance to the residual accommodation of the crystalline lens that remains soft enough for quite some time, even in an elderly patient.

Our principle is, therefore, diametrically opposed to Schachar's and has the advantage of being in line with Helmholtz's theory on accommodation. Moreover, clinical experience shows that we can surgically insert deep intrascleral implants to cause indentation of

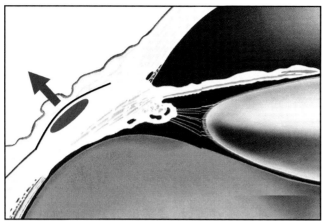

Figure 1. Schachar's theory: The superficial segment theoretically has a left effect. Its position explains why extrusion is easy.

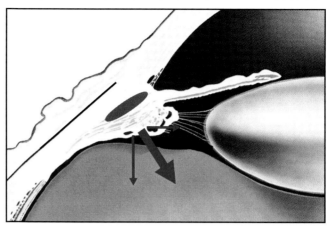

Figure 2. Baikoff's theory: A deep segment can produce an indentation effect of the ciliary body, relaxation of the zonula, and pressure on the vitreous. In addition, it is safe from extrusion.

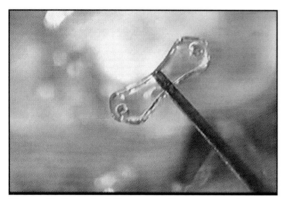

Figure 3. Aspect of the supraciliary segments (courtesy of Pavel Stodulka).

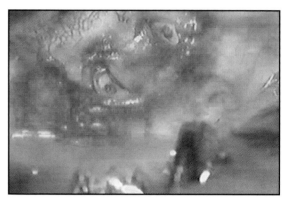

Figure 4. Superficial insertion of a supraciliary segment according to Schachar's theory. Loss of effect after 6 months. The initial effect is due more to an indentation effect than to a lift effect, but the effect is reduced over time because of the thinning of the scleral loop.

the choroid during retinal detachment treatment. We also know that this indentation is permanent and, for several years, can be observed in patients operated on for retinal detachment by carrying out a funduscopic examination. Thus, our aim is to develop supraciliary segments that will indent the ciliary body facing the zonular ring to induce zonular loosening and reduce the large diameter of the crystalline lens (Figure 2).

SURGICAL TECHNIQUE

Anesthesia can be general, locoregional, or topical. A limbal peritomy is carried out in each quadrant between the two right muscles. A loop tunnel is made limited by two 2-mm distant radial cuts. These incisions are measured at a depth of 300 μm with a radial keratotomy knife. A tunnel is created between these two incisions with a disposable 1.25 mm-wide knife. The segments are inserted with their convex side (Figures 3 and 4) facing the inside of the eye, then turned around to fit the circumference of the sclera. The conjunctiva is sealed. The operation is simple and takes about 15 to 20 minutes. Postoperative treatment is prescribed in the form of steroid and antibiotic eye drops.

PRELIMINARY CLINICAL RESULTS

A first generation of supraciliary segments was used on five eyes of three patients.* The patients were close to emmetropia and all suffered from recent or advanced presbyopia. The patients, two men and one woman, were between 41 and 55 years of age. Two right eyes and three left eyes were operated on.

The patients were followed over a period of 6 months with check-ups on day 1, day 7, after 2 weeks, and after 1, 3, and 6 months. Far visual acuity remained unchanged during the observation period—20/20 without correction. Mean refraction was at +0.2 diopter (D) preoperatively and varied only slightly throughout the observation period. Near visual acuity, which on average was J8 preoperatively, reached J3 after 6 months. On day 1, ocular tension rose slightly but came back to normal afterward. There was no postoperative modification of the keratometry and no modification of the

---

*In collaboration with Dr. Pavel Stodulka, Bata Hospital, Zlin, Czech Republic.

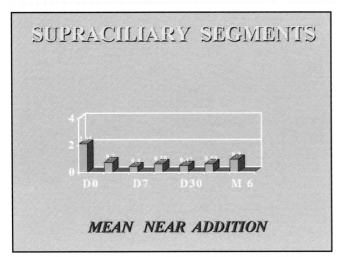

Figure 5. Preoperatively: Addition of +2.00 D. Eight days postoperatively: Addition of +0.4 D. Six months postoperatively: Addition of +0.9 D.

axial length, but perhaps a slight reduction of the anterior chamber depth. To obtain J1 in near vision preoperatively, an addition of 2.05 D was necessary. One week after the intervention, only 0.4 D was necessary and this remained stable during a period of 3 months. At 6 months, there was a loss of effect with an average addition of 0.9 D (Figure 5).

CONCLUSIONS

At the end of this trial, it appeared that the indented supraciliary segments have an effect. This effect decreased after 6 months. On the other hand, the patients' near visual acuity improved significantly. This trial does not establish whether accommodation was effectively restored or whether the results were due to another phenomenon. However, future trials have been scheduled with a modification of the technique. The loss of effect is due to the extrusion of the segments, and photos clearly show the sclera thinning progressively under pressure from the segments.

The aim is to begin a new trial with a completely modified surgical technique. The segments will be inserted in a blind tunnel under the sclera at a depth of 600 µm. The tunnel will be sealed and the segment will have no contact with the scleral surface. We can, therefore, hope to obtain a permanent indentation and improve the effect.

Chapter 13

Anterior Ciliary Sclerotomy With Silicone Expansion Plug Implantation

Effect on Presbyopia and Intraocular Pressure

Hideharu Fukasaku, MD

INTRODUCTION

Recent models of accommodation and presbyopia suggest a surgical approach to the correction of presbyopia. Anterior ciliary sclerotomy (ACS) has been advanced as a possible such correction for presbyopia. We have studied three variations of ACS to demonstrate their effectiveness and safety. Simple ACS and enhanced ACS both showed initial improvement in accommodative amplitude, but rapid regression to preoperative accommodative amplitude was observed. ACS with silicone expansion plug (SEP) implantation showed modest initial improvement in accommodative amplitude that was sustained over the 18 months of study. In addition, a significant and sustained lowering of intraocular pressure (IOP) occurred with ACS with SEP.

Accommodation has until recently been explained by the Helmholtz hypothesis.[1] This hypothesis holds that passive anteroposterior thickening of the lens and relative curvature changes in the anterior and posterior lens surfaces result from zonular relaxation with ciliary muscle contraction (Figure 1). Presbyopia is likewise described as the loss of accommodation due to decreasing elasticity of the lens fibers and capsule.[1-2] Recent work[3-4] suggests a very different model of accommodation. Morphological changes in the lens with accommodative effort are seen as the result of active rather than passive interactions. The three components of the ciliary body—the longitudinal, radial, and circular fibers—act in concert to increase tension in the equatorial zonules while decreasing tension in the anterior and posterior zonules. The result is an active elongation of the lens diameter with peripheral thinning and central thickening due to dynamic internal volume changes (Figure 2). The net result is increased plus refracting power of the eye.

The important difference between the Helmholtz model and the Schachar model is that the latter suggests a more active interaction between the ciliary muscle and the lens/zonule complex. This interaction is an active effort by the ciliary muscle and results in not simply passive relaxation of the lens/zonule complex but a more complicated active differential response of different zonular types, resulting in morphological changes in the lens.

If this recent model of accommodation is correct, then presbyopia may not be explained by simple sclerosis of the lens fibers and capsule, as previously understood. Rather, the decline in accommodative power of the eye may be due to the inability of the lens equator to expand into the posterior chamber. Thornton[5] has described this as "a crowding" of the lens in the posterior chamber as the lens grows.

The lens is ectodermal in origin and grows throughout life, increasing in size in all dimensions. The sclera, on the other hand, is mesodermal in origin and ceases during puberty. There is a discontinuity in growth between the ectodermal lens and mesodermal scleral shell that begins around puberty. The result is an increase in the diameter of the lens and a gradual, progressive narrowing of the space between the lens equator and the ciliary body/sclera or crowding of the lens in the posterior chamber (Figure 3).

The strength of any muscle is dependent on the effective length of pull of that muscle. Decreasing the distance between the equator of the lens and the ciliary body with lens growth decreases the effective length of pull of the ciliary muscle. We visualize this as a loss of ciliary muscle/zonular apparatus "tone" (Figure 4). With the loss of ciliary muscle/zonular apparatus tone, any given accommodative effort results in less pulling on the equatorial zonules and less relaxation of the anterior/posterior zonules, resulting in less change in lens morphology and less accommodative response, or presbyopia. Thus, it is not truly mechanical crowding of the lens in the posterior chamber but a progressive loss of ciliary muscle/zonular apparatus tone that causes presbyopia.

This very appealing model of accommodation/presbyopia suggests a possible surgical correction for presbyopia. If the space between the lens equator and the ciliary body can be expanded, then the length of pull of the ciliary muscle/zonule apparatus should increase and accommodative tone will be restored. Thornton[5] has suggested ACS as a method to safely and effectively expand the globe over the ciliary body and uncrowd the lens (Figure 5).

ANTERIOR CILIARY SCLEROTOMY: EVOLUTION OF A PROCEDURE

As first described,[6] ACS involved eight equally spaced radial incisions of the conjunctiva and sclera overlying the ciliary body in each of the oblique quadrants. Our initial technique[7] modified this to include limbal peritomies overlying the oblique quadrants. This avoided excessive conjunctival bleeding and, more importantly,

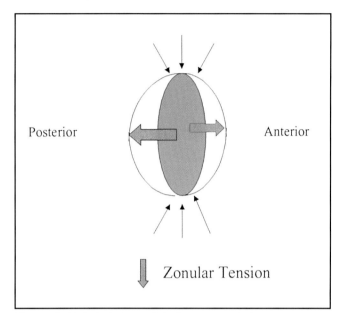

Figure 1. Helmholtz's model of accommodation.

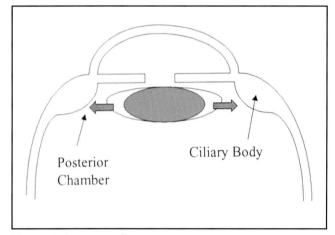

Figure 3. Lens crowding.

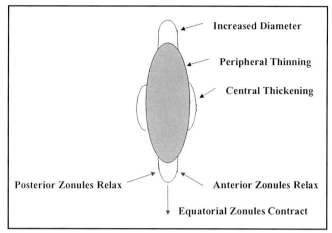

Figure 2. A new model of accommodation.

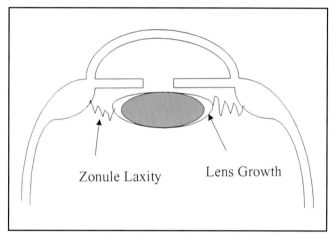

Figure 4. Accommodative tone.

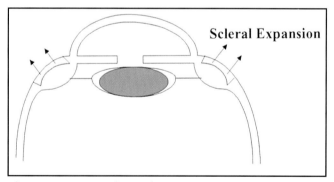

Figure 5. Anterior ciliary sclerotomy (ACS).

allowed accurate measurement of the length and depth of the incision. Incisions through conjunctiva are always difficult to measure due to the conjunctiva's elasticity and compressibility. In addition, we placed two parallel or tandem incisions in each quadrant for a total of eight incisions.

We also introduced the use of ultrasonic biomicroscopy (UBM) to accurately measure the depth of the incision. As with radial keratotomy, an incision of insufficient depth will probably be ineffective; and since one is incising sclera overlying the highly vascular ciliary body and choroid, incisions of excessive depth might prove disastrous. UBM gives us the first accurate method of measuring scleral thickness and is absolutely essential in determining the setting for blade depth prior to incision of the sclera. This allows easy measurement of scleral thickness. We have found scleral thickness to be a consistent 670 microns with very little variation. However, due to the possibility of scleral ectasias or staphylomas overlying the ciliary body/choroid, we continue to perform UBM scleral thickness measurements on all ACS cases.

Initially, our objective was to obtain 95% scleral thickness incisions. Experience with donor sclera indicated that using the

Thornton triple edge diamond knife (Mastel-KOI, T-2241, Rapid City, SD), the blade needed to be set at 600 microns. We further determined that the incision length would be 3.0 mm carried posteriorly starting 1 mm posterior to the surgical limbus to adequately include the sclera overlying the ciliary body and posterior chamber without unnecessarily incising sclera overlying uvea and retina. UBM was used to determine the anteroposterior dimension of the ciliary body.

Initial results were encouraging but limited. After initial postoperative increases of several diopters of accommodation, there was regression; and within several months, only an average of 0.8 diopter (D) increase in accommodation was achieved (simple ACS,

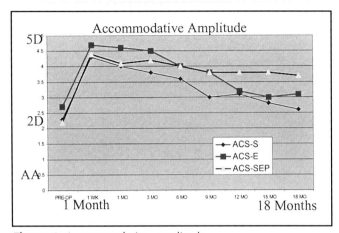

Figure 6. Accommodative amplitude.

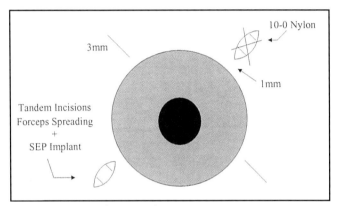

Figure 8. ACS with SEP technique.

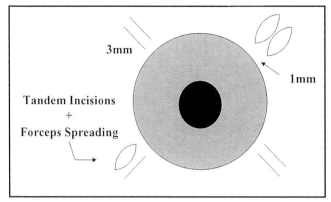

Figure 7. Enhanced ACS technique.

Figure 6). Distance refraction remained stable and there were no postoperative complications such as infection or uveitis. Although the results were limited, all the patients remained enthusiastic about the improvement in their everyday near vision.

To enhance the surgical effect and decrease regression, we increased the sclerotomy depth to full thickness by a spreading dissection technique (Figure 7). Following the incision, we carefully spread the scleral tissue using a specially designed Fukasaku ACS forceps (Katena, Denville, NJ) down to the uveal plane. We termed this *enhanced ACS.* At first, we were quite concerned about our ability to identify this surgical plane since entry into the uvea would surely cause hemorrhage. We found that when approaching the uveal plane there was a distinct bluish blush from the vascular uvea that is easily recognizable. In addition, the subscleral space, usually a potential space, easily opens to become an actual space. We have experienced no hemorrhages in this spreading dissection.

The use of spreading dissection did enhance our results (see Figure 4). We now noted an initial increase in accommodative amplitude of 2.2 D. However, the effect rapidly regressed to near preoperative levels within several months of surgery. Obviously, as the sclerotomy healed any increase in globe diameter was lost.

ANTERIOR CILIARY SCLEROTOMY WITH SCLERAL EXPANSION PLUG IMPLANTATION

The marked regression in effect due to wound contraction and loss of globe expansion found with both simple and enhanced ACS

suggested the addition of a material to keep the incision open. The choice of silicone for the scleral expansion plug was dictated by the need to use a stable, inert material that could be fashioned in the dimensions needed and manipulated surgically. The silicone chosen came from scleral buckle material and was shaped by hand in the operating room. The dimensions chosen, 2.5 mm length and 0.6 mm height, were determined by the estimated incision length of 3 mm and depth of 670 microns. The width of 0.6 mm was calculated based on the desired circumferential expansion of the sclera. Given that the lens diameter change from age 20 to 90 years is 2.5 mm (6.5 to 9.0 mm lens diameter measured on postmortem specimens), there is an average of 0.036 mm per year increase in lens diameter. Hence, a 60-year-old will need to increase globe diameter by 0.72 mm from that of a 40-year-old. This equates to a circumferential expansion of 2.45 mm.

$$\pi \times \text{diameter or } 2 \times 3.41 \times 0.36 = 2.45 \text{ mm}$$

With four silicone plugs to be implanted, each plug width will have to be approximately 0.6 mm.

The silicone expansion plugs fashioned to the above dimensions were implanted in the depth of the sclerotomy. They were then sutured in place through both sclera and plug in a criss-cross fashion using 10-0 nylon (Figure 8). Unlike the original simple ACS technique or our enhanced technique using spreading dissection, we used only single incisions in each oblique quadrant, not tandem incisions.

The fact that there was rapid, marked regression in the gained accommodative amplitude following simple ACS and ACS enhanced only with spreading dissection is not surprising. The effect depends on expansion of the scleral circumference overlying the ciliary body. As the incisions heal, there is wound closure and reduction in scleral circumference back to near preoperative levels. The addition of silicone plugs in ACS-SEP effectively blocked this wound closure and maintained the gained scleral circumferential expansion, hence gaining accommodative amplitude. The fact that the initial gain in accommodative amplitude with ACS-SEP was actually slightly less than either our initial ACS technique or our enhanced ACS technique using spreading dissection is probably due the effect of the sutures holding the SEP in place, tending to close the wound initially. We are now careful not to place any unnecessary tension on these sutures. In addition, we are now using 11-0 Merceline, which should induce less tension and last longer than nylon.

Anterior Ciliary Sclerotomy and Intraocular Pressure

We also noted that in addition to increasing the amplitude of accommodation, ACS-SEP was also associated with a dramatic drop in IOP (Figure 9). Simple ACS and ACS enhanced by spreading dissection, in contrast, caused only a minimal drop in IOP that was lost fairly rapidly. The explanation probably lies in the depth and permanence of the radial incisions. Simple ACS is a shallower incision. No attempt is made to complete a full-thickness sclerotomy. ACS enhanced by spreading dissection, on the other hand, ensures a full-thickness sclerotomy by use of the Fukasaku forceps to dissect down to the uveal plane. This exposes the subscleral space, which is normally an anatomic potential space due to the differential embryological development of the scleral and uveal coats. With dissection, it is possible that we create a limited, localized ciliochoroidal detachment that increases the uveoscleral outflow of aqueous. Traumatic cyclodialysis and surgical ciliochoroidal detachments are known to dramatically increase uveoscleral outflow and can cause hypotony.[7-8] There is no evidence of wound leakage per se, as there is no filtering bleb or Seidel's sign when fluorescein is applied to the conjunctiva overlying the wound.

The loss of IOP lowering effect with ACS enhanced by scleral spreading over a matter of several months probably reflects closure of the incision and hence closure of the ciliochoroidal detachment with decrease in uveoscleral outflow. ACS-SEP, on the other hand, shows negligible loss in IOP lowering effect over many months. This probably represents continued maintenance of the incision separation with the silicone plug and continued ciliochoroidal detachment with ongoing increased uveoscleral outflow.

We have been very satisfied with ACS-SEP and its ability to provide a stable increase in accommodative amplitude. Likewise, patients have been extremely pleased with the results. They report that they are now able to much better attend to such activities of daily living as reading newspapers and product labels. This is despite the modest measured increase in accommodative amplitude of only 1.5 D. We expect that patient satisfaction will increase further with correction of the fellow eye.

Future planned improvements include replacing the criss-cross 10-0 nylon suture with a 11-0 Merceline horizontal mattress suture. We expect that we will be better able to lower the profile of the suture knot to avoid potential conjunctival irritation or erosion and achieve longer suture life. We have also redesigned the expansion plug to be broader at the base (more trapezoidal on end view) to limit forces that might extrude the plug. In addition, we are creating preformed holes in the plug to avoid the time-consuming and difficult task of driving the small cutting needle of a 10-0 or 11-0 suture.

The dramatic and sustained drop in IOP with ACS-SEP suggests a possible role for this procedure in the treatment of glaucoma. The advantage of ACS-SEP in this role is that it seems to affect uveoscleral outflow. Uveoscleral outflow can account for up to 40%

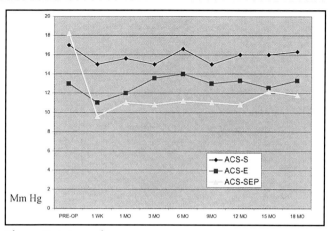

Figure 9. Intraocular pressure.

of total aqueous outflow.[9-10] Thus, unlike betablockers that have little effect on IOP during sleep, stimulation of uveoscleral outflow should help to protect the patient during both day and night. Thus far, IOP reduction has been a serendipitous finding in ACS-SEP, in which we implant expansion plugs in each of the four oblique quadrants. The next logical step will be to attempt to titrate IOP reduction by varying the number of plugs or perhaps the size of the plugs. This study is underway at our facility.

We believe that ACS-SEP is a valuable procedure in the treatment of presbyopia and a procedure that is safe, effective, and well-accepted by patients. Likewise, ACS-SEP promises another treatment modality for glaucoma and we are working on improving its predictability.

References

1. von Helmholtz HH. *Physiological Optics*. New York: Dover Press; 1962:1,143-172,375-415.
2. Fincham EF. The mechanism of accommodation. *Br J Ophthalmol.* 1937;8(Suppl);5-80.
3. Schachar RA. Histology of the ciliary muscle-zonular connection. *Annals of Ophthalmology.* 1996;28(2);70-79.
4. Neider MW, Crawford K, Kaufman PL. In-vivo videography of the rhesus monkey accommodative apparatus. *Arch Ophthalmol.* 1990;69:108.
5. Thornton SP, Shear NA. *Surgery for Hyperopia and Presbyopia.* Baltimore, Md: Williams & Wilkins; 1997:33-36.
6. Fukasaku H. Surgical reversal of presbyopia. Highlights of the 1998 ASCRS meeting. Ophthalmology Interactive; 1998.
7. Pederson JE, Gaasterland DE, MacLellan HM. Experimental ciliochoroidal detachment. Effect on intraocular pressure and aqueous humour flow. *Arch Ophthalmol.* 1979;97:536-541.
8. Toris CB, Pederson JE. Effect of intraocular pressure on uveoscleral outflow following cyclodialysis in the monkey eye. *Invest Ophthalmol Vis Sci.* 1985;26:1745-49.
9. Brubaker RF. Flow of aqueous humor in humans. Invest *Ophthalmol Vis Sci.* 1991;32:3145-66.
10. Reiss GR, Lee DA, Topper J, Brubaker RF. Aqueous humor flow during sleep. *Invest Ophthalmol Vis Sci.* 1984;25:776-8.

Chapter 14

Anterior Ciliary Sclerotomy With Titanium Implants

William Jory, FRCS(C), FRCOphth

INTRODUCTION

One can divide surgical treatment of presbyopia into either true or false categories. The false categories include corneal multi-focal sculpting by lasers, intracorneal multifocal lenses, and the implantation of phakic multifocal implants. There are many studies taking place at this time regarding these false treatments, which treat presbyopia no better than wearing multifocal glasses or contact lenses.

True surgical correction of presbyopia includes ciliary sclerotomy with or without scleral expanders and hinged aphakic lenses as designed by Georges Baikoff, MD.

ANTERIOR CILIARY SCLEROTOMY

Those of us who were doing radial keratotomy in the early and middle 1980s often completed our incisions into the limbus. We noted that these tended to reduce the effect of the myopic correction but increased middle-aged patients' accommodation. From these observations, Dr. Spencer Thornton recognized that there might be a surgical treatment for presbyopia, and in the mid-1990s pioneered anterior ciliary sclerotomy (ACS). As part of an international trial, we commenced this surgery in London in March 1999. The operation consisted of eight scleral incisions starting in the limbus with dissections extending 5 mm posteriorly and deep enough so that the blush of choroid could be visualized. Corrections of up to 2.5 diopters (D) of accommodation were achieved by increasing the scleral circumference just behind the limbus. This allowed the lens more space for accommodative changes. However, over a period of between 4 and 8 months, the effect was largely lost as the incisions healed and the scleral coat retracted to its original circumference.

CHEMICAL ADHESIVES

The answer to this problem had to be in a method of ensuring that the scleral wound edges stayed separate. We have been investigating two lines of possible treatment. The first of these is the installation of chemical adhesives, which have already been used particularly in cardiovascular repair surgery. At this stage, we have not carried out human studies; and although some animal studies have been done, our suggestions are more theoretical than practical at this time.

The first group of chemical adhesives are the acrylics. These can be divided into five types. First, the anaerobic ones are based on acrylic polyester resins. These vary from thin to viscous and have the advantage of low toxicity. The second are the cyanoacrylates, known as tissue glues. These have a fast rate of cure with rapid bonding but are highly toxic. They are very irritating to the conjunctiva. The third type are radiation-cured acrylics. These depend upon radiation to initiate polymerization. Daylight is not sufficient and, therefore, a light-sensitive catalyst is incorporated. However, they are toxic and can cause dermatitis and sensitization, and require ultraviolet radiation for curing. The fourth type consists of two components—an acrylic adhesive plus a catalytic cure initiator. These have low toxicity but require mixing at the site of surgery. Last are the toughened variants, which are flexible but distort under load, reducing their strength-stress and intensity.

The second major group of chemical adhesives that might be suitable are the epoxides. These are thermosetting resins that solidify by polymerization and have low toxicity. There are four types: the single-component heat cured, the single-component radiation, the two-component used with various hardeners, and those toughened with a rubber compound.

In studying the chemistry and biotoxicity of these chemical adhesives, the best candidates appear to be the anaerobic acrylic polyester resins, the two-component acrylic adhesives with a catalytic cure initiator, and the single-component epoxides.

All of these are well-tolerated by the body and can be applied through a broad cannula with syringe into ciliary sclerotomy incisions. Therefore, this would be a rapidly performed procedure, but their permanence is still questionable. There is a tendency for extrusion of such materials from wounds, and this of course would lead to a wearing off of the effect and, therefore, a return of presbyopia.

TITANIUM IMPLANTS

An alternative route would be to insert implants into scleral

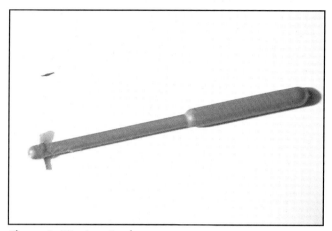

Figure 1. Titanium implant.

incisions. This year, David Jory and I initiated a trial of titanium implants in the United Kingdom (Figure 1) into ciliary sclerotomy incisions. The advantage of titanium is that it has already been used successfully in the sclera in retinal detachment surgery and is very light and strong.

Surgical Procedure

The current procedure is done under local anesthetic. Conjunctival peritomies are done in the four quadrants, and the scleral coat is bare. Using a Pallikaris knife set to achieve an incision depth of 500 microns and with a distance of 3 mm, the incision is created in the limbus in each of the four quadrants and carried posteriorly for 3 mm. Pockets in the scleral incision are then made on each side to fit the lateral wings of the titanium implants (Figure 2). These are inserted with the wings placed in the pockets that have been formed (Figure 3). The conjunctival flaps are then resutured. Antibiotic drops are then instilled and the eye padded until the patient is seen the following day, at which time the patch is removed.

Complications

Two operative complications we have encountered are difficulty in making the scleral lateral pockets at a deep enough layer and the inability of the titanium implant to maintain its position. The operations have been very time-consuming and the titanium implants are therefore being redesigned by the manufacturers, Duckworth and Kent (Herts, England), so that they may stay permanently in place. They can be seen postoperatively, but we believe that the healing process will gradually disguise them as the implants slowly adhere to the sclera. We recognize that titanium implants may be vulnerable to methicillin-resistant *Staphylococcus aureus* (MRSA) but are hopeful that either these titanium implants or suitable chemical adhesives into ciliary sclerotomy incisions may achieve a permanent correction of presbyopia.

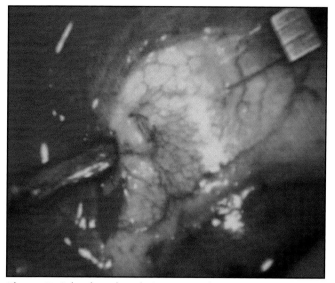

Figure 2. Scleral pockets being created.

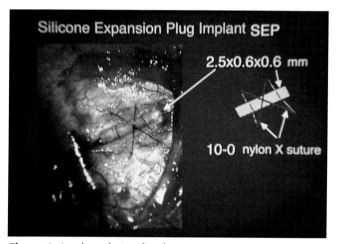

Figure 3. Implants being fixed.

Summary

We would like to emphasize two points. First, we will confuse not only our patients but ourselves if we do not draw a clear distinction between true and false methods of correcting presbyopia. Second, we must be aware that with simple incisions, whether by diamond knife or infrared laser, the effect may wear off. Therefore, claims for surgical correction of presbyopia should be based on its true correction, and the effect should at least last for 2 years and hopefully much longer.

Chapter 15

Clinical Results of Laser Presbyopia Reversal Using the OptiVision Infrared Laser

Vivek Kadambi, MD and J.T. Lin, PhD

INTRODUCTION

Presbyopia is a condition that affects every normal middle-aged individual. Conventionally, this is treated by the use of an additional convex lens spectacle for near work. In the past decade, many attempts have been made to surgically reverse this condition. The Schachar technique[1] (scleral expansion band [SEB]) involves the insertion of implants to expand the sclera, while the Thornton technique[2] (anterior ciliary sclerotomy [ACS]) uses surgical incisions to expand the sclera. Laser presbyopia reversal (LAPR) was first introduced by Dr. J.T. Lin in 1998 and patented by SurgiLight.[3,4] The technique is still evolving, but it may be described in brief as multiple four-quadrant ablative excisions over the sclera overlying the ciliary muscle. One of the fundamental differences between the laser method (LAPR) and the nonlaser scleral expansion method is that the major regression found in the latter is minimal in the former. Tissue healing causes major regression in the SEB and ACS methods.

A prospective study to assess the safety, efficacy, and stability of LAPR is under way at the Clinic of Laser Vision, Bangalore, India.

PATIENT SELECTION

Patients with a history of corneal disease (eg, herpes) or previous ocular procedures including eye muscle surgery; history of ocular pathology or active ocular diseases including corneal scarring, microphthalmia, nystagmus, significant trauma, AIDs, and autoimmune disease; history of systemic diseases including diabetes, rheumatoid arthritis of collagen, vascular diseases; taking medications likely to affect wound healing such as corticosteroids or antimetabolites; history of scleral ectasia; history of retinal detachment or retinopathy; history of corneal dystrophy; or history of glaucoma are excluded. To date, the patients we treated have all had presbyopia of 1.5 diopters (D) or more. They have also had uncorrected vision of less than or equal to 20/40 in both eyes, less than or equal to 1 D of myopia, and less than or equal to 1 D of hyperopia.

MATERIALS AND METHODS

Twelve eyes of six patients underwent LAPR using the IR-3000 OptiVision infrared laser system and fiber optic delivery system manufactured by SurgiLight Inc, Orlando, Fla. The patients were divided into two groups based on age. Group I was between 40 and 50 years old and group II was between 51 and 60 years old. Subjects were selected with preoperative refractive status for distance between –1.0 to +1.5 D. The eyes were thoroughly screened to rule out pre-existing pathology. Preoperative and follow-up examination included refraction, slit lamp examination, funduscopy, intraocular pressure (IOP) measurements, keratometry, corneal topography, and visual fields. The follow-up period was 2 weeks to 3 months.

The procedure was done under infiltration anaesthesia using 4% lidocaine with adrenaline. Topical anesthesia was instilled just prior to infiltration. After making four fornix-based conjunctival flaps in the intermuscular region and achieving hemostasis with bipolar cautery, four pairs of radial ablative scleral excisions were made—one pair in each quadrant. The length of each ablative excision was approximately 4.5 mm in length starting 0.5 mm from the limbus. The separation between the paired ablative excisions was approximately 2.5 mm. The depth of the grooves was about 75% of scleral thickness using the blue hue of the choroid as the endpoint indicator. The peritomy sites were closed with bipolar forceps. The patient was prescribed topical antibiotics and steroids along with analgesic tablets.

CLINICAL PROTOCOL

Anesthesia consists of either a peribulbar (we suggest 4% lidocaine with 50/50 epinephrine/margaine) plus a local anesthetic (we suggest 1% tetracaine applied in a circular ring pledget around the ciliary body for 5 minutes or local injection of 4% lidocaine one quadrant at a time) or a topical ointment applied 20 to 30 minutes prior to surgery. Also place 1% topical proparicaine 5 minutes before procedure. Administer one drop each of an antibiotic and non-

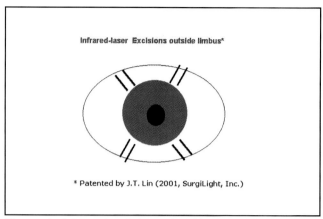

Infrared-laser Excisions outside limbus*

* Patented by J.T. Lin (2001, SurgiLight, Inc.)

Figure 1. Schematic of the eight ablative excision patterns outside the limbus of the eye by an OptiVision IR laser.

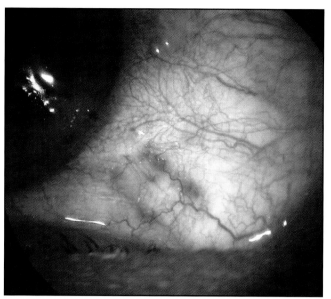

Figure 2. Photo of a pair of ablative scleral excisions in a patient 6 weeks postoperatively.

steroidal anti-inflammatory. During the procedure, drops of tetracaine or lidocaine can be administered as needed.

Prepare the patient as usual for retractive surgery. Insert the lid speculum and place the cornea protector over the cornea (a circular sponge about 6 mm in diameter). After this, follow the steps below:

1. Make eight intermuscular limbal marks using a Mallo marker.

2. Make four fornix-based peritomies at each site.

3. If needed, use bipolar cautery for hemostasis.

4. If needed, use the Mallo marker again to map out two incisions in each quadrant:

    a. 0.5 mm from the limbus (the point where the iris can no longer be seen through the cornea)

    b. Two radially oriented marks (each carried approximately 4.5 mm in length posteriorly over the ciliary body, stopping just anterior to the pars plana)

    c. Approximately 2.5 mm separation between each mark

5. Make two incisions in the quadrant area and ablate the scleral tissue to approximately 80% of scleral thickness (approximately 400 to 500 microns). Watch for the dark blue hue of the choroid as an endpoint.

6. Close the peritomy sites with bipolar forceps.

7. Place one drop Acular and one drop Acuflux.

8. Patch only if needed and instruct the patient to use his or her eyes for normal near and far vision within 24 hours of surgery.

RESULTS

Two treatment groups separated according to age were compared: group I (age 40 to 50) and group II (age 51 to 65). Patients age 40 to 50 showed the greatest improvement, which was hypothesized as due to the amount of elasticity in the ciliary bodies. However, patients age 50 to 65 also showed marked improvement.

The mean preoperative near add in group I was 1.56 D, while in group II it was 2.25 D. The near vision (tested at 35 cm reading distance) in group I with full distance correction was J5 to J10 and in group II between J16 or better. One week post LAPR, all subjects read J3 or better without near addition. All patients reported mild discomfort for 24 to 48 hours postoperatively. Conjunctival hyperemia lasted 2 to 4 weeks. The general observation was that subjec-

tive near vision improvement was noticed about 2 days after the procedure. It continued to improve over 2 to 4 weeks and especially so after the fellow eye was treated. The time interval for treating the fellow eye varied from 1 to 4 weeks. No myopic shift was noted during the follow-up period (maximum 12 months). One case (both eyes) showed regression after 3 months from J3 to J10. No significant change in refraction for distance and no induced astigmatism were noted. In general, there was a tendency for lower IOP readings postoperatively. There were some differences in the manner and speed of conjunctival healing. The scleral scar was visible and quite noticeable in some cases, but there was a tendency for it to decrease with time. No significant complications were encountered. Figure 1 shows the eight ablative excision patterns and Figure 2 shows a patient's eye 6 weeks postoperatively.

DISCUSSION

Accommodation results from the contraction of the ciliary muscle. As aging occurs, there is a relative decrease in functional range of the ciliary muscle. Factors such as hardening of the lens, atrophy of muscle, as well as "crowding of muscle" have been attributed to this. S. Thornton, MD,[2] proposed reversal of presbyopia by ACS. In this technique, an expansion of sclera was achieved by employing radial incisions. H. Fukasaku, MD carried out ACS with the implantation of an SEP. Schachar[1] achieved scleral expansion by insertion of implants. The recent results of A. Glasser, PhD[5] found that there was no accommodation or dynamic change in power for those postoperative presbyopic patients provided by Schachar. Furthermore, all of the above prior techniques showed major regressions from 40% to 90% after 3 to 12 months postoperatively.

SurgiLight's LAPR technique proposed by Dr. Lin involves eight symmetrical partial-thickness radial incisions in the sclera over the ciliary body. This allows for expansion of the sclera and improves the ciliary muscle function. Another hypothesis, presented as the Lin-Kadambi hypothesis, does not credit the scleral expansion to be the prime factor. The hypothesis attributes the increased ciliary muscle functional range to increased elasticity of the scleral ring resulting from the ablation. The absence of significant regression is due to a "fill-in" of the grooves by subconjunctival tissue.

Group II showed less postoperative accommodation than group I. This may be not an accurate reflection of the true picture. We believe that one of the more likely possibilities is that the effect in both age groups may be quite equal, but the higher demand for the near add in the older age group will produce better visual outcomes in younger subjects. Our calculation showed that for a given scleral ablation condition, the overall accommodation is governed by multiple factors: initial lens power (curvature radii), corneal power, anterior chamber depth, and the axial length, in addition to the ciliary muscle and scleral conditions. Although it may be inaccurate to derive any conclusions from the small sample size, it is necessary at this point to consider additional factors that might influence the results in the older age group. These are briefly outlined below:

+ The lenticular "hardening" may negate the effect of increased efficiency of the ciliary muscle-zonular complex.

+ During the procedure, it was generally observed (by V. Kadambi, MD) that the scleral ablation process was somewhat more irregular in the older group. The surgeon subjectively felt nonuniform texture of scleral tissue. Perhaps age-related scleral degeneration may be a contributory factor.

+ The delayed regression noted in one case could be attributed to aggressive healing, but the fact that this case was primarily hyperopic may be an important factor. Unlikely factors may be surgical, such as inadequate depth or width of the ablative grooves. Changes in the pattern of ablation or energy settings are options that may be considered.

As a procedure, LAPR was found to be nonskill-intensive with a short learning curve. Initially, the average surgical time was around 45 minutes. This has been reduced to around 20 minutes. The OptiVision IR-3000 is a solid-state laser system and extremely reliable. The energy output is very stable provided the surgeon ensures that tissue does not char and stick to the tip. All cases demonstrated a significant subjective increase in accommodation. Although the amount of presbyopic reversal is more or less the same in both age groups, the net effect is more demonstrable in the younger age group. It is my feeling that patients older than age 50

may not show uniform results due to the additional factor of lens hardening and decrease of the lens refractive index. More detailed discussion about the Lin-Kadambi hypothesis can be found in Chapter 6.

CONCLUSION

Our initial clinical study demonstrates that LAPR using the OptiVision infrared laser is an effective and safe method to surgically reverse presbyopia and visual recovery is quick; however, long-term follow-up is necessary to evaluate stability of the effect.

REFERENCES

1. Schachar RA. Cause and treatment of presbyopia with a method for increasing the amplitude of accommodation. *Annals of Ophthalmology.* 1992;24(12):445-7,452.
2. Thornton SP. Presbyopia: the new frontier. A report on a procedure to reverse presbyopia: anterior ciliary sclerotomy. 1996.
3. Lin JT. US patent 5144630 and 5520679.
4. Lin JT. US patent 6258082 B1 and 6263879 B1.
5. Fukasaku H. Silicone expansion plug implant surgery for presbyopia. Presented at: American Society of Cataract and Refractive Surgery Symposium; 2000; Boston, Mass.
6. Glasser A, Kaufman P. The mechanism of accommodation in primates. *Ophthalmology.* 1999;106(5):863-72.

BIBLIOGRAPHY

Glasser A, Campbell MC. Biometric, optical and physical changes in the isolated human crystalline lens with age in relation to presbyopia. *Vision Res.* 1999;39:1991-2015.

Helmholtz H. *Helmholtz's Treatise on Physiological Optics.* Vol. 1. Southall JPC, trans. New York: Dover Publications;1962:143.

Lin JT. US Patent No. 6258082 B1 and 6263879 B1.

Lin JT, Mallo S, Rodgers KJA, et al. In: Congress of the ESCRS. 2001;135,144.

Schachar RA, Tello C, Cudmore DP, et al. In vivo increase of the human lens equatorial diameter during accommodation. *Am J Physiol.* 1996;271:R670-6.

SECTION III

Corneal Modifications to Correct Presbyopia

Chapter 16

Presbyopic LASIK

The PARM Technique

Guillermo Avalos, MD and Ariadna Silva, MD

INTRODUCTION

It is known that the range of accommodative amplitude decreases with increasing age such that the nearest point that can be focused gradually recedes, leading (in humans, at least) to the need for optical prostheses for close work such as reading and, eventually, even for focus in intermediate distance. Presbyopia is the age-related normal process of losing accommodation in which the eye is no longer capable of comfortably sustaining the accommodation necessary for clear near vision. It is the most frequent eye problem in the world, with 40% of the population presbyopic. In Latin America there are 115 million people with presbyopia, and every year this number increases by 3 million. It is said that in 2010, there will be almost 145 million people with presbyopia. Even though it is not a cause of legal blindness, the cost associated with loss in productivity is high in the United States.

Wahl et al[1] performed a trial to analyze the emotional and behavioral consequences of age-related visual impairment in descriptive data concerned with subjective well-being, depression, everyday competence, and leisure. They concluded that age-related visual impairment produces a negative impact on emotional and behavioral adaptation in later life. This highlights the need for a range of rehabilitative efforts, including psychosocial elements.

DEFINITION

In presbyopia, the nearest point that can be focused gradually recedes, leading to the need for optical prostheses for close work such as reading and, eventually, even for focus in intermediate distance. For emmetropic people, presbyopia seems to appear practically overnight once they reach their mid 40s. However, the loss of near focus is actually progressive over a person's lifetime whether he or she is emmetropic, myopic, or hyperopic; and the age at which a person requires assistance for near focus will depend in large part on his or her refractive error (Figure 1).

Studies on accommodation in humans have shown that even in the pre-presbyopic eye, there are age-dependent changes in the anterior segment that may be correlated with loss of near vision.

LASER TECHNOLOGY TECHNIQUES

In order to better understand the geometry of the cornea and its topography applied to corneal surgery, it is necessary to review some concepts. First, an axis-based curvature is any directed curvature measured relative to the current axis view. Several axis-based curvatures are used (or at least defined) in corneal topography. Axial and meridional curvatures are oblique and measured in meridional planes, while radial and transverse curvatures are normal. All axis-based curvatures have axial artifacts.

Axial curvature is the radial average of meridional curvature from the axis view to the surface point of interest; in other words, it is the reciprocal of the meridian normal distance from a surface point to the axis view. As axial curvature was the rawest form of mapped Placido data, it formed the original and still the most popular corneal topography map. When compared to meridional maps, axial features are smoother and larger in extent, which is a direct consequence of the radial smoothing via averaging. Meridional curvature is local surface curvature measured in meridional planes. It is generally oblique (not normal), except for asymmetric surfaces. Radial curvature is a local surface curvature measured in radial planes, which are normal surface planes lying perpendicular to traverse planes. Transverse curvature is a local surface curvature measured in transverse planes, which are normal surface planes lying perpendicular to meridional planes. Historically, transverse curvature is also known as sagittal curvature.

The shape of a spheroid (a conoidal surface of revolution) is qualitatively prolate or oblate, depending on whether it is stretched or flattened in its axial dimension. More precisely, a surface of revolution is *prolate* if its meridional curvature decreases from pole to equator, and it is *oblate* if it continually increases. The optical surfaces of the normal human eye, both cornea and lens, are prolate. This shape has an optical advantage in that spherical aberration (the primary aberration of a spherical surface) can be avoided. The prolateness of the anterior cornea reduces but is insufficient to eliminate its spherical aberration.

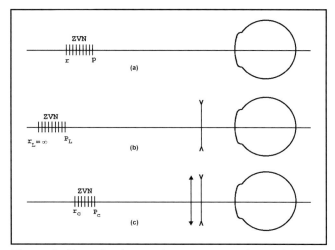

Figure 1. Clear visual zones in an emmetropic eye (a), neutralizing (b), and with add correction (c).

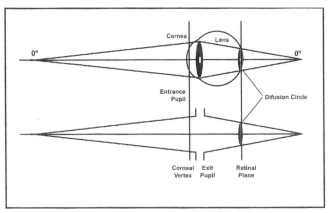

Figure 2. Clear visual zones in an emmetropic eye (a), neutralizing (b), and with add correction (c).

EXCIMER LASER PHOTOREFRACTIVE KERATECTOMY

Using a specially designed mask, Vinciguerra et al[2] developed a procedure for correcting presbyopia with excimer laser photorefractive keratectomy (PRK). A mask consisting of a mobile diaphragm formed by two blunt blades was used to ablate a 10 to 17 µm-deep semilunar-shaped zone immediately below the pupillary center, steepening the corneal curvature in that area (videokeratography controlled) in three patients. After an initial regression of 1 diopter (D) during the first 6 months, the presbyopic correction remained stable for a 1-year follow-up period, enabling uncorrected near vision of J3 in all three eyes. Uncorrected distance visual acuity was not altered. Contrast sensitivity was slightly decreased only at the 11% level. This technique is also in the experimental phase, and more clinical studies are required before it can be used in clinical practice.

LASIK

Every patient treated with an excimer laser is left with an oblate or prolate-shaped cornea depending on his or her degree of myopia or hyperopia. The approach to improve visual quality after laser-assisted in situ keratomileusis (LASIK) is to apply geometric optics and use the patient's refraction, precise preoperative corneal height data, and optimal postoperative anterior corneal shape in order to have a customized prolate shape treatment.

For some patients, standard optical correction for presbyopia is not satisfactory. That is why the latest technology has been under experimentation in order to treat this problem. LASIK is an alternative method for correcting presbyopia. Myopia, hyperopia, and astigmatism are today treated with LASIK by modifying the corneal curvature, which is the rationale for the treatment for presbyopia. Up until today two techniques are under trial for presbyopia: monofocal vision and PARM (Presbyopia Avalos and Rozakis Method).

MONOFOCAL TREATMENT

The main goal of this technique is to make the patient anisometropic so that one eye is used for distance vision and the other for near vision. This treatment is not indicated in all subjects, since its residual consequences are partial loss of stereopsis, astenopia, headache, aniseikonia, and decreased binocularity.

It is possible to increase the myopic effect in the eye for near vision with a posterior LASIK treatment as the presbyopic changes increase, but this will generate more anisometropia with the concomitant astenopia.

Goldberg et al[3] evaluated the outcome of monovision in 432 patients and found that 96% were satisfied and 4% chose enhancement to full distance correction.

Crossed monovision (dominant eye corrected for near) has been done as an alternative option. Jain et al[4] compared this technique with conventional monovision and found no differences in satisfaction between study groups.

Monofocal treatment is indicated for people with low demands on distance and near vision, such as people who drive only in the city, people who do not read, and those who do not perform manual jobs. Therefore, this treatment is not recommended for night drivers, accountants, computer users, engineers, etc. Frequently, patients with monocular vision depend on glasses for different activities, either distance or near vision.

PARM

PARM relates to an apparatus and technique for altering the shape of the cornea to have two concentric vision zones that help a presbyopic patient to focus on near and far items. The objective is to allow the patient to focus on near objects while retaining his or her ability to focus on far objects, taking into account the refractive error of the eye when the treatment is performed. With this LASIK technique, the corneal curvature is modified, creating a bilateral bifocal cornea. The preoperative corneal curvature is the main factor to consider in this type of corrective method. Pachymetry is not fundamental for this treatment, but it is the focusing ability of the eye measured by refractometry. The doctor performing the method next determines an appropriate level of correction that must be applied to the cornea to allow the eye to focus on objects in range (Figure 2). These measurements will determine if the eye is presbyopic plano, presbyopic with spherical hyperopia, or presbyopic with spherical myopia. It may also be determined that any of these three conditions can be combined with astigmatism; in these cases, astigmatism is treated at the same time.

If we have a presbyopic patient of +2.00 D but plano (meaning

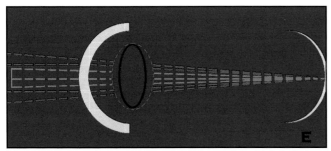

Figure 3. Normal eye focusing by means of accommodation.

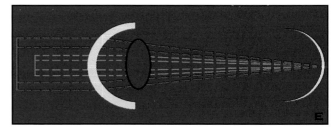

Figure 4. Presbyopic eye. The image of near objects is behind the retina.

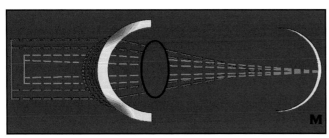

Figure 5. Ablating the periphery, prolate cornea. Now the distance image is in front of the retina.

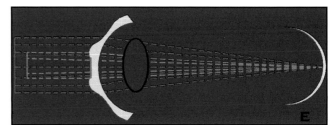

Figure 6. With an ablation done in the central area of the cornea, the distance image is focused on the retina.

that no correction is needed to achieve 20/20 vision other than the correction of presbyopia), a central area of the cornea is selected to perform the initial treatment. In the present context, this central area is a 6-mm optical zone. A flap is then created and the initial treatment is performed by eroding the tissue with a laser beam. The boundaries and definition of the area are determined using a difference of sphere algorithm mathematically that was developed for PARM and defined in a way that the laser can be controlled to remove this tissue.

The preferred treatment for removing this area is to sculpt the cornea with four sequential collapsing crescent-shaped laser beams. This begins with a half-circle-shaped laser applied to the left half of the area. The intensity of the laser and the amount of time it is applied to the central area are determined by a controller designed for PARM that analyzes the zone and determines the time and intensity required for the laser to remove the tissue. The size of the laser gradually collapses until it disappears in the direction from the center corneal area to its edge; the right side corneal area is then treated. Once left and right corneal areas are treated, the doctor changes the laser configuration and treats the top and bottom sections of the central corneal area. Treated cornea now has a steep section (the cornea is thus myopic, prolate) that allows the eye to focus in a range that includes near vision but excludes far vision. With this myopic-shaped cornea, the surgeon now selects a smaller area of the central cornea that is concentric with the previously worked on area; the size of the area is a 4-mm optical zone. The surgeon applies a treatment to this 4-mm zone that allows the cornea to focus on distant objects, thus treating the myopic condition. This treatment is a spherical diopter correction equal to, but negative of, the positive correction applied to the 6-mm zone. In this example, a negative 2.00 D correction is performed in the 4-mm area. The resulting cornea has a central area (oblate) that configures the eye to focus on far objects and a ring-shaped area that allows the eye to focus on near objects. Having undergone this treatment, the presbyopic patient can now focus on near and far objects without the use of implants or reading glasses.

When the eye is hyperopic, PARM is altered to also correct the hyperopia. For instance, the central zone of 6 mm is initially treated with a +2.00 D correction, along with a correction for the hyperopia. For example, in a patient with hyperopia of +3.00 D and presbyopia of +2.00 D, the correction first applied to the central zone of 6 mm is a resulting +5.00 D spherical correction ([hyperopia +3.00 D]+[presbyopia +2.00 D]); the zone of 4 mm is secondly treated with a -2.00 D correction, resulting in the correction of hyperopia in addition to the presbyopia.

When the eye is myopic, the initial correction area includes a combination of the presbyopic and myopic corrections. For example, when the eye is -3.00 D myopic and +2.00 D presbyopic, the presbyopia correction to the central area of 6 mm is a positive 2.00 D correction; the central area of 4 mm is then treated with a negative 5.00 D spherical diopter correction, as suggested by PARM and determined by combining a negative 3.00 D spherical correction from the myopia with a negative 2.00 D spherical correction induced by PARM (Figures 3 to 8).

After the sculpting operations are performed, a topography (Figures 9 to 14) of the sculpted eye may be taken to show the difference in curvature in the 6 mm and 4 mm zones. The surgeon then examines the patient's distance visual acuity and measures near visual acuity. If further errors are found, further sculpting is performed.

As shown, with this LASIK technique (PARM) the corneal curvature is modified, creating a bilateral bifocal cornea. In order to have high-quality vision, corneal keratometry should not be modified up to 48 D. Corneas with more than 48 D produce undesired optical alterations like glare, halos, decreased visual acuity, and decreased contrast sensitivity. For each hypermetropic diopter corrected, the corneal curvature increases in 0.89 keratometric diopters as an average. That is why it is recommended to treat patients with keratometry in the range between 41 to 43 D to obtain postoperative curves under 48 D (see Figures 13 and 14). The corneal flap performed with the microkeratome must be between 8.5 to 9.5 mm in order to have an available corneal surface for treatment of at least

Figure 7. Corneal topography showing the shape of the cornea.

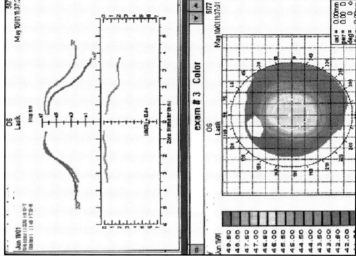

Figure 8. Comparison of the cornea and schematic of the PARM method.

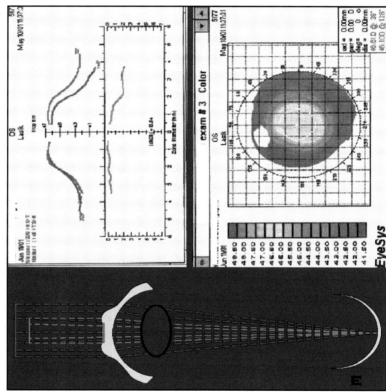

8 mm; this way the laser beam does not touch the hinge of the flap. Pachymetry is not fundamental for this treatment.

PARM has been used to treat patients with 20/20 distance vision and addition of +3.5 D; for hypermetropic patients up to +3.5 D in order to treat the addition for presbyopia, always taking into account the preoperative keratometric measurement.

If astigmatism is present, it is recommended to use 2.50 D as a limit, and in myopic patients a -4.00 D limit. Because of the corneal shape produced after the surgery, there is an induced astigmatism between 0.50 to 0.75 D, which could decrease one or two lines of no corrected visual acuity. The usual LASIK retreatment average for myopia, astigmatism, and hyperopia is 7%; in cases treated for presbyopia it is increased up to 22%, as seen in Avalos' and Rozakis'

patients in the first 2 years of trial. After modifying the nomogram, this retreatment percentage should diminish under the range of 12%. This group has not seen complications from the surgery besides those already reported for regular LASIK technique.

CONCLUSION

In conclusion, PARM provides an effective, safe, inexpensive, and efficient method that eliminates difficulties encountered with prior treatments and obtains new results in the art of presbyopia LASIK surgery.

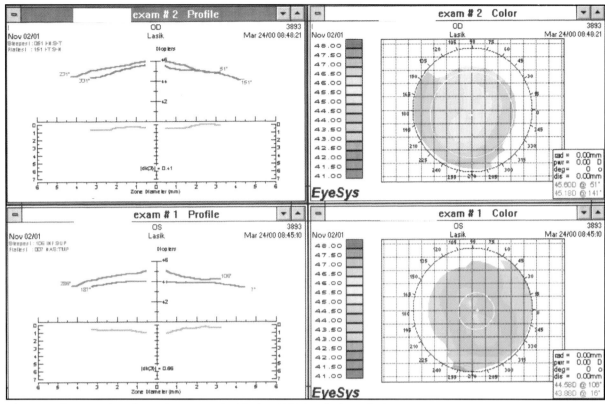

Figure 9. Topography of a patient treated with the PARM technique (before treatment).

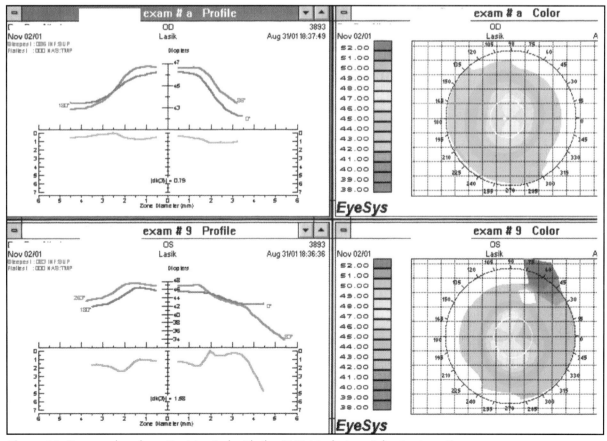

Figure 10. Topography of a patient treated with the PARM technique (after treatment).

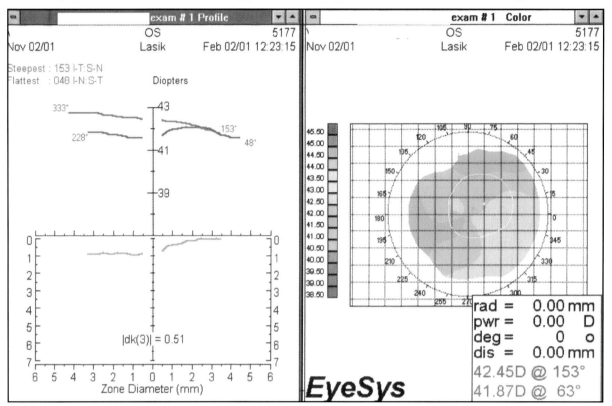

Figure 11. Topography of a patient treated with the PARM technique (before treatment).

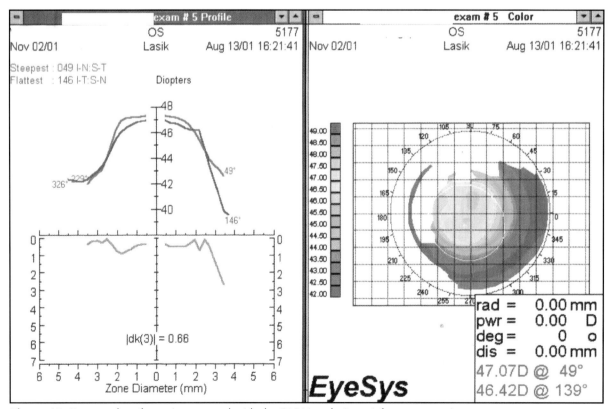

Figure 12. Topography of a patient treated with the PARM technique (after treatment).

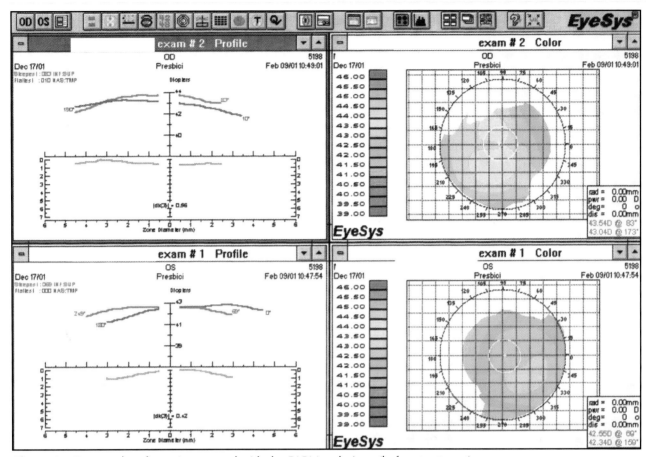

Figure 13. Topography of a patient treated with the PARM technique (before treatment).

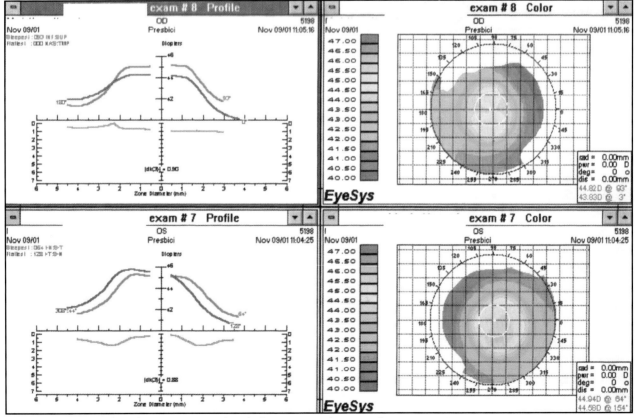

Figure 14. Topography of a patient treated with the PARM technique (after treatment).

REFERENCES

1. Wahl HW, et al. Deteriorating vision in the elderly: double stress? *Ophthalmologie*. 1998;95:389-99.
2. Vinciguerra P, et al. Excimer laser photorefractive keratectomy for presbyopia: 24-month follow-up in three eyes. *J Refract Surg*. 1998;14:31-37.
3. Goldberg DB. Laser in situ keratomileusis monovision. *J Cataract Refract Surg*. 2001;27:1449-55.
4. Jain S, Ou R, Azar DT. Monovision outcomes in presbyopic individuals after refractive surgery. *Ophthalmology*. 2001;108:1430-33.

Chapter 17

Presbyopic LASIK

The Agarwal Technique

Tahira Agarwal, FORCE, DOMS, FICS; Jaiveer Agarwal, FORCE, DO, FICS; Amar Agarwal, MS, FRCS, FRCOphth; Venkatesan Palanivel, MS; and Nishanth Patel, DipNB, DO

INTRODUCTION

Presbyopia is perhaps the true final frontier for the ophthalmologist. Various techniques have been attempted to treat presbyopia, from modifying the sclera and cornea, to modifying the lens. We traveled to Guadalajara, Mexico in October 2000 to perform live phakonit surgeries and no-anesthesia cataract surgery for a conference organized by Dr. Guillermo Avalos. There he taught us a new technique of treating presbyopia using the laser-assisted in situ keratomileusis (LASIK) laser. When we came back to India, we worked on his nomogram and idea, and finally came up with a new formula to treat presbyopia. This new formula and nomogram allowed patients to have presbyopic LASIK and be able to see distance and near without glasses.

NOMOGRAM

The nomogram that we devised has helped us solve the problem of presbyopia. For understanding this, we divided the patients into age ranges of 40 years, 50 years, and 60 years.

To perform this procedure we have to combine hyperopic and myopic LASIK to give the cornea multifocality. So, we first create the LASIK flap with the microkeratome. We use the Hansatome (Bausch & Lomb) with the Bausch & Lomb Chiron 217 excimer machine. Once the flap has been created, we perform a hyperopic ablation of +3. This is done with an optical zone of 5 mm. We then immediately perform a myopic ablation. The myopic ablation is done with the optical zone at 4 mm. We perform a -2 D myopic ablation.

The flap is now cleaned and replaced back in position. The patient is followed up the next day, as in routine LASIK cases. These patients are very happy, as they are able to see both distance and near without glasses. Using the nomogram, we can use this formula for different age groups depending on their respective preoperative refractive powers.

KERATOMETRY

With this LASIK technique the corneal curvature is modified, creating a multifocal cornea. The preoperative corneal curvature is the main factor to consider in this type of corrective method. In order to have high-quality vision, corneal keratometry should not be modified up to 48 D. Corneas with more than 48 D produce undesired optical alterations like glare, halos, decreased visual acuity, and decreased contrast sensitivity.

For each hypermetropic diopter corrected, the corneal curvature increases in 0.89 keratometric diopters as an average; that is why it is recommended to treat patients with keratometry in the range between 41 to 43 D to obtain postoperative curves under 48 D. This point was explained to us very well by Dr. Avalos and we would like to acknowledge his assistance in this.

RESULTS

Five eyes of three patients were included in this preliminary study, and all three patients were informed about the experimental nature of this procedure. The three patients included in this study were hypermetropes and any significant corneal, lenticular, or retinal pathology was ruled out. Preoperative and postoperative uncorrected and best-corrected visual acuity, corneal topography, and pachymetry were the main criteria taken into account to evaluate the efficacy and safety of the procedure. Distant and near uncorrected visual acuity improved after the procedure (Figure 1). Corneal topography (Figures 2a and 2b) also revealed a picture that was in accordance with the improvement in visual acuity.

Figure 1. Comparison of preoperative and postoperative distant uncorrected visual acuity (UCVA).

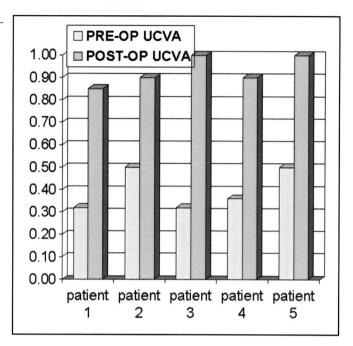

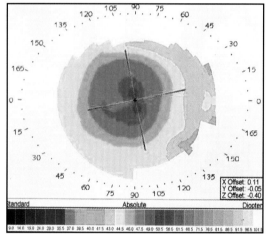

Figure 2a. Postoperative corneal topography of the right eye of a patient in the study.

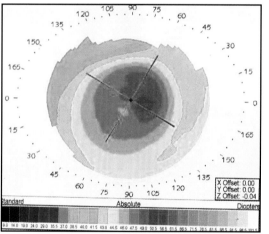

Figure 2b. Postoperative corneal topography of the left eye of a patient in the study.

Chapter 18

Monovision With LASIK

Arthur Cummings, MB, ChB, MMed(Ophth), FCS(SA), FRCS(Ed)

INTRODUCTION

Many patients undergoing corneal refractive surgery today not only want distance vision to be corrected but also want to avoid the need for reading glasses if they are in the presbyopic age range. The procedures for presbyopia are not providing the kind of results that refractive patients have come to expect, and there is no better procedure available at this stage to address presbyopia than monovision.

WHAT IS MONOVISION?

Monovision is the correcting of refractive error so that the distance eye is as close as possible to plano ("zero") and to correct the reading or near eye to a myopic target, normally in the range of -1.00 diopter sphere (DS) to -2.00 DS. In patients who are low myopes, it often results in only one eye having to be corrected; but in patients with hyperopia, astigmatism, or myopia of more than -2.75 DS, it normally requires both eyes to be treated.

THEORY OF MONOVISION

Monovision was first described 40 years ago and has been used most widely with contact lenses. The success of monovision with contact lenses is in the order of 50% to 75%, but it improves when contact lens wearers experiencing problems with the lenses are excluded. The success rate is then in the order of 85%. The success or failure of monovision is largely dependent on a mechanism called *interocular blur suppression*. In those individuals for whom monovision works, the brain suppresses the unwanted image and a clear image dominates. The binocular visual acuity is usually slightly reduced, but this tends to improve over time in those individuals who are adapting to monovision. In those individuals for whom monovision does not work, the brain has difficulty suppressing the unwanted image and there is a consistent ghost image that is very disturbing and unacceptable to most.

TARGET

If the requirement is never to wear spectacles again, the reading eye target needs to be in the range of -2.00 DS. This would allow a person with no accommodation to read at a distance of 50 cm. A person with both eyes corrected to plano, or zero, normally requires reading glasses at age 42 to 45 years due to presbyopia. If the reading eye is corrected to -1.00 DS, the reading glasses are deferred for approximately another 10 years. A target of -0.50 DS adds approximately 5 years to the age before reading glasses are required, and -1.50 DS adds approximately 15 years to the age when reading glasses are required. Typically, the following applies:

Zero/zero: Reading glasses required at 42 to 45 years of age

Zero/-1.00 DS: Reading glasses required at 52 to 55 years of age

Zero -1.50 DS: Reading glasses required at 57 to 60 years of age

Zero/-2.00 DS: Reading glasses most likely never to be needed, although some may use them occasionally at around 65 years of age

WHO IS SUITED FOR MONOVISION?

The following factors are considered when making decisions about monovision:

1. Patients' wishes: Are they stating that they want to see well or are they saying that they do not want to wear glasses again?

2. Age of patient: Monovision is more successful in patients who are already presbyopic.

3. Occupation: People who have variable visual needs during the day, where they are looking in the distance for a period and then up close again, would be particularly bothered by wearing reading glasses. They would find that they were putting them on and taking them off all day (eg, bank clerks, teachers, and general administrative staff). However, those who spend most of the day looking at one particular distance (eg, drivers, computer programmers, etc) usually prefer to see well in the distance and to use reading glasses for near.

4. Sports and hobbies: Our experience has revealed that people participating in sports are slightly less likely to accept monovision than people who do not participate in sports. This correlates with most sports, which require good vision to excel in them.

5. Preoperative best-corrected spectacle acuity.

6. Postoperative uncorrected visual acuity.

PATIENTS' WISHES

When asked why someone is considering refractive surgery, myriad reasons are offered, including wanting to wake up in the morning without having to reach for the glasses, not having to wear glasses for playing sports, etc. No matter how many different reasons are offered, however, there is only one of two possibilities that the patient can be offered, namely:

+ Excellent vision (zero/zero)
+ A solution in which reading glasses are not going to be required at all or at least the need for them is delayed (monovision)

The examiner, therefore, has to listen carefully to what the patient is saying in an attempt to know what it is that he or she really wants—perfect vision with the knowledge that reading glasses are going to be required when he or she approaches the presbyopic age or less than perfect vision with the use of monovision but with the knowledge that he or she is now less dependent, if not totally independent, of all glasses.

AGE

The closer the patient is to age 42, the more likely that monovision is going to be appealing. Correcting a 50-year-old to zero/zero implies excellent distance acuity but also means that the person is going to need reading glasses with immediate effect. This is an unwelcome effect of correcting an older person to zero/zero and needs to be fully explained to the patient beforehand. This person would be interested in a solution in which the need for reading glasses would be eliminated or reduced. On the other hand, a person of age 25 years is usually not very interested in monovision, as he or she is still many years away from becoming presbyopic. If the patient has a zero/zero correction performed, distance acuity is excellent lifelong, and he or she will only require reading glasses at age 42 to 45 years. If the patient chooses monovision at this age, the following applies: the side effects of monovision are inherited immediately, but the benefits are only realized when they reach the presbyopic age. Side effects include increased glare at night and a reduction in overall visual acuity. These are normally not tolerated well when it is realized that the benefits only materialize at a much later stage. The dominant eye is usually corrected for distance; and in the younger patient, he or she is going to continue reading with the zero eye until it becomes more difficult (at around age 42). Only then will he or she start using the myopic eye for reading. The reading eye is therefore carried or is a "spare wheel" without much use in the younger patient.

Another problem occurs with reading specifically: consider the young patient with monovision who is looking in the distance. The one eye can see clearly and the other cannot. In this instance, the brain does not have any difficulty deciding which image to utilize for distance vision. It naturally uses the clear image and suppresses the blurred image. When this same patient is reading, however, both eyes can see at reading distance. The zero eye can still read, as the patient is not yet presbyopic; and the -2.00 eye, for example, is very comfortable at reading distance by design. The problem is, however, that the eyes do not have the same focal distance and cannot see at the same point in space with equal clarity or comfort. The brain has more of a problem suppressing the "unwanted image," as it is a clear image in the first place and patients will often remark that their eyes are tiring easily when reading for prolonged periods. The best way around this problem is to encourage the patient to hold reading material in a position in which one eye is definitely favored over the other rather than a position in which the two eyes are competing to see. If the material is held up closer than usual, the -2.00 eye is at a distinct advantage and the brain has more success at suppressing the other eye. If the material is held farther away, the zero eye gains the upper hand and the brain can more easily suppress the less clear image in the -2.00 eye. This eliminates the competition between the two eyes where the zero eye is continuously trying to accommodate to see well at near and the -2.00 eye is continuously trying to relax accommodation to see near. It needs to be remembered that accommodation is a reflex and that the eyes do not accommodate independent of one another.

OCCUPATION

The manner in which a person spends his or her day is also going to significantly impact the success or lack of success with monovision. Those who require good, uncompromised distance vision tend to do poorly with monovision, as would be expected. These include professional drivers, pilots, game rangers, etc. The same criteria seems to apply for those spending long hours at near, including computer programmers who spend hours at the same distance in front of a computer, solicitors who read continuously for hours on end, etc. The occupations in which monovision has been most successful include teachers, nurses, bank clerks, and general administrative-type work in which the visual needs are varied continuously and constantly throughout the day. In this scenario, the person would have to reach for his or her glasses every time he or she needed to see up close if he or she had a zero/zero correction. With the use of monovision, however, patients do not need an aid for near vision and find that they can spend the day at the office and never need their glasses. This is a very positive change in their lives, where they were used to going around the office and house with their glasses dangling around their necks or in their shirt pockets or handbags.

SPORTS

Golf and tennis appear to be the two sports in which monovision is particularly unsuitable. In all the procedures that I have performed and that others have performed in the clinics in which I have worked, this appears to be a consistent finding. The reasons may be simple—it may be that the vision is simply not good enough and that individuals are now playing less well than before when both eyes were corrected to zero by means of glasses or contact lenses. It may be that they miss some of the second eye's input, resulting in a lesser quality three-dimensional image. Another reason that is probably the likely cause for golfers to change monovision back to zero/zero by means of an enhancement is the following explanation: the dominant eye is normally corrected for distance and the nondominant for near. In a right-eye dominant individual, this would imply that the right eye is corrected. This individual more than likely plays golf right-handed too, and when he or she tees up on the golf course, vision on looking straight ahead is often quite adequate. However, while preparing to hit the shot, he or she is facing the ball and looking over the left shoulder toward the fairway or green. Now the left eye is "leading" and, in fact, the right eye may be seeing nothing more than the bridge of the nose. This implies that the -2.00 eye is now providing the view of the intended shot. Most golfers are not happy with this, understandably.

My experience has shown that most other sportsmen/women tolerate monovision quite well (where balls are involved, slightly less so [football, soccer, rugby, etc] but in other events such as running and swimming, patients are often quite satisfied with the quality of vision). Age plays an important role here too—a 25-year-old soccer player whose vision is quite good with monovision may still decide on zero/zero because of his or her age.

HOBBIES

People who read a lot, sew, or enjoy other hobbies that require fine vision up close will often rather have a zero/zero result and use reading glasses for fine work up close. It needs to be stressed that monovision is better suited to the individual whose needs are varied, and the person who spends hours at the same distance in front of them usually prefers both eyes being corrected to the same target and doesn't mind the glasses as much, as they are not being taken off and put on all the time.

PREOPERATIVE BCVA

Individuals who see very well with their glasses or contact lenses preoperatively are less inclined to accept monovision. The individual with 6/4 (20/12) BCVA is unlikely to accept a monovision result that is perhaps 6/6 (20/20). It is simply not going to be as good as to what he or she is accustomed. Patients with preoperative visual acuity of 6/12 (20/40) or less do not tolerate monovision well in our experience and tend to want both eyes fully corrected so as to maximize the binocular visual acuity.

POSTOPERATIVE UCVA

If the uncorrected visual acuity is poor postoperatively following monovision, then there is a greater likelihood that the patient would be willing to sacrifice the monovision by enhancing the reading eye to zero and then using reading glasses. A contact lens trial is very useful in this instance to make the individual aware of exactly what the implications of his or her decision are going to be.

THE MONOVISION CONSULTATION

Once the initial interview has been conducted, it is usually clear what the individual wants in terms of zero/zero or monovision. Sometimes, however, it is not clear and the patient is open to either suggestion. At this stage of the examination, monovision is demonstrated using the automatic phoropter. The full prescription is entered into the phoropter and then a zero/-2.00 (and sometimes a zero/-1.00) resultant refraction is entered to demonstrate monovision at the push of a button. This immediately reveals the side effects of monovision, and the individual can see the reduction in acuity as well as the increased glare. If he or she is cycloplegic at this stage, the patient can also appreciate the improved reading acuity at 40 cm on the -2.00 eye. A simple comparison is done: the monovision view is compared to the full correction view and rated against one another. We ask the patient to call the full correction view "100%," and this is the reference point for the rest of the test. The monovision view is then compared to this and rated. Although this is a very subjective test and we have never told or shown them what 0% looks like, the test results seem to be very uniform. Historically, this test has an almost 100% record in predicting successful monovision candidates. Any candidate referring to the monovision as "90%" or higher has had a near 100% success rate in terms of monovision. Any patient calling it lower than "80%" has had a near 0% success in adapting to monovision. There are those who refer to it

as being "80%" or "85%," and this group represents a grey area where it works sometimes and other times not. It tends to work in this group for those who are close to age 42 or older, those who expressed a wish to not wear reading glasses, and those with varied visual needs. It tends to work less well for those younger than 37 years of age and in those with more stringent visual requirements.

CONTACT LENS TRIAL

In individuals with simple myopia or hyperopia without significant astigmatism, a contact lens trial is often very useful. Contact lenses are supplied that have a resultant zero/zero refraction as well as contact lenses that provide a monovision refraction (eg, zero/-2.00) A -5.00 patient will get two -5.00 contact lenses to demonstrate full correction with its problems for near work in the presbyopic patient and a -3.00 contact lens for the nondominant eye to demonstrate a zero/-2.00 refraction with its benefits for near work. The contact lens trial is ideal to weigh the two options and make a truly informed decision. It is not always possible due to prescriptions that are unsuitable for contact lens wear (such as high degrees of astigmatism) or in individuals that simply cannot tolerate a contact lens in the eye.

PLANNING

Once it has been established that monovision is to be targeted, the target itself needs to be identified. A target of -2.00 is chosen in more than 90% of cases and -1.00 is chosen by the remainder, almost all of whom would be individuals in their 40s who are intolerant of the zero/-2.00 option but do tolerate the zero/-1.00 option and like the thought of not needing reading glasses immediately. In individuals with -1.00 or -2.00 preoperative refractions of any age, we encourage the practice of treating one eye at a time. In the event that they like the monovision result, they have saved the cost of the second eye's procedure as well as gained the benefits of monovision. In the event that monovision is deemed unsuitable after at least a 6-week postoperative period, the second eye can be corrected to -1.00 or zero, depending on the patient's wishes. The fact that LASIK lends itself so well to enhancement makes one tend to give monovision the benefit of the doubt and try it out, and in the event that it does not work, the reading eye can be enhanced.

If a candidate is prepared to have surgery only if it can be guaranteed that he or she is not going to need glasses at all (ie, that monovision is going to be successful), then a contact lens trial is imperative. If he or she is open-minded about the procedure and doesn't mind the idea of reading glasses, although he or she would prefer to be without them, then monovision can be performed with the knowledge that the enhancement is available should it be necessary. In this latter instance, a contact lens trial is not necessary.

OCULAR DOMINANCE

The dominant eye is normally corrected for distance and the nondominant eye for near. Other authors have found that this can be reversed with good effect ("crossed monovision"), although our clinical outcomes suggest that ocular dominance does play a role and that the dominant eye should be the zero eye.

In our own findings, the rate of monovision success is not influ-

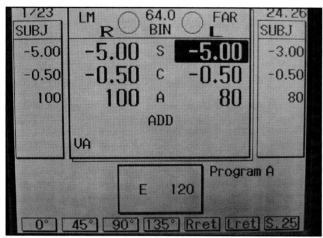

Figure 1. The zero/zero option on the phoropter.

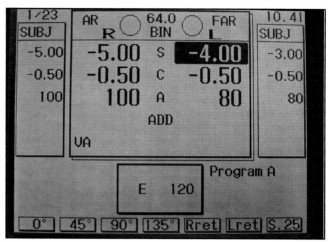

Figure 2. The zero/-1.00 option on the phoropter.

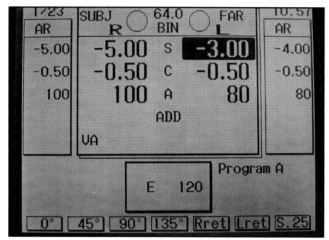

Figure 3. The zero/-2.00 option on the phoropter.

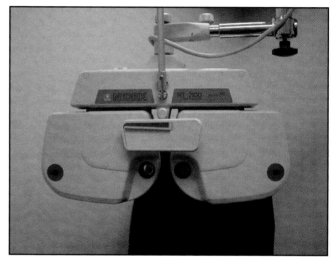

Figure 4. The Nidek RT-2100 automated phoropter (Nidek, Gamagori, Japan).

enced by left or right eye dominance. If the dominant eye is corrected, whether it is the right or left, monovision has the greatest chance of being successful. In our clinic, 79% of people are right eye dominant and 21% are left eye dominant.

The dominance is established by asking the patient which eye he or she uses to take a photograph and by confirming the dominance with a Worth 4-dot test or a finger-pointing test. The contact lens trial is very useful with individuals for whom it is clinically impossible to determine ocular dominance. In these cases, contact lenses are supplied that provide monovision both ways (ie, one set of contact lenses that give zero/-2.00 and a second set of contact lenses that give -2.00/zero). The patient then decides on the eye to be fully corrected based on the lenses that provided the best visual acuity and most comfort.

USING THE AUTOMATED PHOROPTER TO ASSESS MONOVISION SUITABILITY

The automated phoropter can switch between different refractions at the push of a button, and almost instantly the new refraction is in front of the patient. This allows very thorough comparison between different options (eg, zero/zero or zero/-2.00) and

allows an accurate method to compare the different refractions. This "scoring" of a set of monovision lenses against both eyes being fully corrected plays an important role in assessing the suitability of a patient for monovision.

Figures 1 through 3 demonstrate the display on the phoropter unit indicating the zero/zero option (see Figure 1), the zero/-1.00 option (see Figure 2), and the zero/-2.00 option (see Figure 3). Figure 4 is a photograph of the automated phoropter.

ENHANCEMENTS TO ZERO

In the event that monovision is not working out well for the patient, an enhancement can be performed to fully correct the reading eye (to zero). The incidence of enhancement for monovision in our clinic has been 19% for left eye- and right eye-dominant patients.

If the anisometropia is less than or equal to 2.00 DS, the enhancement rate went down to 17.7%. When the anisometropia was more than 2.00 DS, the enhancement rate went up to 25.7% in our series.

In our series, there were two groups of patients undergoing

monovision LASIK. In group 1, the patients had only one eye treated and the untreated eye served as the reading eye. This type of monovision patient accounts for 22% of our monovision treatments. In this group, 24% went on to have the second eye treated, sacrificing the reading eye. In the second group, where both eyes had been treated (78% of our monovision series), 17% proceeded to enhance the myopic eye to zero.

It appears as though economic factors do not play a large role in the success or failure of monovision, as there are costs incurred by the patient when opting to have a previously untreated eye corrected and there are no costs to the patient when having an enhancement performed on a previously treated eye. It would not have been strange to find that the group that had to pay for the second eye's treatment would have been less likely to proceed. This, in fact, was not the case and serves to confirm that when monovision is not working sufficiently well for the patient, he or she is willing to go ahead and treat the second eye despite the additional cost and sacrifice of the reading eye.

In our series, when we considered ideal patients for monovision only, the success of monovision rose to 89%, whereas in the rest of the group it was 72%. The ideal patient had the following characteristics:

+ Already presbyopic (older than 42 years)
+ Rated monovision highly on the phoropter test (almost always higher than 80%)
+ Expressed a wish not to wear glasses at all

Looking at the results for this subset of patients, the average age was 47 years; 93% had expressed a wish not to wear glasses at all. Their success rate for monovision was 89%.

In summary, the most important factors that influenced the success of monovision in our series of monovision LASIK were:

1. Why was the treatment sought in the first place? Was it to see well or was it to get rid of glasses completely?

2. Monovision is more likely to work for the person older than 40 years and even more so for the person older than 50 years of age.

3. The subjective response to the monovision phoropter test also influenced the outcome, with those rating monovision higher than 80% being more likely to adjust to monovision.

4. Monovision was less likely to work if the anisometropia was more than 2.00 D.

5. Females were more likely than males to have monovision performed and were more likely to succeed.

6. Those not participating in sports were slightly more likely to accept monovision than serious sportsmen/women, golfers, or tennis players.

7. Driving, only when done for a living, influenced the success of monovision. Taxi drivers, police car drivers, ambulance drivers, and truck drivers did not adjust well to monovision. On the contrary, people who drove less tended to do quite well with monovision. Eighteen percent of patients needed night driving glasses.

8. Patients were less likely to accept monovision if the preoperative BCVA was less than 6/9 or 20/30.

CONCLUSION

Monovision LASIK is a very useful tool for the patient who does not want to wear glasses, including reading glasses. Monovision LASIK is the most effective method available at the moment to surgically correct presbyopia simultaneously with the refractive error. If careful and thorough patient selection is practiced, the success rate of LASIK monovision should be very high.

BIBLIOGRAPHY

Goldberg D. Laser in situ keratomileusis monovision. *J Cataract Refract Surg.* 2001;27:1449–1455.

Jain S, Ou R, Azar D. Monovision outcomes in presbyopic individuals after refractive surgery. *Ophthalmology.* 2001;8:1430–1433.

Chapter 19

Laser Thermokeratoplasty

Anna Lisa T. Yu, MD; Richard L. Nepomuceno, MD; and
Brian S. Boxer Wachler, MD

Monovision is one of the common methods of correcting presbyopia, a condition in which there is a gradual loss of accommodative response that accompanies aging. Monovision was first proposed by Westsmith four decades ago for contact lens-wearing presbyopes. In monovision, one eye is intentionally corrected for distance vision and the other eye for near vision. The induced anisometropia is usually from 1.00 to 2.00 diopters (D).

Monovision, which is usually achieved through the use of contact lenses, is advantageous in that it provides both distance and near correction independent of gaze position and frees patients from having to wear both distance and reading glasses for most of their daily activities. It also provides a fuller field of view than the various spectacle lens options currently available for presbyopes.[1,2] Furthermore, aniseikonia tends to be relatively insignificant.[3] However, there are some trade-offs with monovision, such as reduced binocular visual acuity, compromised stereopsis, and reduced low-frequency contrast sensitivity.[3]

Ideally, the monovision patient should be able to see clearly at all distances, from far to near. The patient should also be able to suppress the blurred image from either eye depending on the given viewing distance. This is known as interocular blur suppression and prevents the degradation of the good image by the blurred image.[4]

Any compromise in binocular visual functions resulting from monovision should not hinder the patient in performing activities of daily living. It must be kept in mind, though, that monovision patients may occasionally require spectacle correction to optimize vision potential for certain tasks such as night driving or fine near-vision tasks. However, such spectacles should only be needed 15% of the time for monovision to be considered satisfactory.[4]

Several factors have been determined to influence monovision success. Success is more likely if the patient exhibits maximum interocular suppression of blur, does not have significant reduction of stereoacuity, and does not have large esophoric shifts at distance. Patients who demonstrate alternating dominance have a higher chance of success as compared to one who has a strong sighting preference since these patients seem to have a more constant interocular blur suppression.[1] Some psychological and personality traits have also been identified to correlate with monovision success.[5]

For the past several decades, monovision was most commonly achieved using contact lenses, particularly single vision soft contact lenses. This modality has been well-documented in optometric literature. A meta-analysis of 19 contact lens articles by Jain et al showed a mean monovision success rate of 76%. When failures related to contact lens intolerance were excluded, the success rate increased to 81%.[6]

More recently, refractive surgery, namely photorefractive keratectomy (PRK), laser-assisted in situ keratomileusis (LASIK), and laser thermokeratoplasty (LTK), have been used to achieve monovision in presbyopes. Based on a study by Jain et al involving 42 presbyopic myopic patients who underwent refractive surgery to achieve monovision, the success rate was found to be 88%.[7] Wright et al also reported in their study on monovision induced by myopic PRK that 20 out of 21 patients (95%) had binocular visual acuity of 20/25 or better. Patient satisfaction was noted to be high (86%).[8] Unfortunately, there are limited references on monovision and PRK or LASIK, and much less on monovision and LTK. This chapter deals mainly with monovision induced by LTK, as performed in our center.

LTK PROTOCOL

Brian S. Boxer Wachler, MD

PREOPERATIVELY

Patients are started on doxycycline 100 mg by mouth daily for 1 week prior to LTK and kept on the same regimen for 1 week after LTK. This is to stabilize the meibomian glands since the procedure can occasionally induce a flare-up of meibomian-related blepharitis, which can induce astigmatism.

SURGICAL PLANNING

The 6-month or 12-month nomogram is followed for all patients. On occasion, only the 6-mm ring will be utilized for low hyperopic corrections in order to avoid significant myopic overcorrections with the 12-month nomogram. For example, a patient who is +0.75 D or +1.00 D with 20/40 or better uncorrected visual acuity will be treated with the 6 mm ring only. One 6-mm ring is also used for treating a patient to induce "stereovision" (target of −1.00 D or −1.25 D in one eye) who is naturally plano or nearly plano OU. However, these patients may have a higher rate of retreatment.

When treating post-LASIK, post-keratectomy (aborted laser), and post-PRK patients, the attempted correction is divided in half, and only the 6-mm ring is used. Otherwise, using the standard nomogram (two ring treatments) in these patients will result in significant overcorrections.

INTRAOPERATIVELY

1. The patient is positioned at the Sunrise Hyperion laser (Sunrise Technologies, Inc, Fremont, Calif). The patient is then asked to briefly hold his or her eyes open so that the green focusing beams can be focused. This will also allow observation of the degree of angle kappa by observing the visual axis, which is easily assessed by observing the position of the blinking green patient fixation light reflex on the cornea (Purkinje image). This is a very small reflex and usually nasal within the pupil in hyperopic eyes. This location must be mentally imaged because the center of the LTK treatment is on the visual axis, not the pupil center. In other words, the green focusing light must be superimposed slightly inferior (0.25 mm) to the small patient fixation light reflex.

   In some patients, the light reflex will be extremely nasal in the pupil, but the treatment must always be centered on the light reflex even though it appears very nasally decentered on the cornea. The topography will show a centered treatment if this method is followed. Both oculars must be turned clockwise to the maximum to allow better visualization of the faint blinking light.

2. The drying timer is changed to 1 second instead of the default 180 seconds. This is done in the Preferences mode.

3. Topical proparacaine 0.5% (Alcaine) is used for anesthesia. One drop of Alcaine is initially placed on the eye followed by a 1-minute wait, and then a second drop is placed. This is followed by another 1-minute interval, after which the third drop of Alcaine is placed, followed by the last 1-minute interval. It is very important for the patient to keep both eyes closed the whole time during the drops. If the eyes are open, the blink rate is reduced due to the anesthetic, and the cornea will likely desiccate and the epithelium may become irregular from inadvertent desiccation. If irregular epithelium is noted following all the anesthetic drops, then place artificial tears and have the patient keep the eyes closed for 30 minutes. This is usually sufficient to allow normalization of the epithelial surface. The anesthetic routine may then be started from the beginning again. A light-blocking shield should be placed over the fellow eye to eliminate competing images.

4. With 30 seconds left on the last 1-minute interval, press AUTOCAL on the laser, which takes about 30 seconds to get ready. If there is any doubt about a delay after the last anesthetic drop prior to the start of the procedure, an additional anesthetic drop may be given.

5. The cornea and fornix are copiously irrigated with balanced saline solution (BSS) to remove residual anesthetic from the tear film. Place a tissue under the eye to absorb the run-off. This irrigation promotes an even tear film layer.

6. A solid blade eyelid speculum is then inserted, and the patient is instructed to always look straight ahead. (The cornea is no longer wiped, as was done in an older protocol.)

7. The patient is treated with the pause on. The eye tracker is not used.

8. Following the treatment, a dry Merocel sponge is used to remove the epithelial opacities under the slit lamp. This promotes patient comfort. The resulting epithelial defects are completely or nearly healed the following day.

9. The patient receives one drop each of nonsteroidal anti-inflammatory drug (NSAID) and antibiotic immediately after removing the epithelial opacities. A contact lens is not placed on the eye afterward.

POSTOPERATIVELY

1. The patient uses the NSAID twice more on the day of surgery only, and then it is discarded. The antibiotic drop is used four times daily (QID) for 3 days. Artificial tears are used QID for the first month.

2. It is very important, especially during the first week, that the patient does not rub or even squeeze the eyelids so as to minimize trauma to the newly healed epithelium.

3. Fluorescein should not be used during the first week, as it can be associated with an inflammatory reaction around some of the newly epithelialized LTK spots.

4. No steroids are used. Steroids can reverse the effect of the collagen contraction induced by the LTK procedure.

PATIENT SELECTION AND COUNSELING

Careful patient selection and education can prevent a good deal of disappointment and, therefore, are crucial to monovision success. It is important to inquire about occupation, daily home activities, presence of other medical or ophthalmological conditions, hobbies, and sports because patients with occupations requiring good stereopsis or who work in dim lighting conditions may not be very good candidates. Ultimately, the decision rests on the personal preference of the patient.

All patients who choose monovision should be informed about all the possible limitations that monovision may have on visual function, particularly on binocular visual acuity, stereoacuity, and contrast sensitivity. They must also be warned about distance and near ghosting, especially when driving at night. The patient should then be required to sign an informed consent that states all the risks and benefits of monovision.[3,4]

DETERMINATION OF THE DISTANCE EYE

There are different philosophies regarding the selection of the distance vision eye. Typically, the dominant eye is corrected for distance and the nondominant eye for near since the dominant eye is superior for spatial-locomotor tasks such as walking, running, or driving a car; and the nondominant eye is better suited for near vision tasks.[4]

In Dr. Boxer Wachler's practice, eye dominance is determined by use of sighting dominance, which is determined by the "hole test." This test is performed by asking the patient to frame an object in the distance with a triangle created by his or her outstretched arms while keeping both eyes open. The patient is then instructed to bring his or her arms toward the face while keeping the object in

TABLE 1   SUMMARY OF STATISTICS FOR ALL PATIENTS

Number of patients	63
Mean age of patients	53.8 years ±6.6 (SD)
Sex ratio	M:F = 1:1.2
Unilateral treatment	100%
Preoperative mean MRSE*	0.82 D ±0.90 (SD)
Preoperative mean distance visual acuity (logMAR)	0.21 ±0.28 (SD)
Preoperative near visual acuity range (Snellen)	20/40 to 20/250
Preoperative contrast sensitivity (logMAR)	1.28 ±0.28 (SD)

MRSE = manifest refraction spherical equivalent

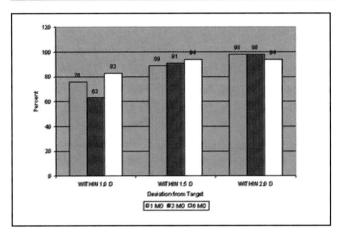

Figure 1. Deviation from target at 1, 3, and 6 months post-LTK.

sight. The eye that is aligned with both the object and hole is the dominant eye.

After determining the dominant eye, a +1.00 D or +1.25 D lens (depending on patient age and manifest refraction) is initially placed over the nondominant eye. The patient is then asked to read the distance vision chart. The test is repeated with the lens over the other eye. The eye that is most comfortable with the plus lens is chosen as the near eye. The patient is then asked to read the near vision chart with the plus lens over the near eye to confirm the findings. The patient's preference ultimately determines which eye is treated.

A monovision trial with a soft disposable single-vision contact lens such as AcuVue (Johnson and Johnson, Jacksonville, Fla) is only done in cases in which the patient experiences inability to suppress blur, which manifests as double vision and visual discomfort. This is also done if the patient's preference is unclear. The trial normally takes 1 week.

DETERMINATION OF THE DEGREE OF ADD POWER

The Sunrise Hyperion LTK system is used to achieve a target of –1.00 D or –1.25 D in the near eye. This approach provides more than adequate vision for the majority of activities in the intermediate range without excessive compromise of binocular visual func-

tion. This approach has been very well tolerated by almost all patients.

RESULTS OF MONOVISION INDUCED BY LTK

From July 2000 until November 2001, a total of 63 patients received monovision treatment using the Sunrise Hyperion LTK system. In this patient population, all received unilateral treatment. Patients were functionally emmetropic and used glasses only for reading. The follow-up schedule was 1 day, 1 week, 1 month, 3 months, 6 months, and 12 months. To date, 44 eyes reached the third month of follow-up, 19 eyes reached the sixth month, but only four eyes had 12 months of follow-up.

For this group, the average age of patients was 53.8 years ±6.6 (standard deviation [SD]) (range: 39 to 76 years). There was no gender predilection. Preoperative distance manifest refraction spherical equivalent (MRSE) for the treated eyes ranged from –0.63 D to +3.75 D with a mean of 0.82 D ±0.90 D. In 53 out of 63 patients (84%), the MRSE fell in the range of ±1.00 D. Mean preoperative distance visual acuity in logMAR was 0.206 (approximately 20/32) ±0.28. Forty-nine out of 63 patients (78%) had Snellen acuities of 20/40 or better. At near, no patient was seeing 20/30 or better preoperatively (Table 1).

The surgical target aimed for in this group ranged from –2.25 D to plano with a mean of –1.14 D ±0.40 (SD). Twenty-three out of 63 patients received one-ring treatments for low hyperopia. The rest received two-ring treatments. There is no significant difference between these two groups except for a slightly higher rate of retreatment (48% for the one-ring group; 30% for two-ring group) and a larger myopic shift in the first 3 months following the two-ring procedure.

Procedural predictability was evaluated at 6 months and showed 83% within 1.00 D and 94% within 2.00 D of intended correction 6 months after LTK (Figure 1).

Stability is shown in Figure 2. As expected, there was an initial large myopic shift of approximately 1.75 D, followed by a slight regression of the refractive effect. There was no significant change in the mean MRSE after the first postoperative month.

Figure 3 shows improvement in uncorrected near visual acuity. Preoperatively, 7 of 63 patients (12%) were seeing equal to or better than 20/60; but at 6 months, 15 out of 19 patients (79%) were 20/60 or better. An acuity of 20/60 or better is sufficient to enable a patient to read magazines and news print.

Uncorrected monocular distance visual acuity at 6 months was slightly poorer, with only 58% of patients achieving a visual acuity

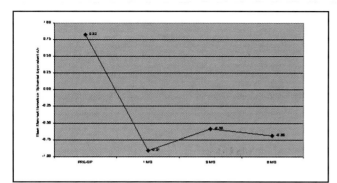

Figure 2. Stability of refraction at follow-up visits.

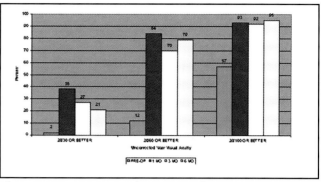

Figure 3. A comparison of pre-LTK and post-LTK uncorrected near visual acuity.

of 20/40 uncorrected or better as compared to the preoperative data, wherein 79% reached this visual acuity. This is mainly due to the resulting myopia (Figure 4).

Few complications were encountered. Table 2 lists these complications and their frequency. Two patients had an induced astigmatism of $\geq$ 2.0 D. One was detected on the first month after the procedure, and the other on the third post-LTK month. These patients subsequently "lost" their induced astigmatism by the sixth post-LTK month. However, two other patients underwent limbal astigmatic keratotomy 3 months and 10 months post-LTK. They had preoperative astigmatism that was compounded by the procedure, thus resulting in decreased distance vision.

For cases of post-LTK inflammation, sterile keratitis, and iritis, the treatment regimen advocated utilizing topical rimexolone 1% four times a day, which was tapered over the course of 1 week. In severe cases, oral methylprednisolone (Medrol, Pharmacia & Upjohn, Peapack, NJ) dose pack is given for 1 week.

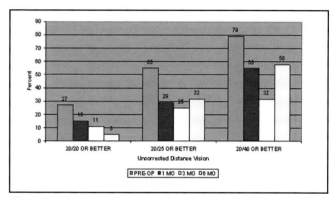

Figure 4. A comparison of uncorrected distance visual acuities.

LTK ENHANCEMENTS

Of the 63 patients treated for monovision, 23 patients received enhancements using the Sunrise Hyperion LTK system. The procedure is usually performed 3 to 6 months after the initial LTK procedure. The enhancement protocol is similar to the initial treatment protocol except that the treatment utilized two rings rotated 22.5 degrees from the initial axis. Currently, the maximum follow-up period is 3 months (Table 3).

CONCLUSION

Based on currently available literature and our experience, monovision achieved through LTK is a reasonable alternative to compensate for presbyopia in properly selected and counseled patients. Although some compromises of visual function exist, these patients can expect a reduced dependence on near vision correction as well as good vision for most viewing distances under most circumstances.

TABLE 2   SUMMARY OF COMPLICATIONS ENCOUNTERED DURING THE STUDY PERIOD

Complications	Number	Percent
Induced astigmatism of $\geq$ 2.0 D	2	3.2
Sterile keratitis of treated LTK spots	1	1.6
Sterile keratitis of treated LTK spots with stromal thinning	2	3.2
Mild iritis	2	3.2
Blepharoconjunctivitis	1	1.6

Note: the induced astigmatism, keratitis with thinning, and iritis occurred in the same two eyes.

TABLE 3   SUMMARY OF PRE-ENHANCEMENT STATISTICS AND POST-ENHANCEMENT OUTCOMES FOR PATIENTS

	Pre-enhancement	Post-enhancement (3 mos)
Number of patients	23	23
Mean manifest refraction spherical equivalent (D)	0.21 D $\pm$ 0.56 (SD)	-0.54 D $\pm$ 0.76 (SD)
Mean distance visual acuity (logMAR)	0.13 $\pm$ 0.12 (SD) (approx 20/25)	0.19 D $\pm$ 0.20 (SD) (approx 20/32)
Near visual acuity range (Snellen)	20/20 to 20/150	20/20 to 20/80
Mean contrast sensitivity (logMAR)	1.23 $\pm$ 0.28 (SD)	0.90 $\pm$ 0.50
Surgical target (D)	1.56 D $\pm$ 0.39 (SD)	—
Mean deviation from target (D)	—	-0.50 D $\pm$ 0.70 (SD)

REFERENCES

1. Erickson P, Schor C. Visual function with presbyopic contact lens correction. *Optom Vis Sci.* 1990;67:22-28.
2. Goldberg DB. Laser in situ keratomileusis monovision. *J Cataract Refract Surg.* 2001;27:1449-1455.
3. Josephson JE, Erickson P, Back A, et al. Monovision. *J Am Optom Assoc.* 1990;61:820-826.
4. Sippel KC, Jain S, Azar DT. Monovision achieved with excimer laser refractive surgery. *Int Ophthalmol Clin.* 2001;41:91-101.
5. Hom MM. Monovision and LASIK. *J Am Optom Assoc.* 1999;70:117-122.
6. Jain S, Arora I, Azar DT. Success of monovision in presbyopes: review of the literature and potential applications to refractive surgery. *Surv Ophthalmol.* 1996;40:491-499.
7. Jain S, Ou R, Azar DT. Monovision outcomes in presbyopic individuals after refractive surgery. *Ophthalmology.* 2001;108:1430-1433.
8. Wright KW, Guemes A, Kapadia MS, et al. Binocular function and patient satisfaction after monovision induced by myopic photorefractive keratectomy. *J Cataract Refract Surg.* 1999;25:177-182.

Chapter 20

Conductive Keratoplasty

Jonathan M. Davidorf, MD; Daniel S. Durrie, MD;
and Ioannis Pallikaris, MD

HYPEROPIA CORRECTION BY NONABLATIVE SURGICAL METHODS

OVERVIEW OF METHODS

Thermal techniques for shrinking peripheral corneal collagen and thereby steepening the central cornea have challenged ophthalmologists for more than 100 years (Table 1). Hot wire thermokeratoplasty used in the 1980s to produce thermal burns that penetrated to 95% of corneal depth in hyperopic eyes showed lack of predictability and stability, and further development was abandoned. More recent techniques have shown positive or mixed outcomes (Table 2).

With increased use worldwide, the benefits and limitations of noncontact holmium YAG (Ho:YAG) laser thermal keratoplasty (noncontact LTK; Sunrise Technologies, Fremont, Calif) become apparent. Refractive regression (impermanence of effect) has been the most notable limitation.[1-10] Another LTK technique, contact Ho:YAG LTK (Holmium 25; Technomed, Baesweiler, Germany) produced higher hyperopic corrections but low predictability and induced astigmatism in initial clinical studies.[11-12] Continuous wave diode LTK (DTK; Rodenstock, ProLaser Medical Systems, Inc, Dusseldorf, Germany), a technology using a similar wavelength as LTK, has shown effective in corneal steepening in animal, cadaver, and blind eyes.[13-15] Finally, conductive keratoplasty (CK; Refractec, Inc, Irvine, Calif), a technique that employs radiofrequency waves to shrink collagen, has shown very promising results for the treatment of hyperopia, presbyopia, and astigmatism, and is the subject of this chapter.[16-19]

COLLAGEN DENATURATION

Collagen, the principal component of corneal tissue, is present as chains wound in tight triple helices and organized into fibrils. Although this conformation provides collagen with great tensile strength and thermal stability, certain temperatures and exposure times will break down its structure and cause denaturation. Exposure time is critical since a specific temperature maintained for a short period may affect collagen, while the same temperature maintained longer will denature collagen.[20-22]

Corneal tissue can be thermally denatured to various degrees: reversible, intermediate (irreversible), and gelatin (irreversible). Reversible changes follow minimal heating of collagen and do not support the contractive forces required to achieve refractive change. Intermediate denaturation is more permanent because the brisk wound healing response[23] may not completely replace the denatured collagen with new collagen. Finally, irreversible denaturation from heating to the gelatin state would bring out a brisk healing response, could cause scarring, and could damage the endothelium.

Thus, the objective of thermokeratoplasty is to deliver sufficient thermal energy to the tissue to achieve intermediate denaturation of collagen while avoiding the gelatin phase. Furthermore, tissue heating should be continuous for the optimal duration to obtain uniform collagen contraction from the anterior to posterior stroma. Under steady-state laboratory conditions, intermediate denaturation occurs with exposure to approximately 65° to 75°C for a specific time period. However, because thermokeratoplasty is a dynamic (not steady-state) process, the state of collagen while undergoing thermokeratoplasty can be inferred, but not exactly defined, through steady-state temperature models.

CONDUCTIVE KERATOPLASTY

MECHANISM OF ACTION

Conductive thermokeratoplasty (CK) is a nonablative, laserless technique conceived by Antonio Mendez, MD[16] in which low-frequency (radiofrequency) energy is applied to the corneal stroma by means of a probe tip inserted into the peripheral cornea at 8 to 32 treatment points (Figure 1). A full circle of CK spots applied to the peripheral cornea produces a "cinching" effect that increases the curvature of the central cornea (Figure 2), thereby decreasing hyperopia. Experiments by Mendez revealed that corneal tissue is heated more homogenously by lower frequencies of energy, and that higher frequencies disperse some of the energy effect at the corneal surface. These findings have been confirmed in studies with the CK technique in the laboratory.[21,22]

The cornea has electrolytic properties and is a good conductor of radiofrequency energy. As the current flows through the tissue immediately surrounding the tip, resistance to this energy creates

TABLE 1	**MILESTONES IN THERMOKERATOPLASTY**

Date	Investigation	Result
1889	Lans, rabbit studies	Radial burns steepened the cornea
1970s	Gasset and Kaufman, keratoconus treatment	Some success
	Aquavella et al, persistent hydrops	Success
1980s	Fyodorov, hot needle keratoplasty treatment of hyperopia	Unpredictable and unstable
	Rowsey Los Alamos Project, treatment of hyperopia	Clinically unsuccessful
1990s	Noncontact holmium laser thermokeratoplasty investigations (Sunrise Technologies, Inc)	Some success in corneal steepening; FDA approval granted in 2000 with stipulation that correction may be temporary
	Mendez, conductive keratoplasty for hyperopia	Some success in denaturing collagen and corneal steepening; procedure later refined by Refractec, Inc
2000	Diode laser thermokeratoplasty (continuous wave) investigations (DTK; Rodenstock, ProLaser Medical Systems, Inc, Dusseldorf, Germany)	Some success with hyperopia treatment; tested outside of United States only
2001	One-year US clinical trial results of safety and efficacy of conductive keratoplasty completed (Refractec, Inc)	Appears effective and safe for treatment of spherical hyperopia

TABLE 2	**NONABLATIVE SYSTEMS FOR REFRACTIVE CORRECTION**

	Sunrise Hyperion Noncontact LTK[1-7]	Conductive Keratoplasty[8-10]	Continuous Wave DTK[11-12]
Manufacturer	Sunrise Technologies Fremont, Calif	Refractec, Inc Irvine, Calif	Rodenstock, ProLaser Inc Dusseldorf, Germany
Approval status	FDA approved for 0.75-3.00 D of spherical hyperopia	Recommended for FDA approval November 2001 for 0.75-3.00 D of spherical hyperopia	Open IDE
Device/energy delivery	Ho:YAG laser, pulsed 226-258 mJ, 5 Hz, noncontact	Radiofrequency energy, 350 kHz, contact probe	CW diode laser, contact device
Wavelength	2.1 μm	Not applicable	1.87 μm
Temp during treatment	Highest temp on corneal surface Significant axial (surface-bottom) temp gradient	Highest temp at center of cylinder Radial (side-to-side) temp gradient No axial (surface-bottom) temp gradient Consistent thermal effect along the probe	Significant axial (surface-bottom) temp gradient
Treatment depth	Wider on surface than in deep stroma	80% of corneal depth based on porcine histology	Not available
Footprint	Conical	Cylindrical	Conical
Number of spots	16 to 32	8, 16, 24, or 32	In development
Nomogram adjustment for increased effect	Increase laser energy/temperature	Increase number of treatment spots	Increase laser energy/temperature
Permanence of effect	Correction decreases over time, although a few eyes retain full correction	Clinical trials demonstrate lasting effect	Not available

heat. Collagen in the area surrounding the tip shrinks and forms a column or cylinder. The CK process is self-limiting because the increasing denaturation of collagen produces increased resistance to the flow of the current. Unlike the direct heat applied in Fyodorov's original "hot needle keratoplasty" technique, radiofrequency current converts to heat; and unlike the pulsed 2.1 µm wavelength infrared energy released by the noncontact laser used in LTK, heat is not applied onto the surface of the cornea.

Because CK radiofrequency treatment has no axial (corneal surface to bottom) gradient, CK-treated tissue is exposed to the same temperature at the tip of the probe (deep in the stroma) as at the top of the probe (the corneal surface). This is in contrast to non-

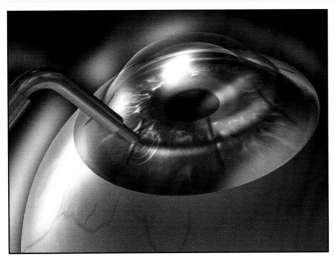

Figure 1. A probe (Keratoplast tip) is inserted into previously marked spots on the midperipheral cornea to release radiofrequency current into the stroma.

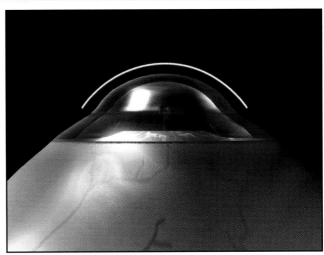

Figure 2. The conductive keratoplasty technique results in a cinching effect that increases the curvature of the central cornea to decrease hyperopia.

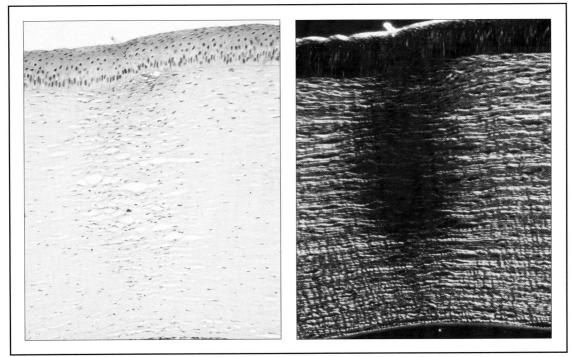

Figure 3. Pig cornea histology 1 week after CK. The CK-treated spot shows a cylindrical footprint approximately 80% of corneal depth.

contact holmium LTK, which has a significant axial gradient and produces the highest temperatures at the corneal surface.

EFFECTS ON THE CORNEA

Histology studies of the pig cornea show that the footprint made by CK is cylindrical and extends deep into the stroma to approximately 80% depth (Figure 3).[21] Striae form between the treated spots, creating a band of tightening that increases the curvature of the central cornea and contributes to a more long-lasting effect (Figures 4 and 5). In contrast, the LTK technique heats tissue in a gradient, generating a cone-shaped footprint to only approximately 50% of corneal depth.[23] A conical footprint is further evidence of the decreasing collagen denaturation from top-down following LTK treatment.

THE CONDUCTIVE KERATOPLASTY DEVICE

Clinical trial results have shown that the conductive keratoplasty procedure using the ViewPoint CK system (Refractec, Inc, Irvine, Calif) successfully treats spherical, previously untreated hyperopia of +0.75 D to +3.00 D.[17] Treatment of astigmatism, presbyopia,[18] refining postcataract outcomes, and over- or undercorrections following laser-assisted in situ keratomileusis (LASIK)[19] have been

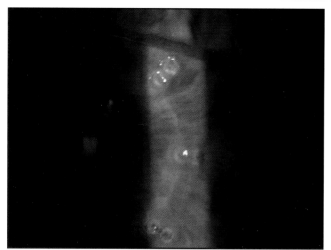

Figure 4. Slit lamp view of treatment spot 1 hour after CK. The pairing of thermal coagulation spots (white-like leucomas) placed at the 6 and 7 mm optical zones can be seen. These spots fade gradually. The striae between treatment zones create a band of tightening around the cornea. They are still visible 12 months postoperatively, suggesting that the effect on the stroma is long-lasting.

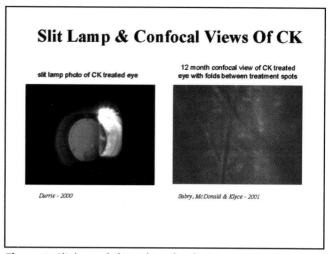

Figure 5. Slit lamp (left) and confocal microscopy (right) views after CK. Retroillumination with the slit lamp shows treatment spots. The arrow points to the bend of the cornea following treatment, resulting in a steeper center and flatter periphery. Confocal microscopy shows folds (striae) between the treatment spots that persist long after treatment and are responsible for the permanence of the treatment.

investigated as potential applications. The system consists of a radiofrequency energy-generating console; a hand-held, reusable, pen-shaped probe attached by a removable cable and connector; and a foot switch that controls release of radiofrequency energy (Figure 6). The energy level defaults to 60% of 1 watt and an exposure time of 0.6 second.

Attached to the probe is the Keratoplast tip (Refractec, Inc; Figure 7), a single-use, disposable, stainless steel, penetrating tip that is 90 μm in diameter and 450 μm long, and delivers the current directly to the corneal stroma. The Keratoplast tip has a proximal bend of 45 degrees and a distal bend of 90 degrees to allow access to the cornea over the patient's brow and nasal regions. At the very distal portion of the tip is a Teflon-coated stainless-steel stop that assures correct depth of penetration.

THE CONDUCTIVE KERATOPLASTY PROCEDURE

PREOPERATIVE EXAMINATION

The examinations preceding a CK procedure should include a manifest and cycloplegic refraction, uncorrected and best spectacle-corrected visual acuity, slit lamp and funduscopic examination, computerized corneal topography, ultrasonic pachymetry, applanation tonometry, and central keratometry.

PATIENT SELECTION

Suitable Patients

Clinical studies have evaluated CK for the treatment of previously untreated spherical hyperopia of up to +3.00 D and ≤ 0.75 D of refractive cylinder, and showed safe, effective, and stable results.

A few smaller studies have evaluated CK for treatment of presbyopia, astigmatism, and over/under LASIK corrections, but guidelines for these indications have not been established. General recommendations for CK treatment include treating only patients with visual acuity correctable to at least 20/40 in both eyes. Hard or rigid gas permeable lenses should be discontinued for at least 3 weeks and soft lenses for at least 2 weeks prior to the preoperative evaluation. Hard contact lens wearers should have two central keratometry readings and two manifest refractions taken at least 1 week apart. The manifest refraction measurements must not differ from the earlier measurements by more than 0.50 D in either meridian. Keratometry mires must be regular.

Unsuitable Patients

Patients with a peripheral pachymetry reading at the 6 mm optical zone of less than 560 μm are not suitable for treatment with conductive keratoplasty. Also unsuitable are those who have had strabismus surgery or are likely to develop strabismus following the CK procedure; have anterior segment pathology; have residual, recurrent, active ocular or uncontrolled eyelid disease or any corneal abnormality; or have signs of progressive or unstable hyperopia. While a history of recurrent corneal erosion or severe basement membrane disease is a relative contraindication, the CK procedure may be preferable to treatment with PRK or LASIK. This has not yet been studied, however.

Other relative contraindications are patients who have a history of herpes zoster keratitis, herpes simplex keratitis, glaucoma, a history of steroid-responsive rise in intraocular pressure (IOP), a preoperative IOP >21 mmHg, or narrow risk angles. Patients with diabetes, diagnosed autoimmune disease, connective tissue disease, an immunocompromised state, current treatment with chronic systemic corticosteroid or other immunosuppressive therapy that may affect wound healing, a history of keloid formation, intractable keratoconjunctivitis sicca, and pregnancy are also considered relatively contraindicated to receive the CK treatment.

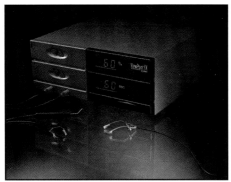

Figure 6. The ViewPoint Conductive Keratoplasty CK system: console, probe, and specula.

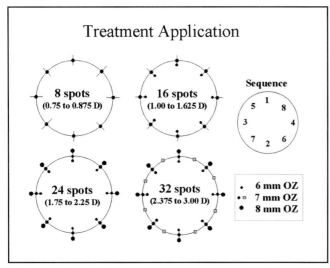

Figure 8. Treatment application. The nomogram is shown within each circle. The application sequence is shown on the right.

PERFORMING THE CK PROCEDURE

TREATMENT METHODS

The surgeon must determine the intended correction (ie, emmetropia or mild myopia for monovision). Administer one drop of topical anesthetic three times at 5-minute intervals, and monitor the patient appropriately for the degree of anesthesia. Do not use pilocarpine.

Insert the CK lid speculum to provide the maximum corneal exposure and an electrical return path. If a lid drape is used, it is important that the drape does not preclude direct contact of the lid speculum and eyelid, otherwise the electrical current return path will be disrupted. Tape the fellow eye closed if it will not be treated. Position the operating microscope or slit lamp biomicroscope over or in front of the eye to be treated. Illumination from the microscope is usually adequate for the procedure.

Inspect the Keratoplast tip under the microscope to ensure it is not damaged or bent prior to application. Mark the cornea with the CK marker while reminding the patient to fixate on the light from

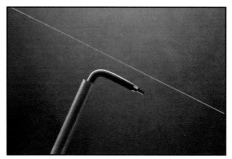

Figure 7. The CK probe (90 μm wide, 450 μm long) with the penetrating Keratoplast tip and coated stop at the distal end. The radiofrequency energy emitted by the CK tip denatures collagen within the targeted treatment zone.

the microscope. Dampen the CK marker with gentian violet or rose bengal stain, center the marker's cross-hair over the visual axis center, and apply light pressure on the marker to make a circular mark with eight intersections on the cornea. If using gentian violet, irrigate with balanced salt solution to remove excess ink. Dry the surface of the cornea thoroughly with a fiber-free sponge to avoid dissipation of applied energy by a wet or damp ocular surface.

Set the appropriate treatment parameters on the console according to the nomogram and sequence of application (Figure 8). Begin treatment at the 7 mm optical zone and continue to the 6 and 8 mm optical zones, if necessary. To treat each spot, place the tip of the delivery probe at the treatment mark on the cornea, perpendicular to the ocular corneal surface. Apply light pressure until the tip penetrates the cornea down to the insulator stop, which prevents further penetration of the tip into corneal tissue.

Depress the foot pedal to apply the radiofrequency energy. A tone will sound as the energy is applied. The default setting for treatment is 350 kHz, 60% power (0.6 watt) for 0.6 second. At each treatment spot, keep the tip in place until the preprogrammed treatment time has been completed (the tone stops). Remove the tip of the delivery probe and repeat the procedure until the full series of spots has been treated according to the treatment plan. Clean the tip with a fiber-free sponge after each treatment spot to remove any tissue debris, taking care not to damage the tip.

POSTOPERATIVE CARE

Following the CK procedure, the surgeon may follow his or her usual refractive surgery postoperative care regimen. Corticosteroids, however, are not recommended. Refractec recommends administration of one drop of a topical ophthalmic antibiotic solution and one drop of an ophthalmic NSAID, continued according to product labeling, for up to 3 days. A bandage contact lens may be used for comfort for 24 to 48 hours postoperatively but is usually not necessary.

CLINICAL STUDIES

PATIENTS AND METHODS

A 2-year, multicenter, prospective clinical trial is being con-

TABLE 3 — EFFICACY VALUES: CK VERSUS LTK

Result	CK Cohort Month 1	CK Cohort Month 6	CK Cohort Month 12	Month 12 Hyperion LTK PMA Cohort*
UCVA 20/20 or better	101/354 (29%)	160/352 (45%)	178/318 (56%)	179/479 (37%)
UCVA 20/25 or better	180/354 (51%)	227/352 (64%)	240/318 (75%)	Not available
UCVA 20/40 or better	281/354 (79%)	316/352 (90%)	294/318 (92%)	407/479 (85%)
MRSE $\leq$ 0.5 D	168/354 (47%)	148/352 (61%)	199/318 (63%)	275/481 (57%)
MRSE $\leq$ 1.0 D	264/354 (75%)	211/352 (88%)	282/318 (89%)	401/481 (83%)
MRSE $\leq$ 2.0 D	333/354 (94%)	232/352 (99%)	316/318 (99%)	474/481 (98%)

*Hyperion LTK Physician Labeling Information, PMA P990078, May 2002.

TABLE 4 — MEAN CHANGE IN REFRACTION OVER TIME: CK VERSUS LTK

Interval (Months)	CK Mean Change in CRSE* (SD) 95% CI	Hyperion LTK Mean Change in MRSE** SD and CI Not Available
3 to 6	0.25 D (0.50), 0.19, 0.31 D	0.30 D
6 to 9	0.11 D (0.41), 0.07, 0.15 D	Not available
6 to 12	Not available	0.36 D
9 to 12	0.11 D (0.35), 0.07 D to 0.15 D	Not available
12-18	Not available	0.25 D
18-24	Not available	0.14 D

Changes are total changes during the interval shown.
CI = confidence interval
*CRSE reported for CK and MRSE for LTK
**Hyperion LTK Physician Labeling Information, PMA P990078, May 2002.

ducted to evaluate the safety, efficacy, and stability of conductive keratoplasty when performed on eyes with +0.75 to +3.00 D of hyperopia and less than 0.75 D of cylinder. Each procedure was performed by one of 13 surgeons at several centers according to methods described in the section entitled "Performing the CK Procedure." All eyes were treated unilaterally at the default setting of 350 kHz, 60% power for 0.6 seconds. No retreatments were performed. Postoperative care and examinations followed the methods described in the Performing the CK Procedure section.

A total of 400 eyes have been treated for low to moderate spherical hyperopia. One-year follow-up data are available from 318 eyes for the variables that indicate treatment efficacy (uncorrected visual acuity [UCVA], best spectacle-corrected visual acuity [BSCVA], manifest refractive spherical equivalent refraction [MRSE], and cycloplegic refractive spherical equivalent [CRSE]). For variables that indicate treatment safety and stability, data are available for 355 eyes.

HYPEROPIA TREATMENT RESULTS

Efficacy

The mean baseline cycloplegic spherical equivalent (SE) refraction of these eyes was +1.86 ± 0.63 D, the median was +1.75 D, and the range was +0.75 to +4.00 D. UCVA preoperatively was 20/40 or worse in 86% of the eyes.

Postoperatively, visual acuity and predictability results were very good (Table 3). Twelve months postoperatively, UCVA was 20/20 or better in 178/318 (60%), 20/25 or better in 240/318 (75%), and 20/40 or better in 294/318 (92%) of the eyes. The procedure was highly predictable. Mean MRSE showed 199/318 (63%) within 0.50 D of intended correction and 282/318 (89%) within 1.0 D at 12 months. Refractive stability was achieved by 6 months since the mean change in MRSE refraction was 0.11 D between months 3 and 6, and also 0.11 D between months 9 and 12. A comparison of MRSE changes of CK versus LTK over time is shown in Table 4.

Safety

Safety variable results are summarized in Table 5. Four of 392 eyes lost >2 lines of BSCVA at 3 months and none lost >2 lines at 12 months. Two lines were lost by 20/392 (5%) at 3 months and 7/355 (2%) at 12 months. However, the loss of 2 lines at 12 months left all seven eyes with very functional vision. Preoperatively, all seven of these eyes had 20/10 to 20/16 BSCVA. Postoperatively, one out of seven eyes had 20/16 BSCVA, three out of seven eyes had 20/20, and three out of seven eyes had 20/25. No eye had BSCVA worse than 20/40 at any follow-up visit. No eye that had 20/20 or better BSCVA preoperatively had worse than 20/25

TABLE 5	SUMMARY OF SAFETY VARIABLES AFTER CK	
	3 Months	12 Months
BSCVA > 2 lines loss	4/392 (1%)	0/355 (0%)
BSCVA 2 lines loss	20/392 (5%)	7/355 (2%)
BSCVA worse than 20/40	0/392 (0%)	0/355 (0%)
Increase > 2.00 D cylinder	8/392 (2%)	1/355 (0.3%)
BSCVA worse than 20/25 if better than 20/20 preoperatively	7/392 (2%)	0/355 (0%)

BSCVA postoperatively. A total of 88% had no change in cylinder at 12 months. One of 355 eyes (0.3%) had a cylinder increase of more than 2.00 D. A total of 6% had 1.00 D of induced cylinder and 4.2% had more than 1.00 D but less than 2.00 D of induced cylinder.

Complications and Adverse Events

No intraoperative complications or adverse events occurred during any of the surgeries. There were no treatment-related adverse events, such as peripheral corneal defect, corneal edema later than 1 week postoperatively, recurrent corneal erosion at 1 month or later, double or ghosting images at any time, foreign body sensation at 1 month or later, or pain at 1 month or later. No haze was seen in 384/390 (98%) of the eyes at 1 month postoperatively, in 96% of eyes at 3 months, in 97% at 6 months, and in 100% at 12 months. The highest level of haze was mild seen in four out of 390 (1%) at month 1 and in one out of 394 (0.25%) at months 3 and 6. There were no occurrences of an uncontrolled IOP increase of > 5 mmHg above baseline. An IOP reading > 25 mmHg was measured in two out of 389 eyes at 6 months and in one eye at 9 and 12 months.

The 12-month results in the ongoing 2-year prospective study of the CK technique for correcting low spherical hyperopia are very encouraging. Postoperative visual acuity and predictability of refraction were excellent, and the stability results surpassed those obtained with the noncontact LTK method. The postoperative refractions appeared to stabilize by the 6-month visit and seem to be stable thereafter. The technique spares the visual axis and has an excellent safety profile.

PRESBYOPIA TREATMENT

Daniel Durrie, MD

Conductive keratoplasty can be very effective for inducing monocular vision to correct presbyopia. A total of 32 eyes of 29 patients were treated in one eye with CK to increase near vision. The amount of myopia induced did not exceed -2.00 D. Patient selection factors were similar to those described in the Suitable Patients section for treatment of hyperopia. The mean age of patients was 52.3 years ±4.3 SD, with a range of 45 to 62 years. The mean preoperative CRSE was +1.39 D ±0.63 D, with a range of +0.75 to +2.38 D. Data on 27 of 32 eyes (84%) was available at 1 month postoperatively and on 16 of 32 (50%) at 3 months postoperatively.

A summary of the efficacy results is shown in Table 6. The percentage of eyes with 20/20 or better binocular distance vision increased from 78% preoperatively to 95% at 1 month and 3

months postoperatively. Acuity of 20/25 or better increased from 88% preoperatively to 100% at 1 month and 3 months. For uncorrected binocular near visual acuity, none of the eyes saw J1+ (20/20 or better) or J1 (20/25 or better) preoperatively, yet 26% had that level of uncorrected binocular acuity postoperatively at 1 month. The percentage increased markedly at month 3 so that 57% saw J1 or better. For J2 or better (20/30 or better), only 3% of the eyes had that level of uncorrected binocular acuity preoperatively, and 52% had that level of acuity 1 month postoperatively.

The postoperative MRSE showed a high degree of accuracy. At 3 months, 88% were within 0.50 D and 1.00 D of intended correction. Seventy-five percent of eyes changed 0.50 D or less from 1 to 3 months postoperatively, and there were no changes after that.

The mean postoperative MRSE showed about 1 D of myopia. Some increase in cylinder was seen at 1 month but diminished to only one out of 16 eyes (6%) having 1.25 D of induced cylinder at 6 months. One eye of 27 was undercorrected by more than +1.00 D, and one out of 27 was overcorrected by less than 1.00 D.

MULTIFOCAL VISION

Conductive keratoplasty has been shown to induce a degree of multifocality in the postoperative cornea. In the multicenter clinical trial, most eyes were emmetropic at 1 year, yet the average patient had more than a 6-line improvement in near vision. These effects can be attributed to the corneal surface changes after the procedure. Small surface leucomas that do not require debridement appear at the treatment spots after CK at the 6, 7, and 8 mm optical zones. These leucomas gradually fade and are not cosmetically visible. However, the striae between the spots are believed to be permanent and responsible for the multifocal effect.

Corneal topography as well as wavefront images of a post-CK cornea show alternating rings of flat and steeper areas (ie, a flat central cornea surrounded by a ring of higher elevation, which is then surrounded by a ring of flatness) (Figure 9). These results resemble the effect that follows implantation of the Array multifocal intraocular lens (Allergan, Inc, Irvine, Calif).

CONCLUSION

The CK technique uses optimal temperature and time exposures of radiofrequency energy to denature corneal collagen in selected treatment spots. Following a full circle of treatment spots, the peripheral cornea flattens and the central cornea steepens. The footprint made in an animal model demonstrated the deep treatment penetration, which is likely to contribute to permanence of

	Preoperatively (N = 32)	Month 1 (N = 27)	Month 3 (N = 16)
TABLE 6 SUMMARY OF MONOVISION STUDY RESULTS			
Binocular Distance UCVA			
≤ 20/20	78%	95%	95%
≤ 20/25	88%	100%	100%
Binocular Near UCVA			
≤ J1	0%	22%	38%
≤ J2	3%	52%	50%
≤ J5	9%	96%	94%
Accuracy of Achieved MRSE Refraction			
± 0.50 D		67%	88%
± 1.00 D		93%	94%
± 2.00 D		100%	100%
Undercorrections > +1.00 D		4%	0%
Overcorrections < -1.00 D		4%	6%
Mean MRSE	+1.39 D	-0.91 D (±0.68)	-0.98 D (± 0.62)
Distance BSCVA			
20/16	63%	33%	38%
20/20	38%	56%	63%
20/25	0%	11%	0%

effect. One-year clinical trial results showed stability of refraction appearing by the 6-month visit. The persistent striae on confocal microscopy confirm the clinical results.

The clinical trial results also suggest that CK may be more stable than LTK, safer than PRK and LASIK, and as effective as LASIK for the treatment of low levels of hyperopia. While both noncontact LTK and CK heat and denature collagen, the better refractive results of CK may be due to the deeper penetration (500 µm for CK, more shallow for noncontact LTK) and CK's resultant cylindrical footprint (versus conical for LTK) of collagen shrinkage. Early results of monovision treatment for presbyopia suggest effective and accurate induction of myopia of up to 2.00 D. The procedure appears to produce a multifocal cornea that allows distance and near vision. The multicenter clinical trial for correction of spherical hyperopia continues for 2 years, and other trials for correction of presbyopia, astigmatism, and for determining specific corneal effects are ongoing.

REFERENCES

1. Koch DD, Kohnen T, McDonnell PJ, et al. Hyperopia correction by non-contact holmium:YAG laser thermokeratoplasty. United States phase IIA clinical study with a 1-year follow-up. *Ophthalmology.* 1996;103:1525-1536.
2. Koch DD, Abarca A, Villareal R, et al. Hyperopia correction by non-contact holmium:YAG laser thermokeratoplasty. Clinical study with two-year follow-up. *Ophthalmology.* 1996;103:731-740.
3. Koch D, Kohnen T, McDonnell P, Menefee R, Berry M. Hyperopia correction by noncontact holmium:YAG laser thermal keratoplasty. United States phase IIA clinical study with a 2-year follow-up. *Ophthalmology.* 1997;104:1938-1947.
4. *Hyperion LTK System Device Labeling, PMA P990078.* Fremont, Calif: Sunrise Technologies; May 2000.
5. Nano HD, Muzzin S. Noncontact holmium:YAG laser thermal keratoplasty for hyperopia. *J Cataract Refract Surg.* 1998;24:751-757.
6. Alio JL, Ismail MM, Sanchez Pego JL. Correction of hyperopia with non-contact Ho:YAG laser thermal keratoplasty. *J Refract Surg.* 1997;13:17-22.

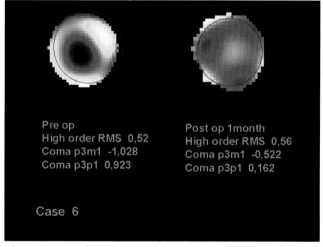

Figure 9. Wavefront image of the cornea before and after CK. The postoperative photo shows a multifocal effect (courtesy of Ioannis Pallikaris, MD).

7. Alio JL, Ismail MM, Artola A, Perez-Santonja JJ. Correction of hyperopia induced by photorefractive keratectomy using non-contact Ho:YAG laser thermal keratoplasty. *J Refract Surg.* 1997;13:13-16.
8. Pop M. Laser thermal keratoplasty for the treatment of photorefractive keratectomy overcorrections: a 1-year follow-up. *Ophthalmology.* 1998;105:926-931.
9. Ismail MM, Alio JL, Perez-Santonja JJ. Noncontact thermokeratoplasty to correct hyperopia induced by laser in situ keratomileusis. *J Cataract Refract Surg.* 1998;24:1191-1194.
10. Durrie DS. Laser thermokeratoplasty for hyperopia and presbyopia. *Rev Ophthalmol.* 2000;8:75-80..
11. Eggink CA, Bardak Y, Cuypers MHM, Deutman AF. Treatment of hyperopia with contact Ho:YAG laser thermal keratoplasty. *J Refract Surg.* 1999;15:16-22.
12. Eggink CA, Meurs P, Bardak Y, Deutman AF. Holmium laser thermal keratoplasty for hyperopia and astigmatism after photorefractive keratectomy. *J Refract Surg.* 2000;16:317-322.

13. Brinkmann R. Koop N, Geerling G, et al. Diode laser thermokeratoplasty: application strategy and dosimetry. *J Refract Surg.* 1998;24:1195-1207.

14. Bende T, Jean B, Oltrup T. Laser thermal keratoplasty using a continuous wave diode laser. *J Refract Surg.* 1999;15:154-158.

15. Geerling G, Koop N, Brikmann R, et al. Continuous-wave diode laser thermokeratoplasty: first clinical experience in blind human eyes. *J Cataract Refract Surg.* 1999;25:32-40.

16. Mendez A, Mendez Noble A. Conductive keratoplasty for the correction of hyperopia. In: Sher NA, ed. *Surgery for Hyperopia and Presbyopia.* Baltimore, Md: Williams & Wilkins; 1997:163-171.

17. McDonald M, Conductive Keratoplasty Investigators Group. Conductive keratoplasty for the correction of low to moderate hyperopia: US clinical trial one-year results. *Ophthalmology.* 2001. Submitted.

18. Durrie D. Treatment of presbyopia: monovision with conductive keratoplasty. Presented at the International Society for Refractive Surgery meeting; Nov 2001; New Orleans, La.

19. Comaish I, Lawless M. Conductive keratoplasty to correct residual hyperopia after previous corneal surgery. *J Cataract Refract Surg.* 2001. Submitted.

20. Pearce J, Thomsen S. Rate process analysis of thermal damage. In: Welch AJ, van Gemert, MJC, eds. *Optical-Thermal Response of Laser-Irradiated Tissue.* New York: Plenum Press; 1995.

21. Chang J, Sodenberg PG, Denham D, Nose I, Lee W, Parel JM. Temperature-induced corneal shrinkage. *Society of Photo-Optical Instrumentation Engineers (SPIE) Proceedings.* 1996;2673:70-76.

22. Goth P, Stern R. Conductive keratoplasty: principles and technology. Presented at American Society Cataract & Refractive Surgery meeting; April 2000; New Orleans, La.

23. Koch DD, Kohnen T, Anderson JA, et al. Histologic changes and wound healing response following 10-pulse noncontact holmium:YAG laser thermal keratoplasty. *J Refract Surg.* 1996;12:623-634.

Lenticular Modifications to Correct Presbyopia

Chapter 21

No-Anesthesia Cataract Surgery With the Karate Chop Technique

Athiya Agarwal, MD, FRSH, DO; Sunita Agarwal, MS, FSVH, DO; and Amar Agarwal, MS, FRCS, FRCOphth

INTRODUCTION

On June 13, 1998 in Ahmedabad, India the first no-anesthesia cataract surgery was performed by the authors at the Phako and Refractive Surgery conference. This was performed as a live surgery in front of 250 delegates. From this, various new concepts in cataract surgery have come about.[1] In the surgery described in this chapter, the karate chop technique was used.

For treating presbyopia, cataract extraction with phacoemulsification is a very good alternative. In such cases, if necessary, one can implant a multifocal or accommodating intraocular lens (IOL). Alternatively, the patient can use one eye for distance and the other for near vision, solving the problem of presbyopia.

NUCLEUS REMOVAL TECHNIQUES

Since the introduction of phacoemulsification as an alternative to the standard cataract extraction technique, surgeons around the world have attempted to make this new procedure safer and easier to perform while assuring good visual outcomes and patient recovery. The fundamental goal of phaco is to remove the cataract with minimal disturbance to the eye using the least amount of surgical manipulations. Each maneuver should be performed with minimal force, and maximal efficiency should be obtained.

The latest generation of phaco procedures began with Dr. Howard Gimbel's "divide and conquer" nuclear fracture technique in which he simply split apart the nuclear rim. Since then we have evolved through various techniques, namely four-quadrant cracking, chip and flip, spring surgery, stop and chop, and phaco chop.

Clear lens removal by phaco is a very good alternative to manage refractive errors. In these cases, because the nucleus is soft one can use only phacoaspiration to remove the nuclei, rather than ultrasound power.

KARATE CHOP

Unlike the peripheral chopping of Nagahara or other stop and chop techniques, we have developed a safer technique called *central anterior chopping* or *karate chop*. In this method, the phaco tip is embedded by a single burst of power in the central safe zone and after lifting the nucleus slightly (to lessen the pressure on the posterior capsule), the chopper is used to chop the nucleus. In soft nuclei, it is very difficult to chop the nucleus. In most cases, one can take it out in one piece. However, if the patient is around 40 years of age, then one might have to chop the nucleus. In such cases we embed the phaco probe in the nucleus, then with the left hand cut the nucleus as if we are cutting a piece of cake. This movement should be done three times in the same place. This will chop the nucleus.

SOFT CATARACTS

In soft cataracts, the technique is a bit different. We embed the phaco tip and then cut the nucleus as if we are cutting a piece of cake. This should be done two to three times in the same area so that the cataract is cut. It is very difficult to chop a soft cataract, so this technique helps in splitting the cataract.

AGARWAL CHOPPER

We have devised our own chopper (Katena). The other choppers, which cut from the periphery, are blunt. Our chopper has a sharp cutting edge and a sharp point. The advantage of such a chopper is that you can chop in the center and need not go to the periphery.

In this method of going directly into the center of the nucleus without any sculpting, the required ultrasound energy is reduced. The chopper always remains within the capsulorrhexis margin and never goes underneath the anterior capsule. Hence, it is easy to work with even small pupils or glaucomatous eyes. Since we do not have to widen the pupil, there is little likelihood of tearing the sphincter and allowing prostaglandins to leak out and cause inflammation or cystoid macular edema. In this technique we can easily go into even hard nuclei on the first attempt.

AGARWAL KARATE CHOP TECHNIQUE

INCISION

The karate chop technique is a modification of the Nagahara chop. The important feature is that we do not chop the periphery.

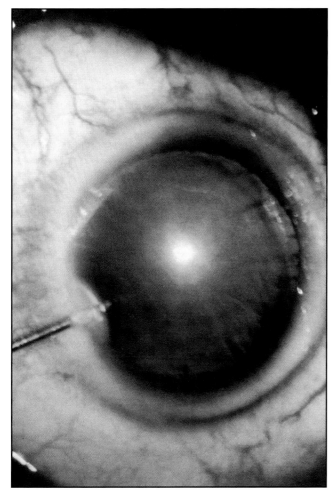

Figure 1. Eye with cataract. Needle enters the eye to inject viscoelastic. This is the most important step in no-anesthesia cataract/clear lens surgery. This gives entry into the eye, through which a straight rod can be passed for stabilization. Note no forceps holds the eye.

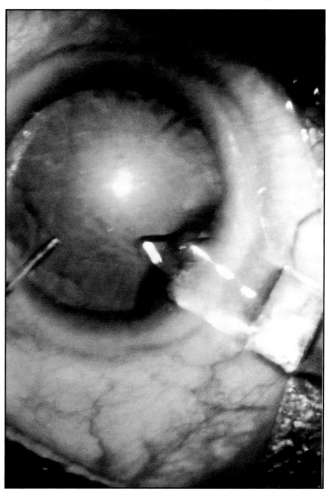

Figure 2. Clear corneal incision. Note the straight rod in the left hand. The right hand is performing the clear corneal incision. This is a temporal incision in which the surgeon is sitting temporally.

A temporal clear corneal section is made. If astigmatism is plus at 90 degrees, then the incision is made superiorly.

First, a needle with viscoelastic is injected inside the eye in the area where the second site is made (Figure 1). This will distend the eye so that when the clear corneal incision is made, the eye will be tense and one can create a good valve. Now use a straight rod to stabilize the eye with the left hand. With the right hand, make the clear corneal incision (Figure 2).

When we first began making the temporal incisions, we positioned ourselves temporally. The problem with this method is that the microscope had to be turned, which in turn would affect the cables connected to the video camera. Further, the theatre staff would be disturbed between the right eye and left eye. To solve this problem, we decided on a different strategy. We have operating trolleys on wheels. The patient is wheeled inside the operation theatre, and for the right eye the trolley is placed slightly oblique so that the surgeon does not change his or her position. The surgeon stays at the 12 o'clock position. For the left eye, the trolley with the patient is rotated horizontally so that the temporal portion of the left eye is at 12 o'clock. This way the patient is moved instead of the surgeon.

CAPSULORRHEXIS

Capsulorrhexis is then performed through the same incision (Figure 3). While performing the rhexis, it is important to note that the rhexis starts from the center and the needle is moved to the right and then downward. This is important because today the concepts of temporal and nasal have changed. It is better to use the terms *superior, inferior, right,* or *left.* If we would start the rhexis from the center and move it to the left, then the weakest point of the rhexis is generally where you finish it. In other words, the point where you tend to lose the rhexis is near its completion. If you have done the rhexis from the center and moved to the left, then you might have an incomplete rhexis on the left-hand side either inferiorly or superiorly. The phaco probe is always moved down and to the left. Every stroke of your hand can extend the rhexis posteriorly, creating a posterior capsular rupture. If we perform the rhexis from the center and move to the right, the flap is pushed inferiorly. If we have an incomplete rhexis near the end, it will be superior and to the right. Any incomplete rhexis can extend and create a posterior capsular tear. In this case, the chances of survival are better.

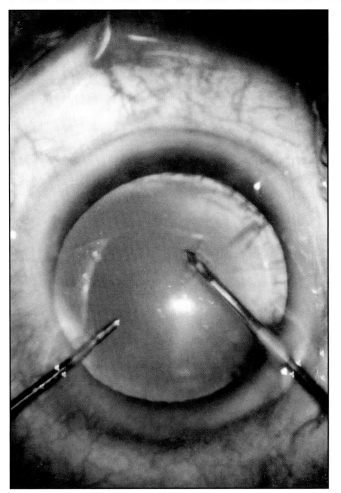

Figure 3. Capsulorrhexis performed with a needle.

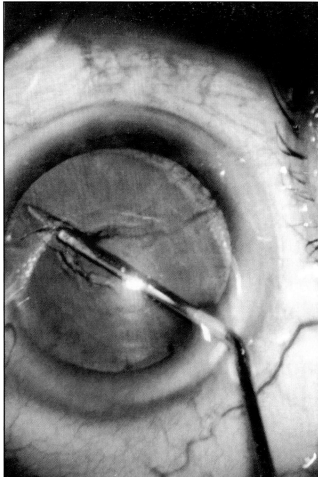

Figure 4. Hydrodissection.

This is because we are moving the phaco probe down and to the left, but the rhexis is incomplete up and to the right.

If you are left-handed, start the rhexis from the center and move to the left and then down.

HYDRODISSECTION

Hydrodissection is then performed (Figure 4). We watch for the fluid wave to determine when hydrodissection is complete. We do not perform hydrodelineation or test for rotation of the nucleus. Viscoelastic is then introduced before inserting the phaco probe.

KARATE CHOP—TWO HALVES

We then insert the phaco probe through the incision slightly superior to the center of the nucleus (Figure 5). At that point, apply ultrasound and see that the phaco tip gets embedded in the nucleus (Figure 6). The direction of the phaco probe should be obliquely downward toward the vitreous and not horizontally toward the iris. This way, only the nucleus will get embedded. The settings at this stage are 70% phaco power, 24 mL/minute flow rate, and 101 mmHg suction. By the time the phaco tip is embedded in the nucleus, the tip has reached the middle of the nucleus. We do not turn the bevel of the phaco tip downward when we do this step, as the embedding is better the other way. We prefer a 15-degree tip, but any tip can be used.

Now stop the phaco ultrasound and bring your foot to position 2 so that only suction is being used—just enough so that when you apply pressure on the nucleus with the chopper, the direction of the pressure is downward. If the capsule is a bit thin, like in hypermature cataracts, be careful not to rupture the posterior capsule and create a nucleus drop. When we lift the nucleus, the pressure on the posterior capsule is lessened. With the chopper, cut the nucleus with a straight downward motion (Figure 7) and then move the chopper to the left when you reach the center of the nucleus. In other words, your left hand moves the chopper like a laterally reversed L. Do not go to the periphery for chopping—do it at the center.

Once you have created a crack, split the nucleus to the center. Rotate the nucleus 180 degrees and crack again so that you get two halves of the nucleus. In brown cataracts, the nucleus will crack but sometimes it will still be attached in the center the nucleus. The nucleus must be totally split in two halves and the posterior capsule should be visible throughout.

KARATE CHOP—FURTHER CHOPPING

Now that you have two halves, you have a shelf to embed the probe. Place the probe with ultrasound into one-half of the nucleus (Figure 8). You can pass the direction of the probe horizontally, as now you have a shelf. Embed the probe, then pull it a little bit. This

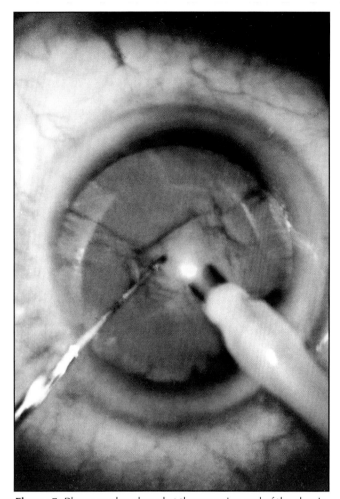

Figure 5. Phaco probe placed at the superior end of the rhexis.

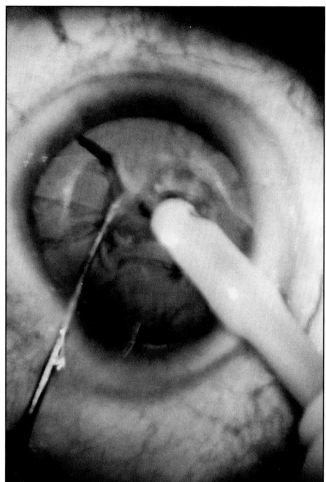

Figure 6. Phaco probe embedded in the nucleus. We started from the superior end of the rhexis and note that it was embedded in the middle of the nucleus. If we had started in the middle, then we would have embedded only inferiorly (ie, at the edge of the rhexis) and chopping would be difficult.

step is important so that you get the extra bit of space for chopping. This will prevent you from chopping the rhexis margin. Apply the force of the chopper downward. Move the chopper to the left so that the nucleus is split. Again, you should see the posterior capsule throughout so that you know the nucleus is totally split. Release the probe, as it will still be embedded in the nucleus. Create three quadrants like this in one-half of the nucleus. Then make another three quadrants in the other half of the nucleus. You now have six quadrants or pie-shaped fragments. The settings at this stage are 50% phaco power, 24 mL/minute flow rate, and 101 mmHg suction. Remember five words: embed, pull, chop, split, and release.

PULSE PHACOEMULSIFICATION

Once all the pieces have been chopped, take out each one by one, and in pulse phaco mode aspirate the pieces at the level of the iris. Do not work in the bag unless the cornea is preoperatively bad or the patient is very elderly. The setting at this stage can be phaco power 50% to 30%, flow rate 24 mL, and suction 101 mmHg.

CORTICAL WASHING AND FOLDABLE IOL IMPLANTATION

The next step is to perform cortical washing (Figure 9). Always try to remove the subincisional cortex first, as that is the most difficult. In Figure 10, note that cortical aspiration is complete. Note

also the rhexis margins. All the time the left hand uses the straight rod to control the movements of the eye. If necessary, use a bimanual irrigation aspiration technique, then inject viscoelastic and implant the foldable IOL. We generally use the plate haptic foldable IOL (Figure 11) with large fenestrations, as we find them superior. Take out the viscoelastic with the irrigation aspiration probe (Figure 12).

STROMAL HYDRATION

At the end of the procedure, inject the balanced saline solution (BSS) inside the lips of the clear corneal incision (Figure 13). This will create a stromal hydration at the wound. This will appear white but disappear after 4 to 5 hours. The advantage of this is that the wound is sealed better.

NO PAD, SUBCONJUNCTIVAL INJECTIONS

No subconjunctival injections or pad are put in the eye. The patient walks out of the theatre and goes home. The patient is seen the next day, and after 1 month glasses are prescribed.

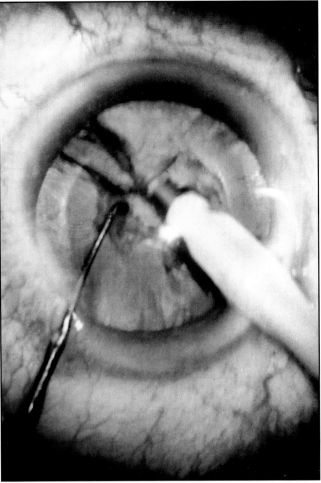

Figure 7. The left hand chops the nucleus and splits it like a laterally reversed L (downward and to the left).

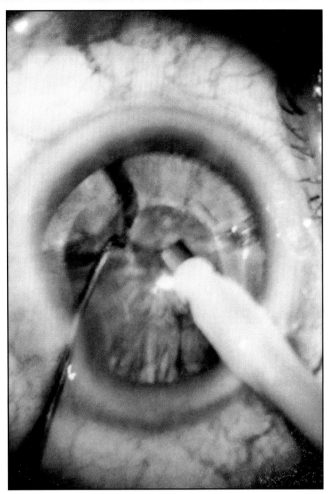

Figure 8. Phaco probe embedded in one-half of the nucleus. The direction must now be horizontal, not vertical, as there is now a shelf of nucleus to embed. Chop and then split the nucleus.

PHACODYNAMICS OF THE PHACO CHOP TECHNIQUE

We should take full advantage of the phaco machine's capability, thereby decreasing physical manipulation of the intraocular tissues. In this phaco chop technique, we use a vacuum of 101 mmHg, about 70% phaco power, and the flow rate is 24 mL/minute.

In this phaco chop technique, the vacuum is most important. It needs to be sufficient to stabilize the nucleus while the chopper is splitting. If the action of the chopper is dislodging the vacuum seal on the phaco tip, the vacuum can be raised from 120 to 200 mmHg. After embedding the phaco needle with mild linear ultrasound power in foot switch position 3, it is important to raise the pedal back to foot switch position 2 while the vacuum builds up. This is because the purpose of ultrasound is to completely embed the aspiration port into the nucleus to obtain good vacuum seal. In foot switch 3, there is risk of adverse heat build-up because the occluded tip prohibits any cooling flow. Also, when manipulating the nucleus by pulling with the embedded tip, the vacuum seal is likely to be compromised by the vibrating needle if it is in foot switch position 3.

ADVANTAGES

The phacoemulsification procedure has been proven to be reasonably safe to the endothelium. As compared to the divide and conquer technique, this phaco karate chop technique eliminates the need for trenching, thereby producing significant reduction in phaco time and power, which in turn decreases endothelial cell damage. Even with increased density of cataract, there is a less pronounced increase in phaco time. Here we utilize the chop to divide the nucleus by mechanical energy. It is safe and effective in nuclear handling during phacoemulsification.

In conventional chop, the disadvantage is that the chopper is placed underneath the anterior capsule and then pulled toward the center. This can potentially damage the capsule and zonules. In phaco chop, we do not go under the rhexis, the vertical element of the chopper remains within the rhexis margin and is visible at all stages. Hence, it is very easy to work with even in small pupils or glaucomatous eyes. The stress is taken by the impacted phaco tip and the chopper rather than transmitting it to the fragile capsule.

By going directly into the center of the nucleus with the phaco tip and not doing any sculpting, we do not need as much ultrasound

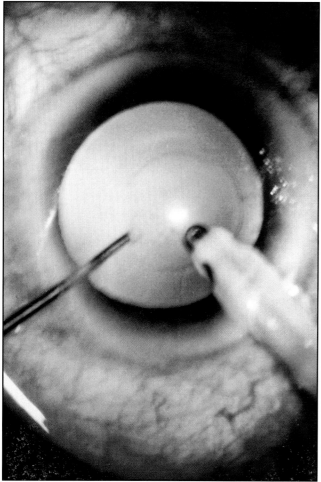

Figure 9. Cortical aspiration is completed. Note the straight rod in the left hand, which helps control movement of the eye.

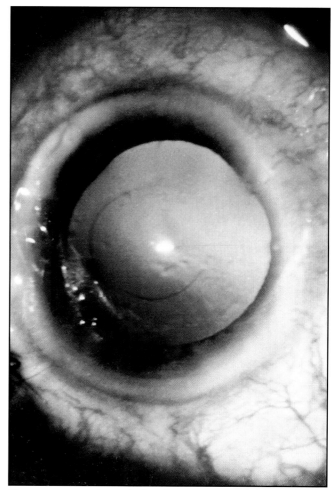

Figure 10. Eye distended with viscoelastic. Note the rhexis margins.

energy as is usually required. It is safe and easy to perform, and we do not have to pass as much BSS (irrigating fluid) through the eye.

DISADVANTAGES

This technique demands continuous use of the left hand and hence requires practice to master it.

TOPICAL ANESTHESIA CATARACT SURGERY

All cases done by the authors were previously done under topical anesthesia. Xylocaine 4% drops were instilled in the eye about three times 10 to 15 minutes before surgery. No intracameral anesthesia was used. It is not advisable to use xylocaine drops while operating. This can damage the epithelium and create more trouble in visualization. No stitches or pad are applied. This is called the no injection, no-stitch, no-pad cataract surgery technique. The authors have now shifted all their cases to the no-anesthesia technique. This is done in both their hospitals in India (Chennai and Bangalore) and their hospital in Dubai, UAE.

NO-ANESTHESIA CATARACT SURGERY

In the past, we had wondered whether topical anesthesia was necessary or not, so we operated on patients without anesthesia. In these patients, no xylocaine drops were instilled. The patients did not have any pain. It is paradoxical because we have been taught from the beginning that we should apply xylocaine. No anesthesia is possible because we do not touch the conjunctiva or sclera. We never use a one-tooth forceps to stabilize the eye. Instead, we use a straight rod, which is passed inside the eye to stabilize it when we are performing the procedure. The first step is very important: we first enter the eye with a needle with viscoelastic and inject the viscoelastic inside the eye. This is done in the area of the side port. We now have an opening in the eye, through which a straight rod can be passed to stabilize it. The anterior chamber should be well maintained and less ultrasound power is used. Techniques such as trenching generate high ultrasound power, which in turn generates heat. This causes pain to the patient.

Following our rules, one can perform no-anesthesia cataract or clear lens extraction surgery.

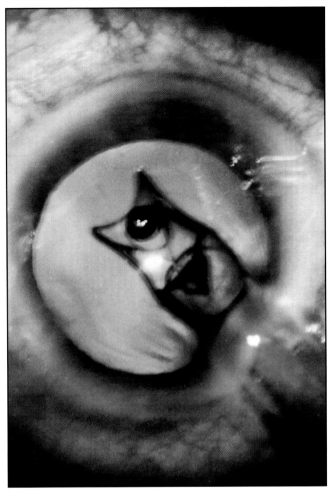

Figure 11. Plate haptic foldable IOL with large fenestrations being implanted.

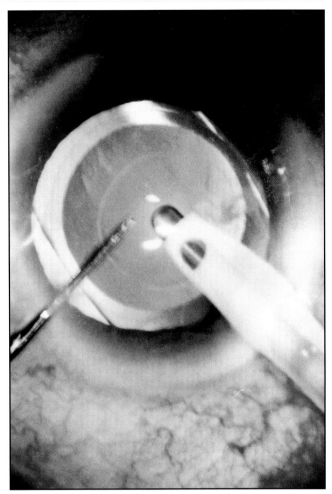

Figure 12. Foldable IOL in the capsular bag. Viscoelastic is removed with the irrigation aspiration probe.

BLURHEX (TRYPAN BLUE) IN MATURE CATARACTS

Various techniques are present that can help one perform the rhexis in mature cataracts:

1. Use a good operating microscope. If the operating microscope is good, one can faintly see the outline of the rhexis.

2. Use an endoilluminator. While one is performing the rhexis with the right hand (dominant hand), in the left hand (nondominant hand) one can hold an endoilluminator. By adjusting the endoilluminator in various positions, one can complete the rhexis, as the edge can be seen.

3. Use a forceps. A forceps is easier to use than a needle, especially in mature cataracts. One can use a good rhexis forceps to complete this step.

4. Use a paraxial light.

With all these techniques, an incomplete rhexis is always a possibility. Many times if the rhexis is incomplete, one might have to convert to an extracapsular cataract extraction to prevent a posterior capsular rupture or nucleus drop.

The solution to this problem is to have a dye that stains the anterior capsule, such as trypan blue. Trypan blue is marketed as Blurhex by Dr. Agarwal's Pharma Ltd. Each milliliter of Blurhex contains 0.6 mg trypan blue, 1.9 mg of sodium monohydrogen orthophosphate, 0.3 mg of sodium dihydrogen orthophosphate, 8.2 mg of sodium chloride, sodium hydroxide for adjusting the pH, and water for injection.

One can inject Blurhex directly or first inject air into the anterior chamber. This prevents water-like dilution of the trypan blue. Then the trypan blue is withdrawn from the vial into a syringe. This is then injected by a cannula into the anterior chamber between the air bubble and the lens capsule. It is kept like that for a minute or two for staining of the anterior capsule. Next, viscoelastic is injected into the anterior chamber to remove the air bubble and trypan blue.

Now, the rhexis is started with a needle (Figure 14), however a forceps can be used instead. We prefer to use a needle, as it gives better control of the size of the rhexis. In the figure, note the left hand holding a rod stabilizing the eye while the rhexis is being performed. The rhexis is continued with the needle. Note the contrast between the capsule, which has been stained, and the cortex, which is not stained. The rhexis is continued and finally completed (Figure 15). When the rhexis is complete, we can see the stained anterior capsule lying in the anterior chamber.

ANTICHAMBER COLLAPSER TO PREVENT SURGE

One of the main pitfalls of phacoemulsification is surge.[1] The problem is that as the nuclear piece gets occluded in the phaco tip

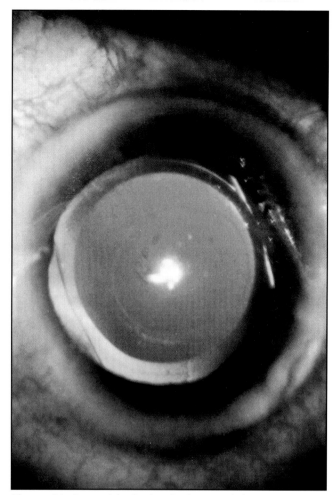

Figure 13. Stromal hydration is done and the case is completed.

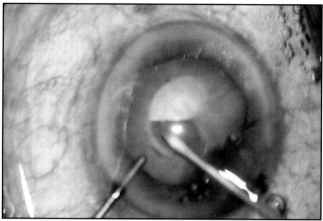

Figure 14. Blurhex (trypan blue) is used to stain the anterior capsule. Note the blue staining of the anterior capsule and the needle performing the rhexis.

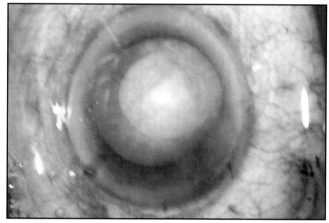

Figure 15. The rhexis is complete. Note the white nucleus in the center and the stained anterior capsule in the periphery.

and we emulsify it, surge occurs. Many people have tried various methods to solve this problem. Some phaco machines, like the Sovereign (Allergan), have been created to solve this problem. Others have tried to use an anterior chamber maintainer to get more fluid into the eye. The problem with the anterior chamber maintainer is that another port has to be made. In other words, we have three ports and if you are doing the case under topical or no anesthesia (as we do in our hospital), it becomes quite cumbersome. Another method to solve surge is to use more phacoaspiration and chop the nuclear pieces with the left hand (nondominant hand). The problem with this, though, is the surgical time increases and if the case includes a hard brown cataract, phacoaspiration will not suffice.

Surge occurs when an occluded fragment is held by high vacuum and is abruptly aspirated with a burst of ultrasound. The fluid from the anterior chamber rushes into the phaco tip and leads to a collapse of the anterior chamber.

One of the authors created a method to solve surge using a device that we call the *antichamber collapser*. We came up with this idea when we were operating cases with phakonit (a new technique in which cataract is removed through a 0.9 mm opening); we wanted more fluid entering the eye. We now routinely use the antichamber collapser to solve the problem of surge.

This method is performed as follows:
1. First, we use two BSS bottles. These are put in the IV stand (Figure 16).
2. Instead of using an IV set for the fluid to move from the bottle to the phaco hand piece, we use a transurethral resection (TUR) set, which is a tubing set used by urologists. The advantage of this is that the bore of the tubing is quite large, so more fluid passes from the infusion bottle to the phaco hand piece. The TUR set has two tubes, which go into each infusion bottle and become one, which then passes into the phaco hand piece.
3. Now we take an air pump (such as what is used in fish tanks) to provide oxygen. The air pump is plugged into the electrical connection.
4. An IV set now connects the air pump to the infusion bottle. The tubing passes from the air pump, and the end of the tubing is passed into one of the infusion bottles.
5. When the air pump is switched on, it pumps air into the infusion bottle. This air goes to the top of the bottle, and because of the pressure, it pumps the fluid down with greater force. With this, the fluid now flows from the infusion bottle into the TUR set to reach the phaco hand piece. The amount of

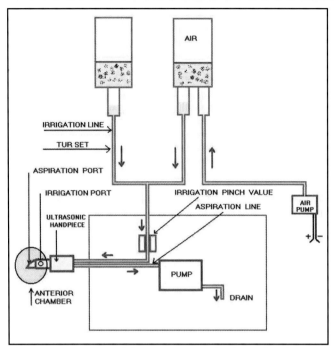

Figure 16. Diagram of the air pump and infusion bottle. Note the two infusion bottles connected to a transurethral resection tubing (TUR) set and the air pump connects to one of the bottles.

fluid now coming out of the hand piece is much greater than what would normally come out and with more force.

6. One can use an air filter between the air pump and the infusion bottle so that the air that is being pumped into the bottle is sterile.

7. This extra amount of fluid coming out compensates for the surge that would occur.

PRESBYOPIA CORRECTION

A popular method of correcting presbyopia and one that we tend to use in our patients is monofocal vision. In this method, one eye is corrected for distance vision and the other for near vision. By this system of refraction, the patient is able to use both eyes and is able to see distance and near without glasses. The near vision eye is about -1.0 to -1.5 D. Sometimes for very fine reading the patient might require reading glasses. The ophthalmologist should explain to the patient that he or she should use both eyes to see, as sometimes he or she might start "checking" each eye individually and complain. Other alternatives are to use a multifocal IOL or accommodating IOL, discussed later in this book.

CONCLUSION

As in any other field, progress is inevitable in ophthalmology, especially in refractive surgery. We have begun to look at refractive surgery as a craft and should constantly try to improve upon it and become better at it. By this, we will be able to provide good vision to more people than any one dared dream just a few decades ago. It also goes without saying that we are and will be forever grateful to all our patients because without their faith, we would never have had the courage to proceed.

Keeping this in mind, we hope and wish that the effectiveness and advantages of this no-anesthesia clear lens extraction technique be realized and practiced, thereby making the technique of phacoemulsification safer and easier, providing good visual outcomes and patient recovery.

REFERENCE

1. Agarwal S, Agarwal A, Sachdev MS, Mehta KR, Fine IH, Agarwal A. *Phacoemulsification, Laser Cataract Surgery & Foldable IOLs.* New Delhi, India: Jaypee Brothers; 1998.

Chapter 22

The Phakonit ThinOptX Rollable Intraocular Lens

Amar Agarwal, MS, FRCS, FRCOphth; Athiya Agarwal, MD, FRSH, DO; and Sunita Agarwal, MS, FSVH, DO

INTRODUCTION

On August 15, 1998 the authors performed the first sub 1 mm cataract surgery by a technique called *phakonit*.[1,2] In this procedure, the cataract was removed through a 0.9-mm incision. The problem with this technique was to find an intraocular lens (IOL) that would pass through such a small incision. Then on October 2, 2001 the authors performed the first case using a phakonit rollable IOL. This was done in their Chennai (India) hospital. The lens used was a special rollable IOL from ThinOptX (Abingdon, Va). This was the first rollable IOL implanted after a phakonit procedure and was thus named the Phakonit ThinOptX Rollable IOL.

PRESBYOPIA

This rollable IOL is also like a foldable IOL, which means presbyopia can be resolved by it. This can be done by giving the patient monofocal vision. In other words, one eye can be corrected for distance and the other for near.

In time, an alternative of such a lens will be to make it either multifocal or accommodating. One advantage is that since the incision size is 0.9 mm, astigmatism will not be created, which again helps in solving the problem of presbyopia. Another future possibility of the lens is to create a presbyopia phakic IOL of the same material.

PRINCIPLE OF PHAKONIT

The term *phakonit* has been given because it is phaco (phako) being done with a needle (n) opening via an incision (i) and with the phaco tip (t).

The problem in phacoemulsification is that we are not able to go below an incision of 1.9 mm. This is because of the infusion sleeve, which takes up a lot of space. The titanium tip of the phaco hand piece has a diameter of 0.9 mm. This is surrounded by the infusion sleeve, which allows fluid to pass into the eye. It also cools the hand piece tip so that a corneal burn does not occur.

The authors separated the phaco tip from the infusion sleeve. The tip was passed inside the eye, and as there was no infusion sleeve present, the size of the incision was 0.9 mm. In the left hand, an irrigating chopper was held, which had fluid passing inside the eye. The left hand was in the same position where the chopper is normally held (ie, the side port incision). The assistant injected fluid (balanced saline solution [BSS]) continuously at the site of the incision to cool the phaco tip. Thus, the cataract was removed through a 0.9 mm opening.

PHAKONIT SURGICAL TECHNIQUE

A specially designed 0.9 mm keratome, an irrigating chopper (Katena), a straight blunt rod, and a 15-degree standard phaco tip without an infusion sleeve are the main prerequisites of this surgery. Viscoelastic is injected with a 26-g needle through the presumed site of side port entry (Figure 1). This inflates the chamber and prevents its collapse when the keratome enters. A straight rod is passed through this site to achieve akinesia and a clear corneal temporal valve is made with 0.9-mm keratome (Figure 2). Katena makes this keratome and the other instruments for phakonit. A continuous curvilinear capsulorrhexis is performed, followed by hydrodissection (Figure 3) and checking the rotation of the nucleus.

After enlarging the side port, a 20-g irrigating chopper connected to the infusion line of the phaco machine is introduced with the foot pedal on position 1. The phaco probe is connected to the aspiration line, and the phaco tip without an infusion sleeve is introduced through a 0.9-mm incision (Figure 4). Using the phaco tip with moderate ultrasound power, the center of the nucleus is directly embedded starting from the superior edge of the rhexis with the phaco probe directed obliquely downward toward the vitreous. The setting at this stage is 50% phaco power, flow rate 24 mL/min, and 110 mmHg suction. When nearly half of the center of the nucleus is embedded, the foot pedal is moved to position 2, as it helps to hold the nucleus due to vacuum rise. To avoid undue pressure on the posterior capsule, the nucleus is lifted slightly, and with the irrigating chopper in the left hand, the nucleus chopped. This is done with a straight downward motion from the inner edge of the rhexis to the center of the nucleus and then to the left in the form of an inverted L shape (Figure 5). Once the crack is created, the nucleus is split to the center. The nucleus is then rotated 180 degrees and cracked again so that it is completely split into two halves.

The nucleus is then rotated 90 degrees and embedding is done in

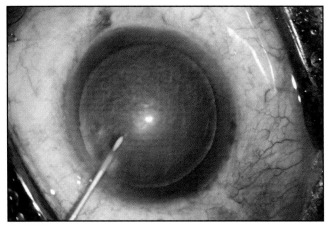

Figure 1. A 26-g needle with viscoelastic enters the side port area. This is for entry of the irrigating chopper.

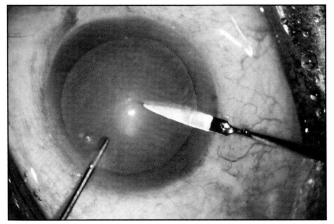

Figure 2. Clear corneal incision made with the keratome (0.9 mm). Note the left hand has a straight rod to stabilize the eye, as the procedure is not performed with anesthesia.

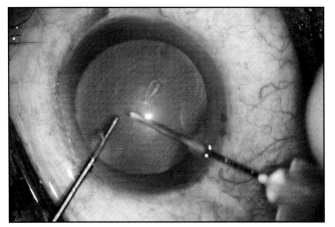

Figure 3. The rhexis is started with a needle.

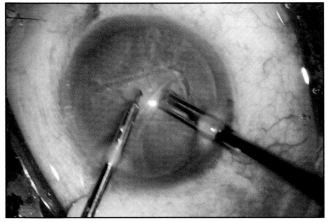

Figure 4. The phakonit irrigating chopper and phaco probe without the sleeve inside the eye.

one-half of the nucleus with the probe directed horizontally (Figure 6). With the previously described technique, three pie-shaped quadrants are created in one half of the nucleus. Similarly, three pie-shaped fragments are created in the other half of the nucleus. With a short burst of energy at pulse mode, each pie-shaped fragment is lifted and brought at the level of iris where it is further emulsified and aspirated sequentially in pulse mode. Thus, the whole nucleus is removed (Figure 7). Note in Figure 7 no corneal burns are present. Cortical wash-up is done with the bimanual irrigation aspiration technique (Figures 8 and 9).

PHAKONIT THINOPTX ROLLABLE IOL

ThinOptX, the company that manufactures these lenses (Figure 10), has patented technology that allows the manufacture of lenses with plus or minus 30 diopters (D) of correction on the thickness of 100 microns. The ThinOptX technology, developed by Wayne Callahan, Scott Callahan, and Joe Callahan, is not limited to choice of material but is achieved by an evolutionary optic and unprecedented nanoscale manufacturing process. The lens is made from off-the-shelf hydrophilic material, which is similar to several IOL materials already on the market. The key to the ThinOptX lens is the optic design and nanoprecision manufacturing. The basic advantage of this lens is that it is ultra thin.

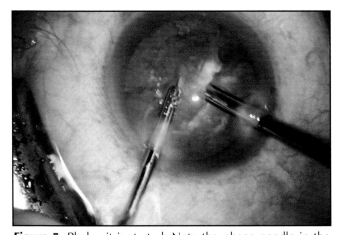

Figure 5. Phakonit is started. Note the phaco needle in the right hand and an irrigating chopper in the left. The crack is created by the karate chop technique. An assistant continuously irrigates the phaco probe area from outside to prevent corneal burns.

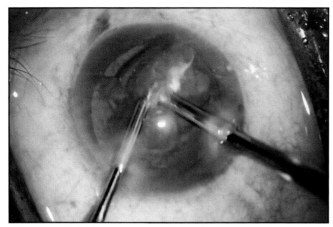

Figure 6. Phakonit, continued. The nuclear pieces are chopped into smaller pie-shaped fragments.

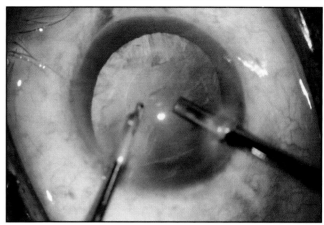

Figure 7. Phakonit is completed. Note the nucleus has been removed and there are no corneal burns.

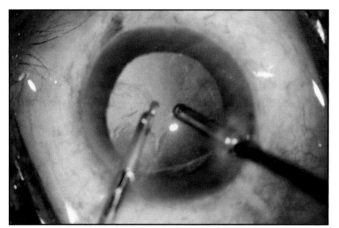

Figure 8. Bimanual irrigation aspiration is started.

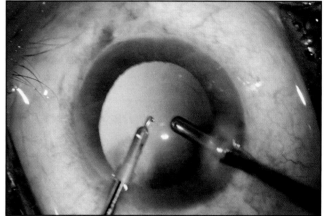

Figure 9. Bimanual irrigation aspiration is completed.

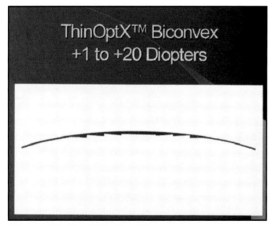

Figure 10. The ThinOptX lens.

ThinLens Optics

Figure 11 illustrates the optical characteristics of the ThinOptX lens. The front surface is a curve that approximates a radius. The back curve is a series of steps with concentric rings. The back surface can be concave, convex, or plano. The combination of steps with the front radius corrects for spherical aberrations. The convex and plano back designs can be used for positive power lenses. The

concave or meniscus back surface is used for negative-powered lenses. In Figure 12, lines intersecting the lens represent parallel light. The light is bent at the intersection of the lens surface in accordance with Snell's law. When light strikes the lens surface, the light is bent toward the central axis. The light travels to the back edge of the lens and again is bent toward the central axis. All the parallel light rays entering the back of the lens come to focus at approximately the same point, therefore the lens is refractive.

GLARE

In the late 1970s, lens companies made lenses with optics that were 5 x 6 mm. The edge for a 20 D lens with a 0.250-mm haptic was .500 mm. The edge was twice as thick as a standard 6-mm lens. Reports of patients with glare and halos in low light conditions began. It is doubtful the pupil was opening to something greater than 5 mm. For light to strike the edge of the lens with the lens in the posterior chamber, it seems the pupil would have to be greater than 5 mm.

In other laboratory work, extreme edge glare was encountered when a light source was placed near a thick, flat piece of plastic. The large edges were covered and never exposed to direct light rays. An extremely small angle of incidence was created. The absorbed light hit the large edge and was reflected back across the sheet of

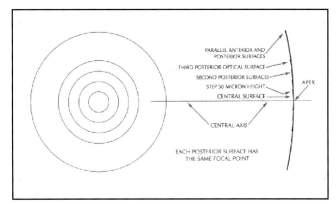

Figure 11. ThinOptX optics.

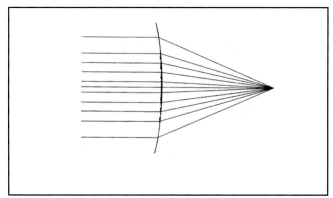

Figure 12. The ThinOptX rollable lens.

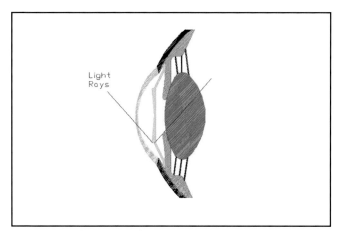

Figure 13. Glare and halos.

plastic to the opposite edge. The light in the lens gave the appearance of a laser generation tube. When the light source was removed, the glare faded away.

A conclusion was reached that much of the light hitting the plastic with small angles of incidence was being absorbed. When the light rays reached the edge, the rays were reflected back across the plastic sheet. The light rays then struck the opposite edge of the plastic sheet and bounced back across the sheet. The same principle seems logical in a lens with a thick edge. This would explain why patients with a high negative lens experience glare in bright sunlight.

Figure 13 illustrates an eye and lens. The light hits the edge of the lens and is reflected unfocused into the eye. With this condition, halo, streaks, and a general loss of contrast would seem logical.

With the ThinOptX technology, each ring has an exposed edge of 50 microns or less. On average, there are three rings per lens plus the outer edge of the lens. The cumulative ring edges are 200 microns. This is much less area than a standard or meniscus lens. This helps patients avoid glare and halos even under low light conditions.

SPHERICAL ABERRATIONS

Spherical aberrations arise from the fact that lenses are most often designed as a portion of a sphere. For a theoretically perfect lens, the radius of the lens surface should increase as the distance from the central axis increases. The lens should be aspheric.

A sphere is not a perfect lens model. The error can be as much as 1.5 D when measured 2 mm from the central optic. The majority of cataract lenses are manufactured with spherical aberrations. The standard aperture on a lens bench is approximately 3 mm. Many lens manufacturers will not have acceptable optics if the apertures were opened to 4 mm.

The ThinOptX lens is manufactured to eliminate most of the spherical aberrations. Each curve on the back has a slightly different radius. The slight change in curvature on each back surface will ensure one focal point.

OTHER ABERRATIONS

Thickness causes a form of aberration due to light rays traveling longer in the thicker portion of the lens. The error is added to spherical aberrations but is small if the lens manufacturer controls the thickness of the lens or compensates for the differences in thickness when measuring the lens. The error is not as much from the

thickness as the fact that most lens benches are calibrated using the back focal length of the lens. A correction factor for thickness is added to determine the lens power. The process can be very accurate if the differences in thickness of the lens are not significant or the lens bench is calibrated between each lens power. The bench should be calibrated even with the same lens power if the lens thickness changes significantly.

The ThinOptX lens is so thin that the error goes away. With a central axis thickness of 50 microns for a meniscus lens and 300 microns for a biconvex or plano optic, there is little error in measuring the lens due to thickness. In fact, with the ThinOptX lens one can measure a lens designed to the same power without adjusting the lens bench. The thinness is one of the reasons that the ThinOptX lens can be manufactured in 0.125 D increments.

FRESNEL LENSES

By definition, the ThinOptX lens is not a Fresnel lens, which is shown in Figure 14. As seen from the figure, the lens has multiple focal points. This makes this lens style diffractive.

The normal lines on the back surface of the Fresnel lens do not originate from the same point; therefore, the back surface of the lens functions as a series of prisms. By selecting the angle, the incoming light rays make the normal line of each prism, and one can choose the focal pattern of the resulting light. One such application is the headlamps of an automobile. The second surface of the ThinOptX lens is designed to assist the front surface in focusing the light at a single point, which by definition is a refractive lens (see Figure 12).

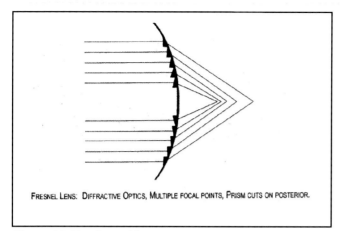

Figure 14. The Fresnel lens.

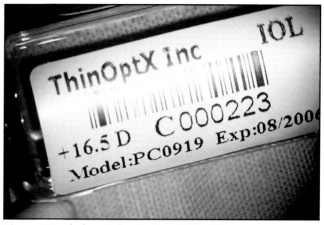

Figure 15. Phakonit ThinOptX rollable IOL in the bottle.

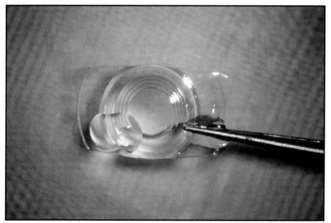

Figure 16. The Phakonit ThinOptX rollable IOL when removed from the bottle.

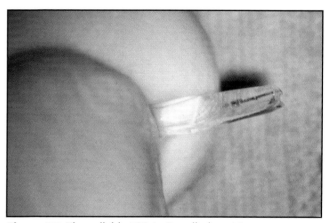

Figure 17. The rollable IOL in its rolled position.

rolled (Figure 17) in a rubbing motion. It is preferable to do this in the bowl of BSS so that the lens remains well-rolled.

The lens is then carefully inserted through the incision (Figure 18). One can then move the lens into the capsular bag (Figures 19 and 20). The tear drop on the haptic should point in a clockwise direction. The smooth optic lenticular surface will be facing posteriorly. The natural warmth of the eye causes the lens to open gradually (Figure 21). Viscoelastic is then removed with the bimanual irrigation aspiration probes (Figure 22). The tips of the foot plates are extremely thin, which allow the lens to be positioned with the foot plates rolled to fit the eye (Figures 23 and 24).

SUMMARY

First, we have to remove the cataract through a sub 1 mm incision. This is possible with the Phakonit technology, as cataracts can be removed through that incision. When we saw the lens, we realized there were certain problems with it. The lens had to be rolled properly. When we rolled the lens with the gloves, the rolling was not good, so we decided to roll it without gloves under the BSS. This gave us excellent rolling. This can be improved by having an instrument that would roll the lens.

We also noticed the size of the lens. The length was acceptable, but the breadth of the lens was too large to go through. We cut the lens vertically on either side. This way the lens became smaller and

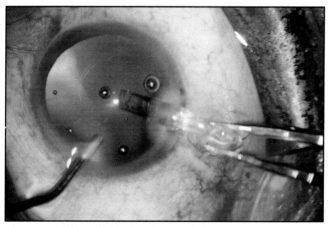

Figure 18. The rollable IOL inserted through the incision.

LENS INSERTION TECHNIQUE

The lens is taken out of the bottle (Figure 15) and held with a forceps (Figure 16). The lens is then placed in a bowl of BSS solution that is approximately body temperature. This makes the lens pliable. Once the lens is pliable, it is taken with the gloved hand, holding it between the index finger and thumb. The lens is then

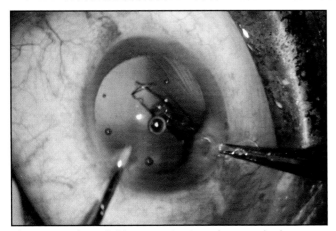

Figure 19. The rollable IOL going into the capsular bag.

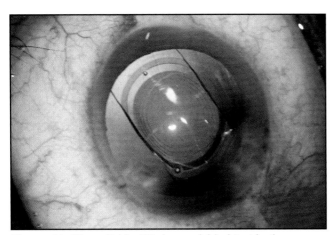

Figure 21. The rollable IOL has unfolded inside the eye on contact with the normal body temperature in the anterior chamber.

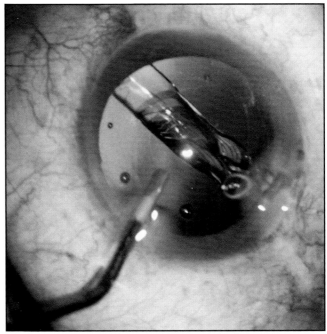

Figure 20. The rollable IOL in the capsular bag.

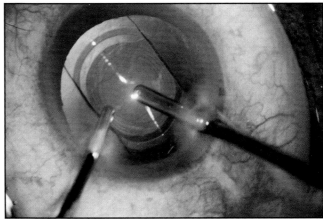

Figure 22. Viscoelastic removed using bimanual irrigation aspiration probes.

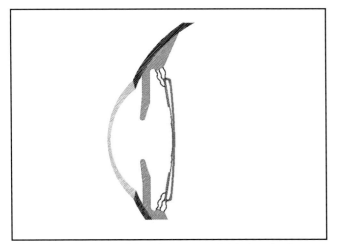

Figure 23. Diagram of the ThinOptX rollable lens in the posterior capsule.

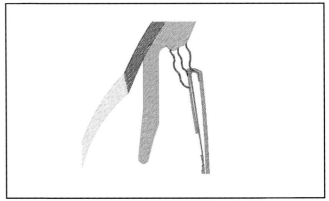

Figure 24. An enlargement of the ThinOptX lens positioned against the equator of the capsule. Note the plate haptics are thin enough to roll or curl, which reduces the pressure on the posterior capsule.

easily maneuverable. The optic size was reduced. ThinOptX now has a special new lens—a rollable IOL with a 5-mm optic for phakonit.

We were worried about the patient having glare and whether the cut edges of the lens would produce problems. When we saw the patient the next day, we noticed the patient had no glare and the lens reacted very well in the eye. This convinced us that the solution was to have a smaller-width lens.

We then checked the patient's topography and astigmatism. There is no point in having a lens go through a 1-mm incision and then still have problems of astigmatism. Phakonit is a tougher surgery to perform than phacoemulsification, so the surgeon should be convinced that it makes sense to shift into a smaller incision. When we saw the patient, there was no astigmatism. In phaco with a foldable IOL, we do see astigmatism. Topography was also done, but we need to perform more cases to document topographic changes in phakonit compared to phacoemulsification.

In conclusion, we need an instrument that will roll the lens and an injector without a cartridge. We are currently using a forceps, which can tear the lens. We have designed an injector that will roll the lens and insert it as well. Ideally, the rollable lens should be an accommodating or multifocal type of IOL so that we not only minimize astigmatism but also solve the problem of presbyopia.

REFERENCES

1. Agarwal S, Agarwal A, Sachdev MS, Mehta KR, Fine IH, Agarwal A. *Phacoemulsification, Laser Cataract Surgery & Foldable IOLs*. 2nd ed. New Delhi, India: Jaypee Brothers; 2000.
2. Boyd BF, Agarwal S, Agarwal A, Agarwal A. *LASIK and Beyond LASIK*. Panama: Highlights of Ophthalmology; 2000.

Chapter 23

The Accommodating Intraocular Lens

J. Stuart Cumming, MD

With careful biometry and by utilizing surgical techniques to reduce corneal cylinder, excellent uncorrected distance vision can be achieved with conventional intraocular lenses (IOLs). It is known that some patients can see well at distance and near postoperatively. This can be due to one or a combination of the following: myopia, corneal cylinder, small pupil, or the optic of the IOL moving forward upon ciliary muscle contraction. A movement of 1 mm of the optic can result in almost 2 diopters (D) of power change within the eye.

The development of an IOL that moves forward and backward along the axis of the eye in response to ciliary muscle contraction and relaxation, and implanted in combination with excellent biometry should allow many patients to function without glasses following cataract surgery.

DEVELOPMENT OF THE ACCOMMODATING AT-45 LENS

EARLY OBSERVATIONS WITH PLATE LENSES

In 1989, some patients I had implanted with plate haptic lenses and who were essentially plano stated that they could read without glasses. These patients were refracted with a maximum plus refraction and their reading ability evaluated in a dimly lit room with good lighting on the reading card. Examining the patients' reading abilities under these circumstances eliminated the possible reasons for pseudoaccommodation: myopia, cylinder, and small pupil. Despite this, a few of these patients could still read J2 or better. Their ability to read after eliminating the pseudoaccommodation factors suggested that perhaps the optic was moving forward, resulting in accommodation.

Ultrasonography was then utilized to scan 10 eyes of these patients, first with a cycloplegic and several days later with pilocarpine. The patients were all older than age 70. The A-scans demonstrated that the optic moved forward 0.7 mm on average following the application of pilocarpine to the eye. This observation suggested that the ciliary muscle may still be functioning in these elderly patients.

Slit lamp examination of patients implanted with plate lenses revealed that the lens optics were located deep within the capsular bag space, which is approximately 5.0 mm front-to-back in elderly patients. The center thickness of the plate lenses was 1.3 mm. At this time, I was implanting the posteriorly vaulted SI-18 lens from Allergan and the uniplanar plate lenses from Staar (VisX Inc, Santa Clara, Calif) and Chiron (Claremont, Calif), and noted that for the same eye the power selection for the plate lens was always between 1.0 and 1.5 D higher than the power selection for the posteriorly vaulted SI-18 lens. This suggested that there were forces acting within the eye that tended to move the optic of a plate lens posteriorly and that of the three-piece loop lens anteriorly. The optics of these two lenses were both made from silicone with the same refractive index of 1.41 and both were 6.0 mm in diameter. The A constants are 117.2 and 119.0 for the SI-18 loop lens and the plate lenses respectively, indicating a more posterior location along the axis of the eye for the plate lens optic.

Measurements of the vitreous cavity length pre- and postoperatively by A scan[1] demonstrated that the plate lens was consistently located in the posterior bag space and that in 50% (six eyes), the vitreous cavity was shortened postoperatively but was never lengthened by more than 0.77 mm, and the spread along the axis of the eye was 1.45 mm. By contrast, the vitreous cavity was only shortened in 20% of the eyes implanted with a loop lens, and its length increased by as much as 2.17 mm. The spread along the axis of the eye was 3.15 mm.

Since the plate lens optic was consistently located up against the vitreous face,[2,3] it was postulated that perhaps constriction of the ciliary muscle caused an increase in vitreous pressure. Adding further support to the supposition is the observation that slit lamp examination of aphakic patients before the introduction of IOLs frequently revealed a bulging of the vitreous face through the pupil upon accommodation.

These observations provoked an extensive literature search, which was conducted in 1989, revealing the following three significant references.

1955: BUSACCA[4]

Busacca, an Italian ophthalmologist practicing in Sao Paulo, Brazil, carefully examined a young, traumatically anaridic patient through the gonioscope, first with a cycloplegic and later with pilocarpine. Busacca made detailed drawings of the relative location and change in shape of the lens, ciliary body, and zonules. These drawings were reduced to a schematic form and overlayed with a grid. Careful examination of the drawings revealed that the ciliary muscle, like any other muscle in the body, redistributes its mass upon constriction and relaxation, that more muscle mass bulked into the vitreous cavity upon constriction, and that the insertion of the zonules into the lens and lens equator were also shown to have moved forward.

1986: COLEMAN[5]

Jackson Coleman cannulized the anterior chamber and vitreous cavities of 10 primates and directly stimulated the ciliary muscle. He demonstrated a simultaneous drop in pressure in the anterior chamber and increase in pressure in the vitreous cavity upon ciliary muscle constriction. These pressure changes can be explained by the observations made in Busacca's drawings showing bulking of the ciliary muscle into the vitreous cavity upon its constriction with reduction of its mass, anterior to the lens.

1986 AND 1991: THORNTON[6,7]

Spencer Thornton investigated in-the-bag implantation of 200 eyes with a polymethylmethacrylate (PMMA) lens with a 6.5 mm optic and loops angulated 7 degrees to give the lens an overall length of 13 mm. Postoperative accommodation of up to 1.5 D was noted in 20% of the eyes. Anterior movement of the optic was demonstrated by A-scans in two eyes upon accommodative effort.

THE FIRST ACCOMMODATING LENS DESIGNS

The first accommodating lens design was manufactured in 1990 and consisted of a plate lens with a 4.5 mm biconvex optic with a groove or hinge across the plate adjacent to the optic (Figure 1). The length of the lens was 10.5 mm, the same length as a standard plate lens. It was reasoned that by increasing the length of the plates, thereby reducing the optic size, there may be a greater mechanical advantage, allowing the optic to have greater movement upon possible changes in the vitreous pressure. Prior to selecting an optic size of 4.5 mm, the optical zone (the distance between the stakes of loop lenses where the loop is staked into the optic) was measured in five lens designs and found to be less than 5.0 mm in all cases.

The first lens was implanted in the United Kingdom on March 12, 1991 in an 85-year-old woman. Atropine 1% was applied at the time of surgery and postoperatively. Paralyzing the ciliary muscle should allow the optic to locate and fixate during fibrosis in the posterior part of the 5.0 mm empty bag space of an elderly patient. Without the atropine, it was postulated that ciliary muscle action, if it were to increase vitreous cavity pressure, may move the optic forward and possibly dislocate one or both of the plates from the capsular bag.

In 1991, Professor Jochen Kammann in Dortmund, Germany agreed to collaborate to clinically evaluate the accommodating lens design. In the early studies, a large capsulorrhexis was performed since it was postulated that the rhexis had to be larger than the optic to allow its forward movement. Ten eyes were implanted and all demonstrated accommodation by the fogging technique.

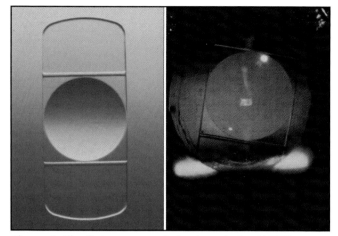

Figure 1. The first accommodating lens design (1990).

However, there was one decentration and more seriously, three lenses dislocated anteriorly; one of the plates of each implanted lens slipped out of the capsular bag and into the sulcus.

The second design (Figure 2), by the addition of centration fixation fingers on the distal ends of the plates, was configured to provide excellent centration and to fixate in the bag, thereby preventing anterior dislocation. The overall length of the lens was 11.5 mm. After designing the lens, a mold had to be made and lenses manufactured of different powers, sterilized, and packaged. After implantation in a limited number of patients, they had to be followed for several months to evaluate any possible complications and the patients' ability to accommodate and read through their distance correction. Changing the lens design and its clinical evaluation was a lengthy process.

The second design was implanted by Professor Kammann in 1993/4 (Figure 3). Twenty-four lenses were implanted. The average accommodative amplitude measured by fogging at 25 months postoperatively was 2.06 D. Centration was perfect; however, there were two anterior dislocations. Two eyes required YAG posterior capsulotomies; however, the accommodative amplitude was unchanged post-YAG.

A-scans were performed on 13 eyes implanted with the second design at an average of 12 months postoperatively, first with a cycloplegic and later with pilocarpine. This study demonstrated an average increase in the vitreous cavity length of 0.95 mm and average decrease in the anterior chamber depth of 1.0 mm upon the administration of pilocarpine, demonstrating anterior movement of the optic upon chemical stimulation of the ciliary muscle. It is estimated that approximately 1.0 mm of movement of a posteriorly vaulting plate lens will change the power of the eye by almost 2.0 D.

Eleven of these 24 eyes, in patients with an average age of 80 years, were examined at an average of 3.5 years postoperatively. The near vision through the distance correction was J3 or better in all cases, and the average accommodative amplitude by fogging was 2.0 D. One of these patients had a YAG posterior capsulotomy 9 months postoperatively.

Between 1994 and 1998, five additional accommodating lens designs were implanted by Professor Kammann. All designs had complications of either decentration or anterior vaulting with the exception of the seventh design (CrystaLens Model AT-45, C & C Vision, Aliso Viejo, Calif).

Second Design
1993/94

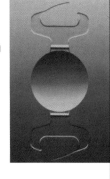

☞ **Implantations: 24**
☞ **Average accommodation**
    2.06 D @ 25 months
☞ **Decentrations: 0**
☞ **Dislocations: 2 (8%)**
☞ **Yag Capsulotomy: 2**
    1 @ 15 months
    1 @ 9 months

Figure 2. Second accommodating lens design (1993/1994).

THE MODEL AT-45

For the seventh design, polyimide loops were molded onto the distal ends of the plates to prevent anterior dislocation of the seventh design, which has an optical zone of 4.5 mm. The overall length of the lens, loop tip-to-loop tip, is 11.5 mm and plate end-to-plate end is 10.5 mm. Grooves or hinges extend across the plate adjacent to the optic. The lens is manufactured from BioSil, a proprietary, high refractive index, third-generation silicone made by C & C Vision.

The first CrystaLenses were implanted in Mexico and Germany in 1998. The design objective was to eliminate the lens dislocations reported with the previous designs while providing distance vision and an adequate accommodative amplitude to perform near and intermediate tasks.

In this trial, patients underwent standard cataract surgery with capsulorrhexis and phacoemulsification. The lens was implanted without folding through a 3.5 to 3.7 mm incision. Use of atropine for a period of 3 weeks following surgery was initially utilized to ensure that the lens was fixated in the most posterior position for distance vision and to provide perfect centration and stability. Since atropine paralyzes the ciliary muscle for 2 weeks, the muscle was paralyzed for 5 weeks. The atropine dosage was reduced over time to one drop instilled by the surgeon immediately following surgery and again on the first postoperative day, thereby eliminating the need for patient compliance. The patients were followed for 6 months with the objective of monitoring for dislocation and decentration.

SUMMARY

The centration of the CrystaLens has been excellent; there have been no dislocations, and the ability of the patients to see at near and intermediate through their distance correction has been variable but observed consistently in all patients, resulting in excellent patient satisfaction in more than 800 implants worldwide. Seventeen YAG capsulotomies have been reported with no effect on the ability of these patients to see at near through their distance correction post-YAG.

Yag Capsulotomy
2nd Design

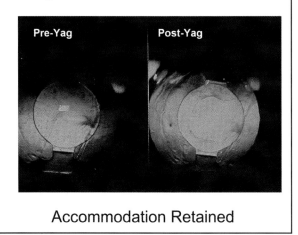

Accommodation Retained

Figure 3. Pre- and post-YAG capsulotomy with the second design, accommodation retained.

Despite the small optic size (4.5 mm), there have been no significant reports of glare with any of the accommodating IOL designs studied. This is probably due to three factors:

1. The deep placement of the optic within the eye
2. Excellent centration
3. The nonreflective nature of the third-generation silicone material BioSil

The results of this initial phase of study of the accommodating lens suggest that good uncorrected near, intermediate, and distance visual acuity can be achieved with the appropriate lens design in postoperative cataract patients. Phase II of the FDA clinical trial is currently under study.

While several approaches have been used with reasonable success to provide near vision in pseudophakic patients, none of the current modalities utilize the natural physiology of the ciliary muscle following cataract removal. The CrystaLens was specifically designed to allow the lens to move forward to provide near and intermediate vision upon ciliary muscle constriction.

Based on the extensive body of clinical data generated by over 30 ophthalmic surgeons who have implanted more than 800 lenses worldwide, the CrystaLens has provided excellent uncorrected vision for both distance, intermediate, and near in the majority of patients, reducing the need for spectacle correction.

REFERENCES

1. Cumming JS, Ritter J. The measurement of vitreous cavity length and its comparison pre- and postoperatively. *Eur J Implant Ref Surg.* 1994;6:261–272.
2. Cumming JS. Postoperative complications and uncorrected acuities after implantation of plate haptic silicone and three-piece silicone intraocular lenses. *J Cataract Refract Surg.* 1997;19:263–274.
3. Kammann J. Vitreous-stabilizing, single-piece, mini-loop, plate-haptic silicone intraocular lens. *J Cataract Refract Surg.* 1998;24:98–106.

4. Busacca A. La physiologie du muscle ciliaire etudiee par la gonio-scopie. *Annales D'Oculistique*. 1955;1–21.
5. Coleman J. On the hydraulic suspension theory of accommodation. *Trans Am Ophthalmol Soc*. 1986;846-868.
6. Thornton S. Lens implantation with restored accommodation. *Current Canadian Ophthalmic Practice*. 1986;4:60–62.
7. Thornton S. *Color Atlas of Lens Implantation*. Baltimore, Md: Williams & Wilkins; 1991:159–162.

Chapter 24

The C & C Vision CrystaLens Model AT-45 Silicone Intraocular Lens

Louis E. Probst, MD

INTRODUCTION

With an estimated 100 million Americans in the presbyopic age group, the surgical options for the correction of presbyopia have generated considerable interest. In fact, everyone will eventually become presbyopic, hence everyone is a potential surgical candidate. In general, this older population has more disposable income and can be more focused on "self improvement" as compared to younger patients with ongoing family concerns. These factors have prompted some to suggest that the ability to correct presbyopia is the "holy grail" of refractive surgery.[1]

EPIDEMIOLOGY OF PRESBYOPIA

Presbyopia is a slow chronic condition of indefinite onset. While the onset of presbyopia can range from early 40s to the early 80s, the prevalence can be considered 100% by the age of 50 if the eye's depth of focus in taken into account.[2] While age of onset has not been associated with gender, presbyopia may be noted sooner in patients of a shorter stature, as they have shorter arms. Early onset of presbyopia has been associated with diabetes, nonprescription drugs, ocular trauma, and living closer to the equator.[3]

OPTIONS FOR THE CORRECTION OF PRESBYOPIA

Despite the enormous market for the surgical correction of presbyopia, there has been variable success with surgical options to date. Many of the proposed procedures have experienced short-lived interest and abbreviated clinical trials. Other procedures, such as monovision correction with laser-assisted in situ keratomileusis (LASIK), laser thermal keratoplasty (LTK), multifocal lenses, and intrastromal lenses offer intermediate solutions by partially restoring the ability to read by altering that optical performance of the eye, rather than actually restoring accommodation. Anterior ciliary sclerostomy and scleral expansion bands attempt to actually restore accommodation by altering the relationship of the crystalline lens, the ciliary body, and the lens zonules.

Monovision can be prescribed with contact lenses or planned when performing LASIK for an associated refractive error. While monovision can be a very successful option, it is always presented as a compromise, as one eye will be used for either distance or near vision. Monovision is poorly tolerated by over 40% of patients[4] and increases the risk of night glare.

LTK was originally performed on the Sunrise Technologies system and now on the Hyperion holmium laser. It is able to correct 1 to 2 diopters (D) of spherical hyperopia. This procedure also induces a degree of multifocality to the cornea, which also improves the patient's near vision and therefore improves reading ability. Unfortunately, regression of this effect invariably occurs over the 1- to 3-year follow-up period.[5] Conductive keratoplasty (CK) is another type of thermal keratoplasty that has recently been tested in clinical trials with promising short-term results.

Multifocal intraocular lenses (IOLs) have been used to correct presbyopia alone by performing a refractive lensectomy or in conjunction with cataract extraction. This lens can be particularly attractive if the patient is also hyperopic. Proper patient selection is extremely important, as detail-oriented patients will be bothered by night glare and loss of contrast sensitively.[6] With explantation rates quoted as high as 10% by some surgeons for the Allergan Array multifocal lens, it is clear that further improvements will need to made for this to become a universally accepted form of presbyopia correction.

Intracorneal hydrogel lenses have been developed by Bausch & Lomb. This would allow a modified monovision with simultaneous near and distance focus in the nondominant eye. A 2-mm hydrogel lens would be inserted into the cornea. Previous studies have indicated that the cornea has a poor tolerance for intrastromal foreign bodies, and intracorneal lenses have been associated with a loss of best-corrected vision and irregular astigmatism, which may limit the success of this procedure.[7]

Anterior ciliary sclerostomy (ACS) has been proposed as another method for the correction presbyopia. Radial cuts in the sclera overlying the ciliary body allow the sclera to extend, which can increase the space between the crystalline lens and the ciliary body. While some initial reports have been good, this procedure has been largely abandoned because of loss of an effect with time.

Scleral expansion bands are the latest proposed procedure for the restoration of accommodation. This procedure is based on the

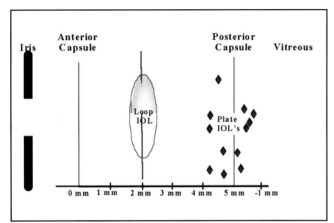

Figure 1. Location of plate haptic IOLs as compared to anterior and posterior lens capsule and the average position of a loop IOL (courtesy of J. Stuart Cumming, MD).

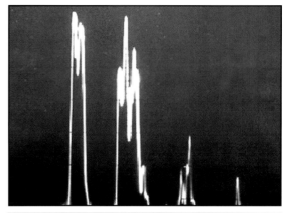

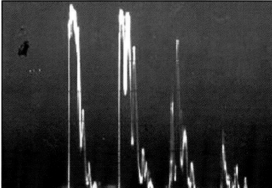

Figure 2. Change in the loop IOL position with ciliary body contraction. Top: A-scan after cycloplegia. Bottom: A-scan after pilocarpine. Note the movement to the left of the second echo indicating anterior movement of the loop IOL (courtesy of C & C Vision, Aliso Viejo, Calif, with permission from J. Stuart Cumming).

assumption that Helmholtz's theories of accommodation are incorrect and that the loss of accommodation is related to the decreased space between the ciliary body, sclera, and the crystalline lens. Experimental and clinical studies do not support this controversial theory of presbyopia; however, the initial reports of the procedure have noted some improvement in accommodation. Unfortunately, the results appear to be inconsistent and short-lived. One particularly concerning result of these clinical trials is the equal improvement in accommodation of the other nonoperated eye, suggesting that the improved accommodation may be more a result of the enhanced accommodative effort from the patient, rather than the surgical effect of the procedure.

THE ROLE OF THE CILIARY BODY IN ACCOMMODATION

Filling of the capsular bag with inflatable endocapsular balloons or in situ cured silicone polymeric gels has been evaluated in animal models to determine whether the accommodative properties of the natural crystalline lens can be replicated.[8-11] These studies presuppose the continued functionality of the ciliary muscle such that removal of a cataractous crystalline lens allows the ciliary muscle to respond to accommodative stimuli.

While there have been conflicting theories on whether the ciliary muscle atrophies with age, it has been shown in a series of published reports that the ciliary muscle not only maintains its strength through the aging process but experiences an increase in force.[12-15] This was demonstrated in a study designed to evaluate the ability of an artificial lens to restore accommodation in the senile eyes of rhesus monkeys, a species that experiences the presbyopic loss of accommodation.[16-18] In this study, the decrease in anterior chamber depth was significantly higher in the operated eyes of each rhesus monkey than in the contralateral control eye, which had not been implanted and failed to demonstrate any accommodative change. Recent studies using magnetic resonance imaging have shown only a slight loss of ciliary muscle contraction with increasing age in patients 80 or more years of age.[19]

Cumming (unpublished data, 2001), through clinical observation, noted that a small number of his cataract patients were able to

see at near through their distance correction after implantation with a plate haptic IOL. Plate haptic lenses are located against the vitreous face and have the ability to slightly flex forward (Figure 1). This observation suggested that there was an apparent ability of the ciliary muscle to move a plate haptic IOL forward and prompted Cumming to appreciate that even in presbyopes, the ciliary muscle may maintain some function and have the ability to move the optic of a carefully designed plate haptic IOL forward upon constriction. This would enable the patient to see at near.

BIRTH OF THE ACCOMMODATING IOL

ACCOMMODATION AND PSEUDOACCOMMODATION

It is known that a certain proportion of patients implanted with standard looped monofocal IOLs appear to have functional near vision without glasses following lens implantation. This effect can be attributed to either accommodation, pseudoaccommodation, or a combination of both. Accommodation would be the result of the optic of the IOL moving forward upon constriction of the ciliary muscle. In 1986, Thornton demonstrated by A-scans that the optic of a three-piece IOL could move forward during constriction of the ciliary muscle in some patients (Figure 2).[20-21]

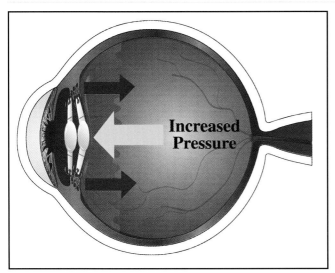

Figure 3. Redistribution of the ciliary muscle mass upon constriction with encroachment into the vitreous cavity (courtesy of C & C Vision, Aliso Viejo, Calif).

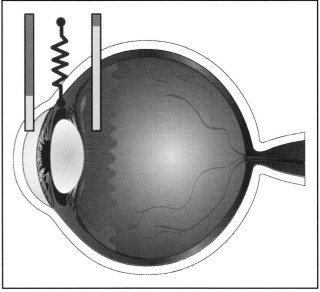

Figure 4. Pressure measurements of the aqueous and vitreous cavities during accommodation indicate a pressure rise in the vitreous cavity with comparatively little change in the aqueous pressure (courtesy of C & C Vision, Aliso Viejo, Calif).

Pseudoaccommodation would be due to one or a combination of the following:

+ Some degree of myopia
+ An aspheric cornea (ie, steep at 90 degrees)
+ A small pupil, resulting in increased depth of focus[22-26]

A literature search revealed that the ciliary muscle, upon constricting, undergoes a redistribution of its mass with encroachment into the vitreous cavity. This could provide vitreous pressure against the posterior lens surface, possibly inducing forward movement of an IOL[27] (Figure 3).

In 1986, Jackson Coleman demonstrated a slight decrease in pressure in the anterior chamber with a simultaneous increase in pressure in the vitreous cavity upon stimulation of the ciliary muscle in 10 primates[28] (Figure 4).

In a population of patients implanted with silicone plate lenses, when near vision was measured through the distance correction at the phoropter (effectively eliminating the pseudoaccommodative effects of myopia, small pupil size, and minus cylinder), a number of patients continued to have good near vision. This suggests that the action of the ciliary muscle alone may have been responsible for the ability of these patients to see at near (JS Cumming, unpublished data).

This hypothesis was further explored by performing A-scan measurements on these few patients who had near vision presumably resulting from action of the ciliary muscle. A-scan measurements were made following cycloplegia with tropicamide and compared to A-scans performed following the administration of pilocarpine. In a group of 10 patients with good distance-corrected near vision, A-scan measurements of the vitreous cavity were approximately 0.7 mm longer following pilocarpine administration than when performed after administration of tropicamide. These data serve to support the ability of the ciliary muscle to move a silicone plate haptic lens forward in a few carefully selected patients, as evidenced by the increased length of the vitreous cavity after treatment with pilocarpine. Further, since the other elements associated with pseudoaccommodation (ie, myopia, small pupil, minus cylinder) were eliminated as factors in providing near vision in these

patients by measuring corrected near acuity at the phoropter, it appeared that near vision may have resulted from action of the ciliary muscle on the vitreous body and lens (JS Cumming, unpublished data).

These findings are consistent with data reported by Hardman et al[29] and Niessen et al.[30] In two similar studies of pseudophakic accommodation, anterior chamber depth was decreased following pilocarpine administration, indicating forward movement of the IOL. While there was a significant difference in anterior chamber depths with pilocarpine as compared to cyclopentolate, the magnitude of this difference was reported to be approximately 0.2 to 0.25 mm, considerably smaller than the 0.7 mm change described previously. Because it has been reported that silicone plate haptic IOLs have a propensity toward posterior positioning or vaulting in the capsular bag, placing the optic up against the vitreous face,[31-33] it can be postulated that the potential magnitude of forward movement of a plate haptic lens is greater than that of a standard looped IOL.

This is further supported by the results of a study comparing the vitreous cavity lengths pre- and postoperatively in eyes implanted with silicone plate haptic lenses to those implanted with silicone multipiece looped lenses.[31] In this study, six (50%) of the 12 eyes implanted with a plate haptic lens had shorter vitreous cavity lengths postoperatively than preoperatively and all were located 0.75 mm or less closer to the position of the posterior capsule prior to surgery. In the eyes implanted with silicone loop lenses, there was shortening of the vitreous cavity in only two of the 10 eyes (20%). This consistent posterior displacement of the plate lens optic places it up against the vitreous face in the capsular bag following implantation and fibrosis, which results in posterior vaulting of the uniplanar plate lens.

Studies published in 1999 by Susan Strenk[34] demonstrated, by high-resolution MRIs (Figure 5), the redistribution of the ciliary body mass invading the vitreous cavity upon accommodation. This confirmed the findings in the drawings made by Busacca in 1955 on an anaridic patient.[27] These MRI images demonstrated ciliary muscle action in all ages, including an 83-year-old patient.

PLATE HAPTIC IOL EXPERIENCE

The concept for an accommodating IOL, a lens that would take advantage of the continued functionality of the ciliary muscle after cataract removal with resulting forward movement of the optic to provide good, consistent near vision, was developed by J. Stuart Cumming, MD. The concept was based on his observations of more than 2000 implanted plate haptic lenses. Cumming observed that these lenses always located in the posterior part of the capsular bag space, which is 5 mm from front to back, immediately after cataract surgery before fibrosis takes place.[31] This was demonstrated by measuring the vitreous cavity length prior to and following cataract surgery after implantation of silicone plate haptic lenses. Thus, the plate haptic design provides the maximal posterior positioning of the lens in the capsular bag space. This would allow the greatest potential forward movement of the lens upon constriction of the ciliary muscle.

Silicone plate lenses with a 6 mm optic were shown to vault posteriorly in the capsular bag space in all of the implanted eyes studied, decreasing the vitreous cavity length in 50% of the eyes.[31] Kammann reported posterior positioning in a substantially greater proportion of eyes (21 of 22, or 96%) implanted with silicone plate lenses with a 5 mm optic.[35] Since the overall haptic/optic length of the lenses in both of these studies was the same (10.5 mm), these data suggested that a smaller optic resulting in longer plate haptics may increase the likelihood of posterior vaulting of the lens with possibly greater potential forward movement of the optic upon ciliary body constriction.

As described above, the posterior position of silicone plate haptic lenses in the capsular bag has been established through pre- and postimplantation measurements of vitreous cavity lengths. For optimal performance of a lens intended to move forward to provide near vision, maximal posterior positioning is desirable. Since it is the action of the ciliary muscle that induces forward movement of the optic of the plate lens in the capsular bag, it was postulated that by eliminating the anterior-biasing force, maximum posterior positioning would be achieved. This was done by paralyzing the ciliary muscle during the early postoperative period when fibrosis of the capsular bag occurs.

On this basis, administration of atropine (1%) at the time of CrystaLens AT-45 silicone multipiece IOL surgery and at the first postoperative day has been proposed as a means of ensuring the maximum posterior positioning and fixation of the lens in the distance-focused and unaccommodated position up against the vitreous face.

Atropine lasts from 10 to 14 days. In addition to maximizing the posterior location of the accommodating IOL, it prevents dislocation during the period of fibrosis and allows excellent centration. During early studies of the initial accommodating lens models, one drop of atropine per day was applied to the eye for 3 weeks. Since patient compliance with this treatment regimen was a concern, a small substudy was conducted to evaluate the need for atropine. The results of this study revealed that atropine administration could

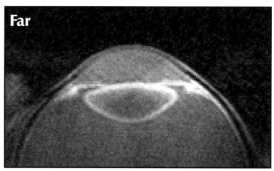

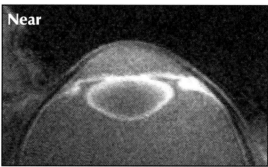

Figure 5. High-resolution MRI of the ciliary muscle. Top: Distance vision. Bottom: Accommodation. Note the posterior protrusion of the ciliary muscle into the vitreous cavity during accommodation[34] (courtesy of C & C Vision, Aliso Viejo, Calif, with permission from Strenk SA, Semmlow JL, Strenk LM, Munoz P, Gronlund-Jacob J, DeMarco JK. Age-related changes in human ciliary muscle and lens: a magnetic resonance imaging study. *Invest Ophthalmol Vis Sci.* 1999;40:1162-1169. © Association for Research in Vision and Ophthalmology).

be reduced to one drop at the time of surgery and one drop on the first day after surgery. This regimen addresses potential patient compliance issues since the surgeon or other personnel are responsible for the administration of atropine.

By allowing the lens to remain in the maximal posterior position, preventing forward movement during the period of fibrosis around the lens haptics, anterior vaulting could be avoided. It was also postulated that ciliary muscle action during the early postoperative period may be a cause of decentration and that centration would be facilitated by paralyzing the ciliary muscle. It occurred to Cumming during his experience with implanting standard silicone plate haptic lenses that because these lenses are only 1.3 mm thick, there is a very large space in front of the lens since the human lens is about 5.0 mm thick in elderly patients. Therefore, a hinge could be placed across the plate haptic near its junction with the optic, and the optic would have space to move anteriorly. The hinge was incorporated to facilitate the forward movement of the optic by minimizing the resistance to the possible pressure exerted on the lens by the forward movement of the vitreous body associated with contraction of the ciliary muscle.

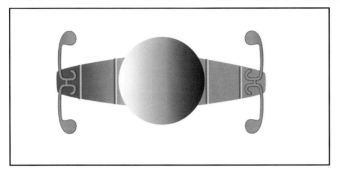

Figure 6. CrystaLens schematic.

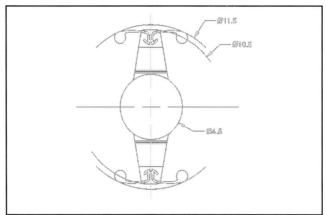

Figure 7. CrystaLens design and measurements.

DEVELOPMENT OF THE CRYSTALENS

DESCRIPTION

The C & C Vision CrystaLens (Figure 6) is a modified plate haptic lens manufactured from a high refractive index (RI = 1.430), third-generation nonreflective silicone material (BioSil), which contains an ultraviolet (UV) filter. The lens is hinged adjacent to the optic and has small looped polyimide haptics, which have been shown to fixate firmly in the capsular bag.[36] The grooves across the plates adjacent to the optic make the junction of the optic with the plate haptic the most flexible part of the haptic/optic design. The overall length of the lens is 11.5 mm (loop tip-to-loop tip measurement), while the overall length as measured from the ends of the plate haptics is 10.5 mm. The optic is biconvex and 4.5 mm in diameter. The A-constant is 119.0, and the lens is designed for placement into the capsular bag.

PRECLINICAL STUDIES

Extensive preclinical testing of the CrystaLens was conducted in accordance with internationally recognized standards for permanent implants. The CrystaLens IOL met all requirements for biocompatibility of medical devices. In addition, the CrystaLens was subjected to rigorous optical and mechanical testing in accordance with the guidelines of the US Food and Drug Administration (FDA) for IOLs. In each test, 10 sterile, finished lenses each of low (18.5 D), midrange (23.0), and high diopters (25.0) were evaluated. Compression force at 10 mm (immediate and after decay), axial displacement (immediate and after force decay), and angle of contact were all characterized for the CrystaLens in accordance with FDA guidelines as well as internationally recognized standards for IOLs (Figure 7).

DURABILITY OF THE CRYSTALENS

The third-generation silicone material (BioSil) used in the manufacture of the CrystaLens has been extensively evaluated to determine its ability to withstand the multiple flexions that will result from the repeated changes of focus during normal functioning of an eye implanted with this lens. A movement of 1 mm can provide up to 2 D of added power, which is equivalent to the power of a standard bifocal in a pair of glasses. The number and extent of accommodative cycles that the eye experiences during the course of a day is difficult to estimate. However, in an analysis conducted by Arthur P. Little, it was estimated that the average frequency of accommodation is probably on the order of 20 to 120 per hour (one cycle every 3 minutes to one every 30 seconds). Assuming that an average person is awake 16 hours per day, the range would be from 20 cycles per hour (120,000 per year) to 120 cycles per hour (720,000 per year). With a fatigue lifetime exceeding 20 million cycles, it has been roughly estimated that the CrystaLens should last a minimum of 30 years and probably much longer.

DISTANCE-CORRECTED NEAR VISION: AT-45 IOL VS MULTIFOCAL AND MONOFOCAL IOLS

Previous IOL studies have reported the distance-corrected near vision results, which make for interesting comparisons. Steinert et al[37] reported the results for the Array multifocal silicone IOL (Allergan Surgical, Irvine, Calif) from a multicenter trial involving 456 patients. Eighty-six percent of eyes were able to read 20/30 (J3) or better uncorrected as compared to 96% of the eyes implanted with the AT-45 IOL.[38] In this same study, the monofocal control group had an uncorrected near vision of 20/30 in just 49% of eyes. A similar study of 671 patients with the previous model of the multifocal IOL found that 50% of eyes with the multifocal IOL and 26% of eyes with the standard monofocal lens had an uncorrected near acuity of 20/30 or better.[39] These results were very similar to the distance-corrected near vision results (Table 1). These studies suggest that the AT-45 performs better for distance-corrected near vision when compared to the other IOL alternatives.

POTENTIAL COMPLICATIONS ASSOCIATED WITH THE AT-45 IOL

Breakthrough technology is rarely introduced without clinical challenges. As previously discussed, the early models of the accommodating IOL were associated with unacceptable rates of dislocations and decentrations. The design changes in the later modes of the lens have improved the safety profile of the lens significantly. Centration has been excellent, there have been no dislocations, and the ability of the patients to see at near and intermediate through their distance correction has been variable but observed

TABLE 1	COMPARISON OF UCNA AND DCNA FOR THE AT-45, MULTIFOCAL, AND MONOFOCAL IOLs			
	AT-45 Accommodating IOL[38]	Array Multifocal IOL[37]	Monofocal IOL[37]	Monofocal IOL[39]
Eyes J3 or better UCNA	96%	86%	49%	38%
Eyes J3 or better DCNA	97%	81%	48%	37%

UCNA = uncorrected near acuity; DCNA = distance-corrected near acuity

consistently in all patients, resulting in excellent patient satisfaction in more than 800 implants worldwide.

GLARE AND LOSS OF CONTRAST SENSITIVITY

Glare and contrast sensitivity were tested in a comparative study reported at the American Society for Cataract and Refractive Surgery (ASCRS) 2001 meeting in San Diego, Calif, conducted by Michael Colvard, MD, one of the principal investigators in the US multicenter clinical trial of the CrystaLens. Glare and contrast sensitivity were measured in 10 CrystaLens-implanted eyes (mean age = 75.7 years), 10 eyes (average age = 72 years) implanted with a silicone multifocal IOL with a 6.0 mm optic, and 10 eyes (mean age = 75.3 years) implanted with a 6.0 mm monofocal acrylic IOL. The mean follow-up was 1 year. Test results were independently analyzed by leading contrast vision expert Arthur Ginsburg, PhD of the Vision Science Research Group in San Ramon, Calif.

Since the patients were all in the older cataract age group, the pupils in the AT-45 group all measured 6.0 mm or less. The AT-45 IOL performed at the same level as the monofocal silicone IOLs and better than the multifocal Array IOL on the contrast sensitivity testing. Similarly, the AT-45 and the monofocal IOL patients reported no severe halos on glare testing, while the two patients in the Array group reported this problem. One patient in the AT-45 IOL group complained of moderate difficulty with night driving compared to none in either of the other groups. Therefore, it appears that the small 4.5 mm optic does not introduce major glare problems in patients with pupils 6.0 mm or less, however the night driving problem requires further study.

Zaldivar reported two eyes with halos from a total of 25 eyes with 1 to 6 months follow-up (R. Zaldivar, unpublished data). Infrared analysis of these eyes indicated that the halos were noted only in the eyes with fibrosis of the anterior capsule.

Despite the small 4.5 mm optic size, there have been minimal reports of glare with any of the accommodating IOL designs studied. This is probably due to three factors:

1. The deep placement of the optic within the eye
2. Excellent centration
3. The nonreflective nature of the third-generation silicone material

Stephen Slade, MD, the medical monitor for the C & C Vision US multicenter clinical trial of the CrystaLens, postulates that the lens is so retroplaced that its 4.5 mm optic is actually equivalent to a 5.8 or 5.9 mm optic of a lens located in the anterior capsular bag space.

OPACIFICATION OF THE POSTERIOR CAPSULE

Opacification of the posterior capsule was noted in two of the 28 eyes followed for 2 years by Chayet (AS Chayet, unpublished data, 2001). YAG capsulotomies were performed without complications or a loss on the near vision. Seventeen YAG capsulotomies have been reported worldwide with no effect on the ability of these patients to see at near through their distance correction post-YAG.

LONG-TERM EFFECTIVENESS

Although results of ongoing clinical trials are still preliminary, visual performance following implantation of the CrystaLens has been excellent. As previously reported, in the 11 eyes (average patient age = 80 years) implanted by Professor Kammann with the second design, distance and near vision remain unchanged from previous examinations 3.5 years after implantation, and all patients read J3 or better through their distance correction. A-scans on 11 of these eyes before and after pilocarpine demonstrated anterior movement of the optic of approximately 1.0 mm 12 months postoperatively. In the multicenter clinical trials conducted in Mexico, 14 bilateral patients (average age = 71 years) implanted with the CrystaLens by Arturo Chayet, MD, 100% (14/14) of the patients are seeing 20/40 or better uncorrected distance and J3 or better at near; 70% (11/14) had 20/30 or better uncorrected distance and J3 or better at near 2 years after surgery. In the US multicenter clinical trials, 98% (41/42) of the patients are seeing 20/25 or better with their corrected distance vision and 93% (39/42) J3 or better through their distance correction at near 11 months or longer after surgery. In addition, A-scans have demonstrated anterior movement of the optic, and retinal wavefront power maps have shown power changes of up to 3.0 D.

THEORETICAL CONCERNS

Potential complications that have not been reported but could occur include "hinge fatigue" and capsular fibrosis. Hinge fatigue would result after years of accommodation that could result in a loss of the flexibility of the AT-45 hinge or perhaps a breakdown at the hinge location. Hinge fatigue has not been noted to be a problem with the international experience with the AT-45 IOL during up to 3.5 years of follow-up. Capsular fibrosis could result in anterior movement of the IOL, causing a shift in the refraction to -2.5 D of myopia. Conversely, a decrease in the diameter of the capsular bag could result in posterior lens movement and subsequent hyperopia. To date, shifts in the postoperative refraction due to lens movement have not been reported.

CONCLUSIONS

While several approaches have been used with reasonable success to provide near vision in pseudophakic patients, none of the current modalities utilize the natural physiology of the ciliary muscle following cataract removal. The C & C Vision CrystaLens IOL was specifically designed to allow the lens to move forward to provide near and intermediate vision upon ciliary muscle constriction.

Irrespective of the possible mechanistic basis for the translational movement of the accommodating IOL in the eye, the early clinical findings following lens implantation show that an IOL designed to move forward and backward upon ciliary muscle constriction and relaxation provides substantial functional distance, intermediate, and near vision in pseudophakic patients. Subsequent clinical studies on the CrystaLens have demonstrated excellent near and intermediate visual acuity measured through the distance correction without an add. In nearly all implanted eyes, the uncorrected and distance-corrected near acuity improved substantially in these cataract patients. Uncorrected distance visual acuities were also excellent, with more than 90% of patients having distance acuities of 20/40 or better. Based on the extensive body of clinical data generated by over 30 ophthalmic surgeons who have implanted more than 800 lenses worldwide, the CrystaLens has provided excellent uncorrected vision for both distance, intermediate, and near in the majority of patients, reducing their need for spectacle correction.

REFERENCES

1. Lindstrom RL. The future of refractive surgery. II Horizon Technology. *Refractive Eyecare for Ophthalmologists*. 2001;May:5-10.
2. Hamasaki D, Ong J. Marg E. The amplitude of accommodation in presbyopia. *American Journal of Optometry and Archives of the American Academy of Optometry*. 1956;30:3-14.
3. Miranda MN. The environment in the onset of presbyopia. In: Stark LW, Obrecht G, eds. *Presbyopia*. New York: Fairchild Publications; 1987:19-27.
4. Erickson DB, Erickson P. Psychological factors and sex differences in acceptance of monovision. *Percept Mot Skills*. 2000; 91(3Pt2):1113-9.
5. Attia W, Perez-Santonja JJ, Alio JL. Laser in situ keratomileusis for recurrent hyperopia following laser thermal keratoplasty. *J Refract Surg*. 2000;16(2):163-9.
6. Leyland M, Zinicola E. Multifocal versus monofocal intraocular lenses after cataract extraction. *Cochrane Database Syst Rev*. 2001;3:31-69.
7. Steinert RF, Storie B, Smith P, et al. Hydrogel intracorneal lenses in aphakic eyes. *Arch Ophthalmol*. 1996;114(2):135-41.
8. Nishi O, Nakai Y, Yamagda Y, Mizumoto Y. Amplitudes of accommodation of primate lenses refilled with two types of inflatable endocapsular balloons. *Arch Ophthalmol*. 1993;111:1677-1684.
9. Hara T, Sakka Y, Sakanishi K, et al. Complications associated with endocapsular balloon implantation in rabbit eyes. *J Cataract Refract Surg*. 1994;20:507-512.
10. Parel J, Gelender H, Trefers W, Norton E. Phaco-ersatz: cataract surgery designed to preserve accommodation. *Graefes Arch Clin Exp Ophthalmol*. 1986;224:165-173.
11. Haefliger E, Parel J, Fantes F, et al. Accommodation of an endocapsular silicone lens (phako-ersatz) in the nonhuman primate. *Ophthalmology*. 1987;94:471-477.
12. Fisher R. The force of contraction of the human ciliary muscle during accommodation. *J Physiol*. 1977;270:51-74.
13. Fisher R. The mechanics of accommodation in relation to presbyopia. In: Stark L, Obrecht G, eds. *Recent Research and Reviews from the Third International Symposium*. New York: Professional Press; 1987:42-4.
14. Fisher R. The mechanics of accommodation in relation to presbyopia. *Eye*. 1988;2:646-649.
15. Fisher R. The ciliary body in accommodation. *Transactions of the Ophthalmology Society UK*. 1986;105:208-219.
16. Glasser A, Kaufman PL. The mechanism of accommodation in primates. *Ophthalmology*. 1999;106:863-872.
17. Bito L, DeRousseau C, Kaufmann P, Bito J. Age dependent loss of accommodative amplitude in rhesus monkeys: an animal model for presbyopia. *Invest Ophthalmol Vis Sci*. 1982;23:23-31.
18. Haefliger E, Parel J. Accommodation of an endocapsular silicone lens (phako-ersatz) in the aging rhesus monkey. *Journal of Refractive Corneal Surgery*. 1994;10:550-555.
19. Strenk SA, Semmlow JL, Strenk LM, Munoz P, Gronlund-Jacob J, DeMarco JK. Age-related changes in human ciliary muscle and lens: a magnetic resonance imaging study. *Invest Ophthalmol Vis Sci*. 1999;40(6):1162-1169.
20. Thornton S. Lens implantation with restored accommodation. *Current Canadian Ophthalmic Practice*. 1986;4:60–62.
21. Thornton S. *Color Atlas of Lens Implantation*. Baltimore, Md: Williams & Wilkins; 1991:159–162.
22. Huber C. Planned myopic astigmatism as a substitute for accommodation in pseudophakia. *American Intraocular Implant Society*. 1981;7:244.
23. Huber C. Myopic astigmatism as a substitute for accommodation in pseudophakia. *Doc Ophthalmol*. 1981;52:123.
24. Nakazawa N, Ohtsuki K. Apparent accommodation in pseudophakic eyes after implantation of posterior chamber intraocular lenses. *Am J Ophthalmol*. 1983;96:435-438.
25. Trindade F, Oliveira A, Frasson M. Benefit of against-the-rule astigmatism to uncorrected near acuity. *J Cataract Refract Surg*. 1997;23:82–85.
26. Percival S. Prospectively randomized trial comparing the pseudoaccommodation of the AMO Array multifocal lens and a monofocal lens. *J Cataract Refract Surg*. 1993;19:26–31.
27. Busacca A. La physiologie du muscle ciliaire etudiee par la gonioscopie. *Annales D'Oculistique*. 1955;1–21.
28. Coleman DJ. On the hydraulic suspension theory of accommodation. *Transactions of the American Ophthalmology Society*. 1986;84:846-68.
29. Hardman Lea S, Rubinstein M, Snead M, Haworth S. Pseudophakic accommodation? A study of the stability of capsular bag supported, one piece, rigid tripod, or soft flexible implants. *Br J Ophthalmol*. 1990;74:22-25.
30. Niessen A, De Jong L, Van der Heijde G. Pseudoaccommodation in pseudophakia. *European Journal of Implant amd Refractive Surgery*. 1992;4:91-94.
31. Cumming JS, Ritter J. The measurement of vitreous cavity length and its comparison pre- and postoperatively. *European Journal of Implant amd Refractive Surgery*. 1994;6:261–272.
32. Colin J. Clinical results of implanting a silicone hapticanchor-plate intraocular lens. *J Cataract Refract Surg*. 1996;2:1286–1290.
33. Cumming JS. Postoperative complications and uncorrected acuities after implantation of plate haptic silicone and three-piece silicone intraocular lenses. *J Cataract Refract Surg*. 1997;19:263–274.
34. Strenk SA. Age-related changes in human ciliary muscle and lens: a magnetic resonance imaging study. *Invest Ophthalmol Vis Sci*. 1999;40:6.
35. Kammann J. Vitreous-stabilizing, single-piece, mini-loop, plate-haptic silicone intraocular lens. *J Cataract Refract Surg*. 1998;24:98–106.
36. Kent D, Peng Q, Isaacs R, Whiteside S, Barker D, Apple D. Mini-haptics to improve capsular fixation of plate haptic silicone intraocular lenses. *J Cataract Refract Surg*. 1998;24:666–671.
37. Steinert RF, Aker BL, Tentacost DJ, et al. A prospective comparative study of the AMO Array zonule-progressive multifocal silicone intraocular lens and monofocal intraocular lens. *Ophthalmology*. 1999;106:1243-1255.

38. Cumming JS, Slade SG, Chayet AC, et al. Clinical evaluation of the model AT-45 silicone accommodating intraocular lens. *Ophthalmology.* 2001;108:2005-2010.
39. Lindstrom RL. Food and Drug Administration study update. One year results from 671 patients with the 3M multifocal intraocular lens. *Ophthalmology.* 1993;100:91-7.

BIBLIOGRAPHY

Coleman DJ. Unified model for the accommodative mechanism. *Am J Ophthalmol.* 1970;69:1063-79.

Coleman DJ, Fish SK. Presbyopia, accommodation, and the mature cataract. *Ophthalmology.* 2001;108-1554-1551.

Donders FC. *On the Anolomolies of Accommodation and the Refraction of the Eye.* London: New Sydenham Society; 1864:25-26.

Fincham E. The mechanism of accommodation. *Br J Ophthalmol.* 1937;8:1-9.

Glasser A, Campbell MCW. Biometric, optical and physical changes in the isolated human crystalline lens with age in relation to presbyopia. *Vision Res.* 1999;39:1991-2015.

Glasser A, Campbell MCW. Presbyopia and the optical changes in the human crystalline lens with age. *Vision Res.* 1998;38(2):209-229.

Koretz JF, Handelman GH. Modeling age-related accommodative loss in the human eye. *Math Model.* 1986;7:1003-1014.

Schachar RA. Zonular function: a new hypothesis with clinical implications. *Annals of Ophthalmology.* 1994;26:36-8.

Schachar RA, Cudmore DP. The effect of gravity on the amplitude of accommodation. *Annals of Ophthalmology.* 1994;26:65-70.

Thornton SP. Anterior ciliary sclerostomy (ACS), a procedure to reverse presbyopia. In: Sher N, ed. *Surgery for Hyperopia and Presbyopia.* Baltimore, Md: Williams & Wilkins; 1997:33-36.

Tschering MHE. *Physiological Optics: Dioptrics of the Eye, Functions of the Retina, Ocular Movements, and Binocular Vision.* 2nd ed. Philadelphia, Pa: Keystone; 1904:160-89.

Von Helmholtz H. Uber die akkommodation des auges. Albreckt von Graefes. *Arch Ophthalmol.* 1985;1:89.

Werblin TP. Discussion of Cumming JS, Slade SG, Chayet AC, et al. Clinical evaluation of the model AT-45 silicone accommodating intraocular lens. *Ophthalmology.* 2001;108:2011.

Chapter 25

The HumanOptics Akkommodative 1CU Intraocular Lens

Restoring Accommodation in the Pseudophakic Patient

Gregory J. Pamel, MD

Surgical treatments addressing presbyopia in the human eye have involved multiple modalities with variable results. These have included scleral expansion surgery using silicone bands,[1,2] laser presbyopia reversal using a solid-state laser,[3] photorefractive keratectomy,[4] implantation of multifocal posterior chamber IOLs,[5,6] and corneal inlays.[7]

In the cataract patient population, multifocal and bifocal implants[5,6] have been used to provide improvement in near vision after surgery without true restoration of accommodation. Experimental techniques, such as "phaco ersatz," involve endocapsular cataract surgery with the injection of a pliable silicone polymer.[8,9] This technique is currently being studied as a method to restore pseudophakic accommodation. The C & C Vision AT-45 accommodating lens, currently undergoing US clinical trials, has shown early success in restoring accommodation in the pseudophakic patient.[10]

HumanOptics is a company based in Erlangen, Germany and has developed a novel, pseudophakic intraocular foldable implant—the HumanOptics Akkommodative 1CU lens—designed to correct both distance and near vision based on Helmholtz's theory.

According to Helmholtz,[11,12] accommodation occurs when the ciliary muscle contracts, resulting in relaxation of the zonular attachments to the natural crystalline lens. With the relaxation of the zonules, the lens assumes a more spherical shape, leading to an increase in the dioptric power of the lens and resulting in near objects coming into focus on the retinal plane. When accommodation ceases, the relaxation of the ciliary muscle results in an increase in tension in the zonules with a resultant flattening in the shape of the lens and a subsequent reduction in its dioptric power. This brings distant objects into focus on the retinal plane.

MECHANISM OF ACTION OF THE AKKOMMODATIVE 1CU IMPLANT

The principle behind the Akkommodative 1CU lens is based on the fact that the ciliary muscle continues to function even after the removal of the natural crystalline lens. Ultrasound and magnetic resonance imaging studies have shown that ciliary muscle contraction continues to take place in most patients, even in those over the age of 80.[2,13] Presbyopia is mainly caused by age-related changes in the lens and lens capsule. The lens hardens as it ages and the lens capsule loses its elasticity. Both of these factors lead to a lens that loses its ability to change shape as it ages.[11]

The Akkommodative 1CU was developed on the basis of the work done by Khalil Hanna, MD using finite element computer models. It is a hydrophyllic acrylic lens with a refractive index of 1.46 with an integrated ultraviolet (UV) inhibitor. The lens has four square edge dynamic transition elements with an overall diameter of 9.8 mm and a biconvex optic of 5.5 mm (Figure 1). It comes in a diopter (D) range of +16 to 26.0 D, in 0.5 D increments. The lens functions by dynamic transition elements that enable the optical power of the lens to change during accommodation.[14-16]

With the Akkommodative 1CU inserted into the bag, stimulus of accommodation leads to contraction of the ciliary muscle and relaxation of the zonules. The resultant mechanical energy stored in the capsular bag is transmitted to the implant during accommodation (Figure 2). This leads to a specific posterior deformation of the implant that increases its optical power, allowing near objects to focus on the retina. When accommodation ends, the ciliary muscle relaxes and zonular tension increases (Figure 3). The capsular bag is stretched and the Akkommodative IOL returns to its unaccommodative state. This results in distant objects being focused on the retina.

SURGICAL TECHNIQUE

Preoperatively, calculation of the implant power is done using standard A-scan biometry.

Intraoperatively, a continuous curvilinear capsulorrhexis is performed through a 3 mm scleral tunnel incision. Two stab incisions are made under viscoelastic to allow a lens hook to unfold the wings of the haptics in the capsular bag after implantation.

The implant is inserted through a 3.2 mm incision using a foldable injector. A small amount of viscoelastic is injected into the tunnel and onto the loading chamber of the cartridge (Figure 4). The lens comes packaged in a sterile container filled with saline. After the lens is removed from the saline, it is placed in the loading chamber of the cartridge with the hooks located at the extremities of the haptics and facing up.

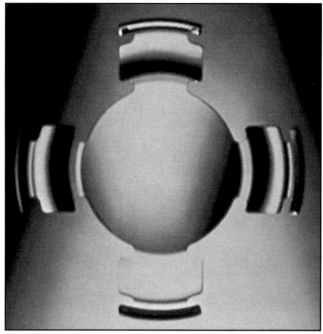

Figure 1. The HumanOptics Akkommodative 1CU lens.

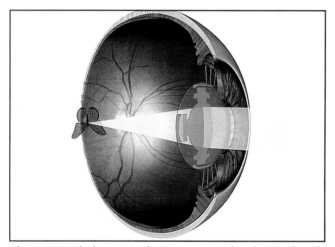

Figure 3. With the eye in the unaccommodated state, the ciliary muscle relaxes and the zonules contract, resulting in a posterior displacement of the Akkommodative 1CU IOL. This allows objects at distance to be focused on the retina.

The lens is placed in the cartridge so that the folding axis is respected. The folding axis positions the haptics on either side of the center of the loading chamber. A forceps is used to apply parallel pressure to fold the lens, and the cartridge is then closed. The forceps are slowly removed and used to place the haptics into the loading chamber. The wings of the haptics are then closed and the cartridge is placed in the injector (Figure 5). The cartridge must be in the correct position so that the tunnel runs parallel to the tip of the injector. The lens is ready to be injected into the eye by slowly depressing the plunger of the injector to force the lens in the tunnel of the cartridge.

Once the tip of the cartridge is placed within the anterior chamber, the lens is injected into the capsular bag and allowed to unfold. The optic will unfold slowly, but the haptics will usually require

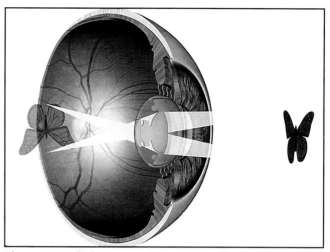

Figure 2. With the eye in the accommodative state, the ciliary muscle contracts and the zonules relax, resulting in a forward displacement of the Akkommodative 1CU IOL. This allows near objects to be focused on the retina.

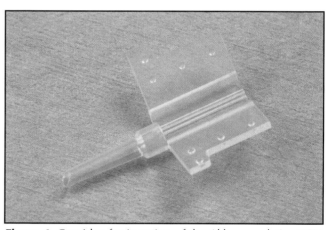

Figure 4. Cartridge for insertion of the Akkommodative 1CU IOL.

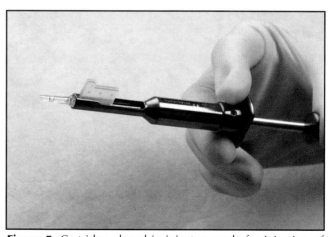

Figure 5. Cartridge placed in injector, ready for injection of the Akkommodative 1CU IOL.

TABLE 1   *RESULTS OF THE AKKOMMODATIVE 1CU AFTER 6 MONTHS**

	Far Distance Acuity		
	Range	*Mean*	*Average*
BCDVA	0.63 to 1.25	1.0	1.0
UCDVA	0.4 to 1.0	0.4	0.61
	Near Distance Acuity		
NVA with BCDVA	0.2 to 0.6	0.3	0.34
Near point accommodation (D)	0.5 to 2.2		1.69
Near point accommodation (cm)	39 to 200		59

*University of Erlangen-Nuremberg, first 12 patients implanted with Akkommodative 1CU by Dr. Michael Küchle
BCDVA = best-corrected distance visual acuity; UCDVA = uncorrected distance visual acuity; NVA = near visual acuity

unfolding, which can be achieved by injecting viscoelastic on the optic or by using a lens hook. The lens hook is used to unfold the wings of the haptics into the capsular bag, creating four-point fixation of the implant.

INITIAL RESULTS

To date, more than 300 Akkommodative 1CUs have been successfully implanted in Germany, Italy, France, and Japan.[15] Most of the lens implantations have been performed by Küchle at the University Eye Hospital in Erlangen-Nuremberg. These lenses have been implanted after approval was granted from the human studies committee at the University of Erlangen-Nuremberg. This meant that only one eye received the implant for the initial study.[15]

HumanOptics reported the results in their own publication of the first 12 patients with 6 months follow-up who had the 1CU implanted by Küchle at the University of Erlangen-Nuremberg.[14] As Table 1 indicates, near point of accommodation ranged from 0.5 to 2.2 D with a mean of 1.69 D. Best-corrected distance visual acuity ranged from approximately 20/30 to 20/16. Near visual acuity when distance acuity was best corrected averaged 0.3 to 0.4 on the Birkhäuser reading charts and J2-3 in patients ranging in ages from 45 to 87 years old. Unlike Jaeger cards, Birkhäuser reading charts require the patient to read actual text as opposed to random letters. These values of accommodation and reading vision will most likely change when both eyes of the same patient receive the implant.

Küchle et al independently reported the first six patients with 1CU HumanOptics IOLs with at least 3 months follow-up.[17] There were no intraoperative complications with successful in-the-bag implantation and good centration in all cases. The lens underwent rigorous biocompatibility testing in accordance with international standards and passed all tests. Tyndallometry revealed lower cell and flare results than other IOLs.

Investigators at University of Erlangen-Nuremberg used static and dynamic methods of measuring accommodation with this implant.[18] Objective static methods included ultrasound biomicroscopy, autorefraction, wavefront analysis, and the measurement of the anterior chamber depth using the Zeiss IOL Master. Subjective static methods included subjective refraction techniques measuring the eye in the accommodative and unaccommodative

states after pharmacological stimulation with pilocarpine and atropine, respectively. Dynamic methods of measuring accommodation include objective dynamic streak retinoscopy and subjective measurements of near point of accommodation and defocus techniques using minus spheres.[18]

Ultrasound biomicroscopy demonstrated forward movement of the 1CU during accommodation. Wavefront aberrometry was used to demonstrate a change in higher-order aberrations from the unaccommodative to the accommodative state. While the phakic eye was accommodating to a near target, the implanted eye underwent wavefront measurements.[18] Future studies will need to be done to assess the reliability of this method of measuring accommodation.

An alternative way of objectively measuring accommodation is using the Zeiss IOL Master. This instrument can measure anterior chamber depth in the accommodative and unaccommodative state. Accommodation was induced by instilling pilocarpine 2%, waiting 30 minutes, and then measuring anterior chamber depth. The unaccommodative state was induced by instilling atropine 1%, waiting 30 minutes, and then measuring the anterior chamber depth. A change of anterior chamber depth of 1.35 mm was measured from the unaccommodative to the accommodative state in the initial series of 12 patients who received the implant in one eye only. This resulted in 1.65 D of accommodation per millimeter of change in anterior chamber depth.[14,18]

Streak retinoscopy was used to measure accommodation. A difference between retinoscopic near and distance refraction of 0.625 to 1.875 D was measured in this group of patients.[17] Subjective measurement of accommodation was carried out using the defocus minus sphere method. With best-corrected visual acuity at distance, minus spheres were placed in front of the eye in 0.5 D increments until the 20/40 line became blurred. With this method, near points of accommodation ranged from 0.5 to 2.2 D. Using the push-up method, near points of accommodation between 40 to 100 cm were measured in all patients. A larger prospective study involving 33 eyes was submitted for publication at the time of this writing. Similar results were reported by Küchle in this group of patients.[19]

Capsular opacification rates have yet to be determined in this small series of patients. However, preliminary reports from the company indicate that in 40 patients with greater than 1 year of follow-up, there were no lens epithelial cells noted in the optical zone, causing opacification of the capsule.[15]

The Akkommodative 1CU IOL appears to show great promise from early studies to be a novel way to restore some accommodative function in pseudophakic patients. Additional larger multicenter clinical trials will need to address several issues and will begin after the time of this publication in seven sites in Europe. Standardized measurements of accommodation need to be performed in these larger, multicenter clinical trials both monocularly and binocularly to determine the effectiveness of this lens in those respective conditions. Posterior capsular opacification rates will need to be determined, although preliminary reports from the company indicate that they are low. Lens centration, contrast sensitivity, and subjective glare and halo measurements will also have to be studied in these larger series of patients.

REFERENCES

1. Matthews S. Scleral expansion surgery does not restore accommodation in human presbyopia. *Ophthalmology*. 1999;106:873-877.
2. Schachar RA. Cause and treatment of presbyopia with a method for increasing the amplitude of accommodation. *Annals of Ophthalmology*. 1992;24:445-447.
3. Angelucci D. Laser retreatment designed to reverse presbyopia. *Eye World*. 2001;6:5.
4. Vinciguerra P, Nizzola GM, Nizzola F, Ascarii A, Azzolini M, Epstein D. Zonal photorefractive keratectomy for presbyopia. *J Refract Surg*. 1998;14(2Suppl):18-21.
5. Allen ED, Burton RL, Webber SK, et al. Comparison of a diffractive and a monofocal intraocular lens. *J Cataract Refract Surg*. 1996;22:446-451.
6. Gray PJ, Lyall MG. Diffractive multifocal intraocular lens implants for unilateral cataracts in prepresbyopic patients. *Br J Ophthalmol*. 1992;76:336-337.
7. Keates RH, Martines E, Tennen DG, Reich C. Small-diameter corneal inlay in presbyopic or pseudophakic patients. *J Cataract Refract Surg*. 1995;21:519-521.
8. Haefliger E, Parel JM. Accommodation of an endocapsular silicone lens (phaco-ersatz) in the aging rhesus monkey. *J Refract Corneal Surg*. 1994;10:550-555.
9. Nishi O, Nishi K, Mano C, Ichihara M, Honda T. Controlling the capsular shape in lens refilling. *Arch Ophthalmol*. 1997;115:507-51.
10. Cumming, JS, Slade SG, Chayet A. Clinical evaluation of the model AT-45 silicone accommodating intraocular lens: results of feasibility and the initial phase of the food and drug administration clinical trial. *Ophthalmology*. 2001;108:200-209.
11. Glasser A, Kaufman PL. The mechanism of accommodation in primates. Presented at the ESCRS Congress; Sept 2001; Amsterdam.
12. Southall JPC, trans. *Helmholtz's Treatise on Physiological Optics*. 3rd ed. New York: Dover Publications; 1962.
13. Strenk SA, Semmlow JL, Strenk LM, Munoz P, Gronlund-Jacob J, DeMarco JK. Age-related changes in human ciliary muscle and lens: a magnetic resonance imaging study. *Invest Ophthalmol Vis Sci*. 1999;40:1162-1169.
14. Medner A, ed. *HumanOptics Scientific Newsletter*. 2001;1:1-4.
15. HumanOptics Corp. Personal communication; Nov 2001.
16. Küchle M, Gusek GC, Langenbucher A, Seitz B. First and preliminary results of a new posterior chamber intraocular lens. Available at: http://www.onjoph.com/global/artikel/pciol-body.html. Accessed Sept 2000.
17. Küchle M, Langenbucher A, Gusek-Schneider G, Steitz B, Hanna K. First implantation of a new, potentially accommodative posterior chamber intraocular lens. *Klinische Monatsblätter für Augenheilkunde*. 2001;218:603-608.
18. Langenbucher A. Personal communication; Nov 2001.
19. Küchle M. Personal communication; Nov 2001.

BIBLIOGRAPHY

Coleman DJ, Fish SK. Presbyopia, accommodation, and the mature catenary. *Ophthalmology*. 2001;108;1544-1551.
Tamm E, Lütjen-Drecoll E, Jungkunz W, Rohen JW. Posterior attachment of ciliary muscle in young, accommodating old, presbyopic monkeys. *Invest Ophthalmol Vis Sci*. 1992;32:1678-1692.

Chapter 26

Refractive Lens Exchange With a Multifocal Intraocular Lens

*I. Howard Fine, MD; Richard S. Hoffman, MD;
and Mark Packer, MD*

Excimer laser refractive surgery is growing in popularity throughout the world but has its limitations. Patients with extreme degrees of myopia and hyperopia are poor candidates for corneal refractive surgery, and presbyopic patients must rely on reading glasses or monovision in order to obtain the full range of visual function. These limitations in laser refractive surgery have led to a resurgence of intraocular modalities for the correction of refractive errors.

Advances in small-incision cataract surgery have enhanced this procedure from one primarily concerned with the safe removal of the cataractous lens to a procedure refined to yield the best possible postoperative refractive result. As the outcomes of cataract surgery have improved, the use of lens surgery as a refractive modality in patients without cataracts has increased in popularity. The removal of the crystalline lens and replacement with a pseudophakic lens for the purposes of reducing or eliminating refractive errors has been labeled with many titles. These titles include *clear lensectomy,*[1,2] *clear lens phacoemulsification,*[3] *clear lens replacement, clear lens extraction,*[4-12] *clear lens exchange, presbyopic lens exchange,* and *refractive lens exchange.* Since these procedures may be performed in older patients with significant nuclear sclerosis but normal spectacle-corrected visual acuity, the term *clear lens* may not be appropriate to describe lens exchange surgery that many older individuals are undergoing. Similarly, a *clear lens exchange* in a young, highly hyperopic patient may be performed for refractive purposes but not necessarily to address pre-existing presbyopia, thus *presbyopic lens exchange* would not be an appropriate term for this group of patients. The term *refractive lens exchange* appears to best describe the technique of removing the crystalline lens and replacing it with a pseudophakic lens in any aged patient for the purpose of reducing or eliminating refractive errors and/or addressing presbyopia.

MULTIFOCAL LENSES

Perhaps the greatest catalyst for the resurgence of refractive lens exchange has been the development of multifocal lens technology. High hyperopes, presbyopes, and patients with borderline cataracts who have presented for refractive surgery have been ideal candidates for this new technology.

Multifocal intraocular lens (IOL) technology offers patients sub-stantial benefits. The elimination of a presbyopic condition and restoration of normal vision by simulating accommodation greatly enhances the quality of life for most patients. The only multifocal IOL available for general use in the United States is the Array (Allergan Surgical Products, Irvine, Calif). The advantages of astigmatically neutral clear corneal incisions have allowed for increased utilization of multifocal technology in both cataract and refractive lens exchange surgery.

LENS DESIGN

The principle of any multifocal design is to create multiple image points behind the lens. The goal of the Array lens is to enable less reduction in visual acuity for a given amount of defocus by improving the depth of field. The Array is a zonal progressive IOL with five concentric zones on the anterior surface (Figure 1). Zones 1, 3, and 5 are distance-dominant zones, while zones 2 and 4 are near dominant. The lens has an aspherical component, and each zone repeats the entire refractive sequence corresponding to distance, intermediate, and near foci. This results in vision over a range of distances. The lens uses 100% of the incoming available light and is weighted for optimum light distribution. With typical pupil sizes, approximately half of the light is distributed for distance, one-third for near vision, and the remainder for intermediate vision. The lens utilizes continuous surface construction, and consequently there is no loss of light through defraction and no degradation of image quality as a result of surface discontinuities. The lens has a foldable silicone optic that is 6.0 mm in diameter with haptics made of polymethylmethacrylate and a haptic diameter of 13 mm. The lens can be inserted through a clear corneal or scleral tunnel incision that is 2.8 mm wide, utilizing the Unfolder injector system (Allergan Surgical Products).

CLINICAL RESULTS

The efficacy of multifocal technology has been documented in many clinical studies. Early studies of the one-piece Array documented a larger percentage of patients who were able to read J2 print after undergoing multifocal lens implantation compared to patients with monofocal implants.[13,14,15] Similar results have been documented for the foldable Array.[16] Clinical trials comparing mul-

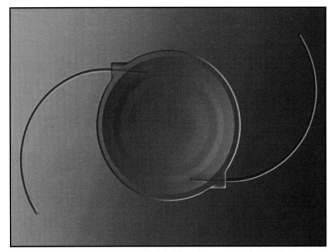

Figure 1. The Array AMO foldable silicone multifocal intraocular lens.

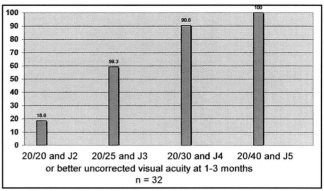

Figure 2. Clinical results of bilateral Array implantation following refractive lens exchange, percentage of patients.

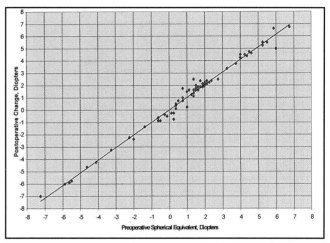

Figure 3. Scattergram demonstrating reduction of spherical equivalent in refractive lens exchange eyes, preoperative spherical equivalent versus postoperative change in spherical equivalent.

tifocal lens implantation compared to monofocal lens implantation in the same patient also revealed improved intermediate and near vision in the multifocal eye compared to the monofocal eye.[17,18]

Many studies have evaluated both the objective and subjective qualities of contrast sensitivity, stereoacuity, glare disability, and photic phenomena following implantation of multifocal IOLs. Refractive multifocal IOLs such as the Array were found to be superior to diffractive multifocal IOLs by demonstrating better contrast sensitivity and less glare disability.[19] The Array does produce a small amount of contrast sensitivity loss equivalent to the loss of one line of visual acuity at the 11% contrast level using Regan contrast sensitivity charts.[14] This loss of contrast sensitivity at low levels is only present when the Array is placed monocularly and has not been demonstrated with bilateral placement and binocular testing.[20] In addition to relatively normal contrast sensitivity, good random-dot stereopsis and less distance and near aniseikonia were present in bilaterally placed patients compared to unilateral implants.[21]

One of the potential drawbacks of the Array lens has been the potential for an appreciation of halos around point sources of light at night in the early weeks and months following surgery.[22] Most patients will learn to disregard these halos with time, and bilateral implantation appears to improve these subjective symptoms. Concerns about the visual function of patients at night have been allayed by a driving simulation study in which bilateral Array multifocal patients performed only slightly worse than patients with bilateral monofocal IOLs. The results indicated no consistent difference in driving performance and safety between the two groups.[23] In a study by Javitt et al, 41% percent of bilateral Array subjects were found to never require spectacles compared to 11.7% of monofocal controls. Overall, subjects with bilateral Array IOLs reported better overall vision, less limitation in visual function, and less use of spectacles than monofocal controls.[24]

A small recent study reviewed the clinical results of bilaterally implanted Array multifocal lens implants in refractive lens exchange patients.[25] A total of 68 eyes were evaluated, comprising 32 bilateral and four unilateral Array implantations. One hundred percent of patients undergoing bilateral refractive lens exchange achieved binocular visual acuity of 20/40 and J5 or better, as measured 1 to 3 months postoperatively. Over 90 percent achieved uncorrected binocular visual acuity of 20/30 and J4 or better, and

nearly 60 percent achieved uncorrected binocular visual acuity of 20/25 and J3 or better (Figure 2). This study included patients with preoperative spherical equivalents between 7 diopters (D) of myopia and 7 D of hyperopia, with the majority of patients having preoperative spherical equivalents between plano and +2.50. Excellent lens power determinations and refractive results were achieved (Figure 3).

PATIENT SELECTION

Specific guidelines with respect to the selection of candidates and surgical strategies that enhance outcomes with this IOL have been developed. Allergan recommends using the Array multifocal IOL for bilateral cataract patients whose surgery is uncomplicated and whose personality is such that they are not likely to fixate on the presence of minor visual aberrations such as halos around lights. There is obviously a broad range of patients who would be acceptable candidates. Relative or absolute contraindications include the presence of ocular pathologies other than cataracts that may degrade image formation or may be associated with less than adequate visual function postoperatively despite visual improvement following surgery. Pre-existing ocular pathologies that are frequently looked upon as contraindications include age-related macular degeneration, uncontrolled diabetes or diabetic retinopathy, uncontrolled glaucoma, recurrent inflammatory eye disease, retinal detachment risk, and corneal disease or previous refractive surgery in the form of radial keratotomy (RK), photorefractive keratectomy (PRK), or laser-assisted in situ keratomileusis (LASIK). However, a recent study has revealed comparable distance acuity outcomes in Array and monofocal patients with concurrent eye disease such as macular degeneration, glaucoma, and diabetic retinopathy.[26]

Utilization of these lenses in patients who complain excessively, are highly introspective, or fussy should be avoided. In addition, conservative use of this lens is recommended when evaluating patients with occupations that include frequent night driving and occupations that put high demands on vision and near work such as engineers and architects. Such patients need to demonstrate a strong desire for relative spectacle independence in order to be considered for a refractive lens exchange with Array implantation.

In our practice, patient selection has been reduced to a very rapid process. Once someone has been determined to be a candidate for refractive lens exchange, the patient is asked two questions. The first question is, "If an implant could be placed in your eye that would allow you to see both distance and near without glasses under most circumstances, would that be an advantage?" Patients are then asked, "If the lens is associated with halos around lights at night, would it still be an advantage?" If they do not think they would be bothered by these symptoms, they can receive a multifocal IOL. If concern over halos or night driving is strong, then these patients may receive monofocal lenses with appropriate informed consent regarding loss of accommodation and the need for reading glasses, or consideration of a different refractive surgical procedure.

Prior to implanting an Array, all candidates should be informed of the lens' statistics to ensure that they understand that spectacle independence is not guaranteed. Approximately 41% of the patients implanted with bilateral Array IOLs will never need to wear glasses, 50% wear glasses on a limited basis such as driving at night or during prolonged reading, 12% will always need to wear glasses for near work, and approximately 8% will need to wear spectacles on a full-time basis for distance and near correction.[23] In addition, 15% of patients were found to have difficulty with halos at night and 11% had difficulty with glare compared to 6% and 1% respectively in monofocal patients.

Finally, the patient's axial length and risk for retinal detachment or other retinal complications should be considered. Although there have been many publications documenting a low rate of complications in highly myopic clear lens extractions,[1,3,8-10] others have warned of significant long-term risks of retinal complications despite prophylactic treatment.[27,28] With this in mind, other phakic refractive modalities should be considered in extremely high myopes. If refractive lens exchange is performed in these patients, extensive informed consent regarding the long-term risks for retinal complications should naturally occur preoperatively.

PREOPERATIVE MEASUREMENTS

The most important assessment for successful multifocal lens use, other then patient selection, involves precise preoperative measurements of axial length in addition to accurate lens power calculations. There are some practitioners who feel that immersion biometry is necessary for accurate axial length determination. However, applanation techniques in combination with the Holladay 2 formula yield accurate and consistent results with greater patient convenience and less technician time. A newer device that is now available, the Zeiss IOL Master, is a combined biometry instrument for noncontact optical measurements of axial length, corneal curvature, and anterior chamber depth that yields extremely accurate and efficient measurements with minimal patient inconvenience. The axial length measurement is based on an interference-optical method termed *partial coherence interferometry*, and measurements are claimed to be compatible with acoustic immersion measurements and accurate to within 30 microns. The Quantel Axis II immersion biometry unit is also a convenient and accurate device for axial length measurements. The device yields quick and precise axial length measurements using immersion biometry without requiring the patient to be placed in the supine position. Regardless of the technique being used to measure axial length, it is important that the surgeon use biometry that he or she feels yields the most consistent and accurate results.

When determining lens power calculations, the Holladay 2 formula takes into account disparities in anterior segment and axial lengths by adding the white-to-white corneal diameter and lens thickness into the formula. Addition of these variables helps predict the exact position of the IOL in the eye and has improved refractive predictability. The SRK T and the SRK II formulas can be used as a final check in the lens power assessment; and for eyes with less than 22 mm in axial length, the Hoffer Q formula should be utilized for comparative purposes.

SURGICAL TECHNIQUE

The multifocal Array works best when the final postoperative refraction has less than 1 D of astigmatism. Therefore, it is very important that incision construction be appropriate with respect to size and location. A clear corneal incision at the temporal periphery that is 3 mm or less in width and 2 mm long is highly recommended.[29] Each surgeon should be aware of his or her usual amount of surgically induced astigmatism by vector analysis. The surgeon must also be able to utilize one of the many modalities for addressing preoperative astigmatism. Although both T and arcuate keratotomies at the 7 mm optical zone can be utilized, there is an increasing trend favoring limbal relaxing incisions for the reduction or elimination of pre-existing astigmatism.[30,31]

In preparation for phacoemulsification, the capsulorrhexis must be round in shape and sized so that there is a small margin of anterior capsule overlapping the optic circumferentially (Figure 4). This is important in order to guarantee in-the-bag placement of the IOL and prevent anterior/posterior alterations in location that would affect the final refractive status. Hydrodelineation and cortical cleaving hydrodissection are very important in all patients because they facilitate lens disassembly and complete cortical clean-up.[32] Complete and fastidious cortical clean-up will hopefully reduce the incidence of posterior capsule opacification whose presence, even in very small amounts, will inordinately degrade the visual acuity in Array patients. It is because of this phenomenon that patients implanted with Array lenses will require YAG laser posterior capsulotomies earlier than patients implanted with monofocal IOLs.

Minimally invasive surgery is very important. Techniques that produce effective phacoemulsification times of less than 20 seconds and average phacoemulsification powers of 10% or less are highly advantageous and can best be achieved with power modulations (burst mode or two pulses per second) rather than continuous phacoemulsification modes.[33,34] The Array is inserted easiest by means of the Unfolder injector system. Complete removal of all viscoelastic from the anterior chamber and behind the lens will reduce the incidence of postoperative pressure spikes and myopic shift from capsular block syndrome.

COMPLICATIONS MANAGEMENT

When intraoperative complications develop, they must be handled precisely and appropriately. In situations in which the first eye has already had an Array implanted, complications management must be directed toward finding any possible way of implanting an Array in the second eye. Under most circumstances, capsule rupture will still allow for implantation of an Array as long as there is an intact capsulorrhexis. Under these circumstances, the lens haptics are implanted in the sulcus, and the optic is prolapsed posteriorly through the anterior capsulorrhexis. This is facilitated by a capsulorrhexis that is slightly smaller than the diameter of the optic in order to capture the optic in essentially an in-the-bag location. If full sulcus implantation is utilized, then appropriate change in the IOL power will need to be made in order to compensate for the more anterior location of the IOL within the eye. When vitreous loss occurs, a meticulous vitrectomy with clearing of all vitreous strands must be performed.

It is important to avoid iris trauma since the pupil size and shape may impact the visual function of a multifocal IOL postoperatively. If the pupil is less than 2.5 mm, there may be an impairment of near visual acuity due to the location of the rings serving near visual acuity. For patients with small postoperative pupil diameters affecting near vision, a mydriatic pupilloplasty can be successfully performed with an argon laser.[35] Enlargement of the pupil will expose the near dominant rings of the multifocal IOL and restore near vision in most patients.

TARGETING EMMETROPIA

The most important skill to master in the refractive lens exchange patient is the ultimate achievement of emmetropia. Emmetropia can be achieved successfully with accurate IOL power calculations and adjunctive modalities for eliminating astigmatism. With the trend toward smaller astigmatically neutral clear corneal incisions, it is now possible to more accurately address pre-existing astigmatism at the time of lens surgery. The popularization of limbal relaxing incisions by Gills and Nichamin[30,31] has added a useful means of reducing up to 3.50 D of pre-existing astigmatism by placing paired 600 micron-deep incisions at the limbus in the steep meridian. When against-the-rule astigmatism is present, the temporal groove of the paired limbal relaxing incisions can be utilized as the site of entry for the clear corneal incision. This is a simple and practical approach for reducing pre-existing astigmatism at the time of surgery, and since the coupling of these incisions is one to one, no alteration in the calculated lens power is needed.

REFRACTIVE SURPRISE

On occasion, surgeons may be presented with an unexpected refractive surprise following surgery. These miscalculations in lens power can be disappointing to both the surgeon and patient but,

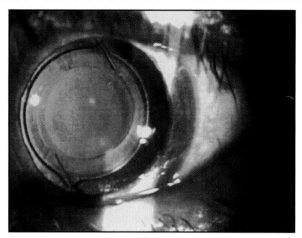

Figure 4. The Array multifocal intraocular lens in situ. Note the capsulorrhexis overlapping the edge of the lens optic.

happily, the means for correcting these refractive errors are increasing. When there is a gross error in the inserted lens, the best approach is to perform a lens exchange as soon as possible. When smaller errors are encountered or lens exchange is felt to be unsafe, various adjunctive procedures are available to address these refractive surprises.

One of the simplest techniques to address residual myopia following surgery is a two-, three-, or four-cut RK with a large optical zone. RK is still a relatively safe procedure with little likelihood for significant hyperopic shift with conservative incision and optical zone placement. When residual hyperopia is present following cataract surgery, holmium:YAG laser thermal keratoplasty (LTK, Sunrise Technologies) is an option for reducing hyperopia and appears to work best in older patients and those with 1 to 2 D of refractive error. Another option for reducing 0.5 to 1.0 D of hyperopia involves rotating the IOL out of the capsular bag and placing it in the ciliary sulcus to increase the functional power of the lens. LASIK can also be performed to eliminate myopia, hyperopia, or astigmatism following surgery complicated by unexpected refractive results.

An interesting and simple intraocular approach to the postoperative refractive surprise involves the use of IOLs placed in the sulcus over the primary IOL in a piggyback fashion. Staar Surgical now produces the AQ5010V foldable silicone IOL that is useful for sulcus placement as a secondary piggyback lens. The Staar AQ5010V has an overall length of 14.0 mm and is available in powers between –4.0 to +4.0 D in whole diopter powers. In smaller eyes with larger hyperopic postoperative errors, the Staar AQ2010V is 13.5 mm in overall length and is available in powers between +5.0 to +9.0 D in whole diopter steps. This approach is especially useful when expensive refractive lasers are not available or when corneal surgery is not feasible.

POSTOPERATIVE COURSE

If glasses are required after surgery in a patient implanted with a multifocal IOL, the spherical correction should be determined by over-plusing the patient to a slight blur and gradually reducing the power until the best acuity is reached. Patients are able to focus through the near portions of their IOL, thus it is possible to over-minus a patient if care is not taken to push the plus power. When using this defocusing technique, it is critical to stop as soon as distance acuity is maximized to avoid over-minusing the patient. The cylinder power should be the smallest amount that provides the best acuity. If add power is necessary, the full add power for the required working distance should be prescribed.

If patients are unduly bothered by photic phenomena such as halos and glare, these symptoms can be alleviated by various techniques. Weak pilocarpine at a concentration of 0.125% or weaker will constrict the pupil to a diameter that will usually lessen the severity of halos without significantly affecting near visual acuity. Similarly, brimonidine tartrate ophthalmic solution 0.2% (Alphagan, Allergan) has been shown to reduce pupil size under scotopic conditions[36] and can also be administered in an attempt to reduce halo and glare symptoms. Another approach involves the use of over-minused spectacles in order to push the secondary focal point behind the retina and thus lessen the effect of image blur from multiple images in front of the retina. Polarized lenses have also been found to be helpful in reducing photic phenomena. Perhaps the most important technique is the implantation of bilateral Array lenses as close in time as possible in order to allow patients the ability to use the lenses together, which appears to allow for improved binocular distance and near vision compared to monocular acuity. Finally, most patients report that halos improve or disappear with the passage of several weeks to months.

FINAL COMMENTS

Thanks to the successes of the excimer laser, refractive surgery is increasing in popularity throughout the world. Corneal refractive surgery, however, has its limitations. Patients with severe degrees of myopia and hyperopia are poor candidates for excimer laser surgery, and presbyopes must contend with reading glasses or monovision to address their near visual needs. The rapid recovery and astigmatically neutral incisions currently being used for modern cataract surgery have allowed this procedure to be used with greater predictability for refractive lens exchanges in patients who are otherwise not suffering from visually significant cataracts. The increased accuracy and safety of small-incision cataract surgery is now creating an incentive for borderline cataract patients to opt for surgery sooner than later in order to reap the refractive benefits of relative spectacle independence. Many of these patients are more than willing to pay for refractive lens exchanges rather than wait for their cataracts to become visually significant to a level where private insurance or government insurance will cover the costs.

As this procedure becomes more popular, it will create a win-win situation for all involved. First, patients can enjoy a predictable refractive procedure with rapid recovery that can address all types and severities of refractive errors in addition to addressing presbyopia with multifocal or accommodative lens technology. Second, surgeons can offer these procedures without the intrusion of private or government insurance and establish a less disruptive relationship with their patients. Finally, government can enjoy the decreased financial burden from the expenses of cataract surgery for the ever-increasing ranks of aging baby-boomers, as more and more of these patients opt for lens exchanges to address their refractive surgery goals, ultimately reaching Medicare coverage as pseudophakes.

Successful integration of refractive lens exchanges into the general ophthalmologist's practice is fairly straightforward since most surgeons are currently performing small-incision cataract surgery for their cataract patients. Essentially, the same procedure is performed for a refractive lens exchange differing only in removal of a relatively clear crystalline lens and simple adjunctive techniques for reducing corneal astigmatism. Although any style of foldable IOL can be used for lens exchanges, multifocal IOLs currently offer the best option for addressing both the elimination of refractive errors and presbyopia. Refractive lens exchange with multifocal lens technology is not for every patient considering refractive surgery but does offer substantial benefits especially in high hyperopes, presbyopes, and patients with borderline or soon to be clinically significant cataracts who are requesting refractive surgery. Appropriate patient screening, accurate biometry and lens power calculations, and meticulous surgical technique will allow surgeons to maximize their success with this procedure.

REFERENCES

1. Colin J, Robinet A. Clear lensectomy and implantation of low-power posterior chamber intraocular lens for the correction of high myopia. *Ophthalmology.* 1994;101:107-112.
2. Siganos DS, Pallikaris IG. Clear lensectomy and intraocular lens implantation for hyperopia from +7 to +14 diopters. *J Refract Surg.* 1998;14:105-113.
3. Pucci V, Morselli S, Romanelli F, et al. Clear lens phacoemulsification for correction of high myopia. *J Cataract Refract Surg.* 2001;27:896-900.
4. Ge J, Arellano A, Salz J. Surgical correction of hyperopia: clear lens extraction and laser correction. *Ophthalmology Clinics of North America.* 2001;14:301-13.
5. Fine IH, Hoffman RS, Packer P. Clear-lens extraction with multifocal lens implantation. *Int Ophthalmol Clin.* 2001;41:113-121.
6. Pop M, Payette Y, Amyot M. Clear lens extraction with intraocular lens followed by photorefractive keratectomy or laser in situ keratomileusis. *Ophthalmology.* 2000;107:1776-1781.
7. Kolahdouz-Isfahani AH, Rostamian K, Wallace D, Salz JJ. Clear lens extraction with intraocular lens implantation for hyperopia. *J Refract Surg.* 1999;15:316-323.
8. Jimenez-Alfaro I, Miguelez S, Bueno JL, Puy P. Clear lens extraction and implantation of negative-power posterior chamber intraocular lenses to correct extreme myopia. *J Cataract Refract Surg.* 1998;24:1310-1316.
9. Lyle WA, Jin GJ. Clear lens extraction to correct hyperopia. *J Cataract Refract Surg.* 1997;23:1051-1056.
10. Lee KH, Lee JH. Long-term results of clear lens extraction for severe myopia. *J Cataract Refract Surg.* 1996;22:1411-1415.
11. Gris O, Guell JL, Manero F, Muller A. Clear lens extraction to correct high myopia. *J Cataract Refract Surg.* 1996;22:686-689.
12. Lyle WA, Jin GJ. Clear lens extraction for the correction of high refractive error. *J Cataract Refract Surg.* 1994;20:273-276.
13. Percival SPB, Setty SS. Prospectively randomized trial comparing the pseudoaccommodation of the AMO Array multifocal lens and a monofocal lens. *J Cataract Refract Surg.* 1993;19:26-31.
14. Steinert RF, Post CT, Brint SF, et al. A progressive, randomized, double-masked comparison of a zonal-progressive multifocal intraocular lens and a monofocal intraocular lens. *Ophthalmology.* 1992;99:853-861.
15. Negishi K, Nagamoto T, Hara E, et al. Clinical evaluation of a five-zone refractive multifocal intraocular lens. *J Cataract Refract Surg.* 1996;22:110-115.
16. Brydon KW, Tokarewicz AC, Nichols BD. AMO Array multifocal lens versus monofocal correction in cataract surgery. *J Cataract Refract Surg.* 2000;26:96-100.
17. Vaquero-Ruano M, Encinas JL, Millan I, et al. AMO Array multifocal versus monofocal intraocular lenses: long-term follow-up. *J Cataract Refract Surg.* 1998;24:118-123.
18. Steinert RF, Aker BL, Trentacost DJ, et al. A prospective study of the AMO Array zonal-progressive multifocal silicone intraocular lens and a monofocal intraocular lens. *Ophthalmology.* 1999;106:1243-1255.

19. Pieh S, Weghaupt H, Skorpik C. Contrast sensitivity and glare disability with diffractive and refractive multifocal intraocular lenses. *J Cataract Refract Surg.* 1998;24:659-662.

20. Arens B, Freudenthaler N, Quentin CD. Binocular function after bilateral implantation of monofocal and refractive multifocal intraocular lenses. *J Cataract Refract Surg.* 1999;25:399-404.

21. Haring G, Gronemeyer A, Hedderich J, de Decker W. Stereoacuity and aniseikonia after unilateral and bilateral implantation of the Array refractive multifocal intraocular lens. *J Cataract Refract Surg.* 1999;25:1151-1156.

22. Dick HB, Krummenauer F, Schwenn O, et al. Objective and subjective evaluation of photic phenomena after monofocal and multifocal intraocular lens implantation. *Ophthalmology.* 1999;106:1878-1886.

23. Featherstone KA, Bloomfield JR, Lang AJ, et al. Driving simulation study: bilateral Array multifocal versus bilateral AMO monofocal intraocular lenses. *J Cataract Refract Surg.* 1999;25:1254-1262.

24. Javitt JC, Wang F, Trentacost DJ, et al. Outcomes of cataract extraction with multifocal intraocular lens implantation—functional status and quality of life. *Ophthalmology.* 1997;104:589-599.

25. Packer M, Fine IH, Hoffman RS. Refractive lens exchange with the Array multifocal lens. *J Cataract Refract Surg.* In press.

26. Kamath GG, Prasas S, Danson A, Phillips RP. Visual outcome with the Array multifocal intraocular lens in patients with concurrent eye disease. *J Cataract Refract Surg.* 2000;26:576-581.

27. Rodriguez A, Gutierrez E, Alvira G. Complications of clear lens extraction in axial myopia. *Arch Ophthalmol.* 1987;105:1522-1523.

28. Ripandelli G, Billi B, Fedeli R, Stirpe M. Retinal detachment after clear lens extraction in 41 eyes with axial myopia. *Retina.* 1996;16:3-6.

29. Fine IH. Corneal tunnel incision with a temporal approach. In: Fine IH, Fichman RA, Grabow HB, eds. *Clear-Corneal Cataract Surgery and Topical Anesthesia.* Thorofare, NJ: SLACK Incorporated; 1993:5-26.

30. Gills JP, Gayton JL. Reducing pre-existing astigmatism. In: Gills JP, ed. *Cataract Surgery: The State of the Art.* Thorofare, NJ: SLACK Incorporated; 1998: 53-66.

31. Nichamin L. Refining astigmatic keratotomy during cataract surgery. *Ocular Surgery News.* 1993;April 15.

32. Fine IH. Cortical cleaving hydrodissection. *J Cataract Refract Surg.* 1992;18:508-512.

33. Fine IH. The choo-choo chop and flip phacoemulsification technique. *Operative Techniques in Cataract and Refractive Surgery.* 1998;1(2):61-65.

34. Fine IH, Packer M, Hoffman RS. The use of power modulations in phacoemulsification: choo choo chop and flip phacoemulsification. *J Cataract Refract Surg.* 2001;27:188-197.

35. Thomas JV. Pupilloplasty and photomydriasis. In: Belcher CD, Thomas JV, Simmons RJ, eds. *Photocoagulation in Glaucoma and Anterior Segment Disease.* Baltimore, Md: Williams & Wilkins; 1984:150-157.

36. McDonald JE, El-Moatassem Kotb AM, Decker BB. Effect of brimonidine tartrate ophthalmic solution 0.2% on pupil size in normal eyes under different luminance conditions. *J Cataract Refract Surg.* 2001; 27:560-564.

Chapter 27

Presbyopic Phakic Intraocular Lenses

Georges F. Baikoff, MD

EVOLUTION OF THE CONCEPT OF IMPLANTS

Since 1987, we have witnessed the development of angle-supported or iris-supported anterior chamber implants. These implants were one piece made entirely of polymethylmethacrylate (PMMA). More recently, posterior chamber implants made of soft material have appeared. It is clear today that the advantages of angle-supported implants such as the Nuvita type are numerous: facility of insertion, excellent tolerance, absence of endothelial damage, absence of cataracts, no inflammatory response. However, they can induce some pupillary ovalization, especially if the implants are oversized, and they have to be inserted through a 5.5 to 6 mm incision, which can be a source of astigmatism. There is a regular rise in the number of induced cataracts related to the use of posterior chamber phakic intraocular lenses (IOLs) (10% to 20%). In time and depending on the age of the subjects, cataracts are more often observed. On the other hand, posterior chamber implants have the advantage of being able to be inserted through a small self-sealing incision that heals rapidly and does not induce astigmatism.

ANGLE SUPPORT

It is time to develop an angle-supported anterior chamber implant combining the advantages of the two techniques (Figure 1). This is how the GBR/Vivarte (Ciba Vision, Duluth, Ga) implant was born—the first foldable angle-supported implant capable of being inserted through a small 3.2-mm self-sealing incision. The haptics are in PMMA, the three foot plates in hydrophilic acrylic, and an optic diameter of 5.5 mm in hydrophilic acrylic. The optical part is bifocal. The central part favors distant vision, and an intermediate rim (+2.5 diopters [D] addition) gives the near vision (Figures 2 and 3).

SIZING THE INTERNAL DIAMETER OF THE ANTERIOR CHAMBER

The second problem to be solved is the adaptation of the lens to the anterior segment. In fact, in order to avoid pupillary ovalization, it is essential to choose the most suitable lens for the anterior segment. Two systems are under study: a plastic sizer used preoperatively and an optical digital sizer used preoperatively to measure the internal diameter of the anterior chamber. The optical digital sizer is still at the development stage, but we believe that it will be available in the very near future and be extremely precise. Nevertheless, it is essential to check the diameter of the implant to be used at the beginning of surgery by inserting the plastic sizer into the anterior chamber. Beforehand, the center of the cornea is marked with the same type of marker used for radial keratotomy (RK), and the plastic sizer is inserted into the anterior chamber. The projection of the cornea center onto the plastic sizer is observed through the microscope, and in this way we know the diameter of the anterior chamber. Currently, implants are available in 0.5-mm diameter graduations. If there is a doubt, it is preferable to use a slightly smaller implant rather than a slightly larger one. A slightly smaller implant can rotate in the anterior chamber without causing endothelial damage, whereas an implant that is too large will put tension on the iris root and be the cause of pupillary ovalization.

Other techniques for measuring the internal diameter of the anterior segment are being tested. They are the wide-angled ultrasound biomicroscope (UBM) and ocular coherence tomography (OCT). The precision of these two techniques should be in the region of about 10 microns. These optical and ultrasonographic techniques should allow us to preoperatively measure the internal diameter of the anterior segment in a very precise way and, therefore, only order one implant per eye.

FOLDING AND UNFOLDING

The third point to be developed is the folding system that allows the implant to open up inside the anterior chamber parallel to the iris. Today, two types of folders exist, allowing the implant to be folded into three parts (N folding) or into four parts (M folding). A precise protocol must be followed in order to ensure that they are securely inserted into the anterior chamber.

SURGICAL TECHNIQUE

Anesthesia can be general, local-regional, or topical. A 3.2 mm self-sealing corneoscleral incision is made with a routine precalibrated phako knife. One or two side ports can be made to facilitate manipulations in the anterior chamber. Immediately after having made the incision, viscoelastic is injected into the anterior chamber

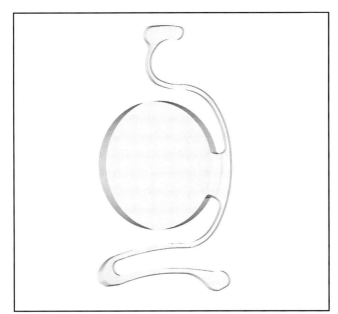

Figure 1. The GBR implant.

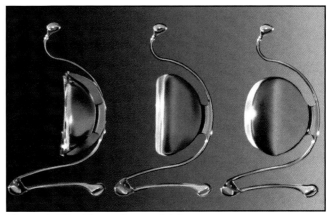

Figure 2. The Vivarte lens unfolding.

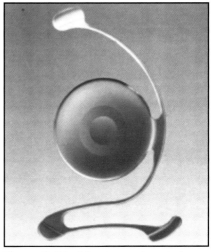

Figure 3. The Vivarte presbyopic lens.

to increase the pressure and obtain an anterior chamber as deep as possible. The implant is folded in the N or M folder, then held with the holding forceps and inserted into the anterior chamber. The foot plates of the leading haptic are inserted first beginning with the knee. The optic is then inserted through a 3.2-mm incision, and once it is completely inserted in the anterior chamber the forceps are opened slightly to enable the implant to open up slowly. The implant unfolds like an accordion, parallel to the iris plane. Risk of endothelial contact is almost zero. The trailing haptic is inserted into the anterior chamber, and the foot plate is placed in the angle with a Leister hook. The viscous is evacuated; it is important to check that the incision is watertight, then the operation is over (Figures 4 to 11).

Standard postoperative treatment includes steroids and antibiotic eye drops for 1 month.

RESULTS

Eight eyes received refractive presbyopic implants.[1,2] All patients were emmetropic before the operation and needed an addition of + 2.50 D in order to read J1. They were approximately 55 years of age, without astigmatism. Follow-up was between 1 month and 2 years. Two patients were immediately explanted because the lenses were oversized. They recuperated to their initial acuity. Out of the six other patients, five recuperated 20/20 without correction after surgery; one recuperated 20/25. All the patients read J1 without correction. Apart from early postoperative hypertonia due to the viscous, ocular tension was normal long-term and no complications were observed with the anterior segment (Figures 12 and 13).

EVOLUTION OF OPTICAL PRINCIPLES

We have seen that refractive implants are capable of correcting myopia, hypermyopia, and astigmatism in certain cases. It is perfectly clear today that the new ophthalmological frontier lies with the surgical correction of presbyopia. The GBR/Vivarte presbyopic implant is the first refractive implant in the world destined to correct presbyopia. It consists of a bifocal lens favoring distance vision in the center with an intermediary optical zone for near vision. Today the lens is available with an addition of +2.50 D that will enable compensation of emmetropic patients between 50 and 60 years old.

The first results showed that in 80% of the cases, the patients maintained their far visual acuity, and in near visual acuity they were able to read J1 or Parinaud 2 without correction. In the future, it will be possible to correct ametropias from −3 to +3 D.

Important: This implant is intended to correct presbyopia in emmetropic patients without astigmatism. The existence of preoperative astigmatism would greatly jeopardize the results.

One can imagine that the future of optical evolution lies in a wider range of corrections, refractive and diffractive systems, as well as multifocal systems. One can also imagine being able to correct presbyopic patients who have been previously treated for ametropia by laser-assisted in situ keratomileusis (LASIK) or photorefractive keratectomy (PRK).

However, it is important that this type of surgery be used only if the angle is open and the anterior chamber depth is equal to or over 3 mm.

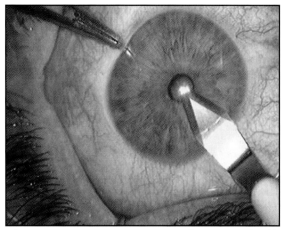

Figure 4. GBR surgery: 3.2 mm clear corneal self-sealing incision.

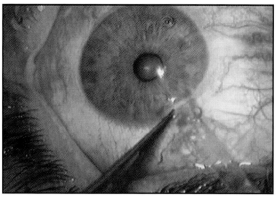

Figure 5. GBR surgery: Introduction of the plastic sizer to evaluate the internal diameter of the anterior chamber.

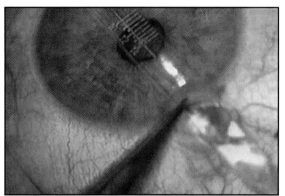

Figure 6. GBR surgery: Introduction of the plastic sizer to evaluate the internal diameter of the anterior chamber.

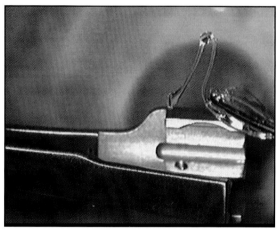

Figure 7. GBR surgery: The folding process.

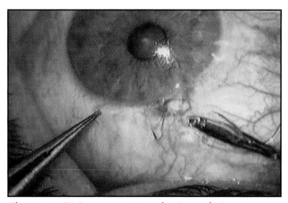

Figure 8. GBR surgery: Introduction of Vivarte.

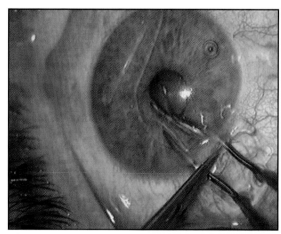

Figure 9. GBR surgery: Unfolding of the lens.

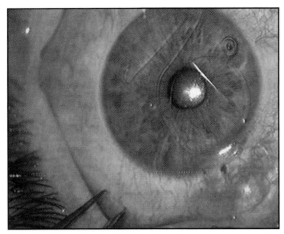

Figure 10. GBR surgery: No iridectomy is needed.

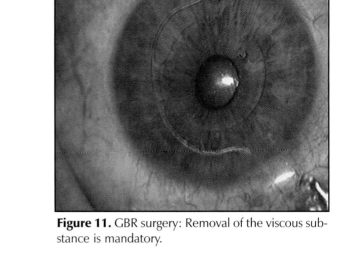

Figure 11. GBR surgery: Removal of the viscous substance is mandatory.

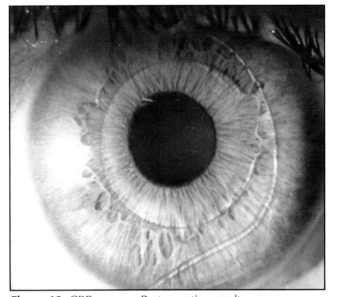

Figure 12. GBR surgery: Postoperative results.

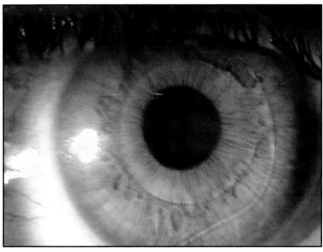

Figure 13. GBR surgery: Postoperative results.

CONCLUSION

Supraciliary segments have been proven effective to a certain degree but will have to be better defined in the future. Their effect is not permanent, and when faced with the extrusion of certain segments, a significant regression in presbyopia correction has been observed.

The theoretical advantage of these segments lies in the fact that they can be removed—even exchanged—should one desire. In the case of extrusion, it was noted that the eyes more or less returned to their initial state. Finally, as there is no creation of a multifocal system on the crystalline lens, the patients did not suffer from side effects after surgery. The segments should therefore be well-tolerated in dim light with no effect on contrast sensitivity.

Presbyopic phakic implants have the advantage of being effective. Their effectiveness depends on the additional optical power of the intermediary zone of the lens, which can be easily determined or controlled. As long as the lens is well-tolerated in the anterior segment, its effect is permanent; but the lens can be removed or exchanged in the case of adverse reaction. The lens can also be removed through a small incision should the patient develop a cataract and require surgery.

In the future, it is possible to imagine that these lenses could be constantly adapted to the patient during his or her life, that the patient could exchange the lens for better optical quality implants as well as multifocal, diffractive, or other types of implants. Today, lenses have the disadvantage of creating side effects due to the concentric optical lens. Patients suffer from halos in dim light, but this is generally well-tolerated. Halos must not be considered a serious phenomenon because patients prefer the discomfort due to halos rather than the discomfort due to presbyopia. As far as patients are concerned, the small side effect of the implant in night vision is the least of their worries.

REFERENCES

1. Volkva PE. University Hospital, BRNO, Czech Republic.
2. Clinique Monticelle, Marseille, France.

Index

Build Your Library

Along with this title, we publish numerous products on a variety of topics. We are sure that you will find the below titles to be an essential addition to your library. Order your copies today or contact us for a copy of our latest catalog for additional product information.

CUSTOMIZED CORNEAL ABLATION: THE QUEST FOR SUPERVISION

Scott MacRae, MD; Ronald Krueger, MD; and Raymond A. Applegate, OD, PhD

416 pp., Hard Cover, 2001, ISBN 1-55642-488-4, Order #64884, $215.00

This book presents most of the new technologies available to achieve customized corneal ablation. It will teach you how to combine these technologies with your current techniques and then move beyond standard LASIK into the world of "SuperVision." Astronomy, mathematics, basic science, and optics have joined ophthalmology in the quest for SuperVision, where 20/20 is no longer the standard of excellence. For the first time this information is available in one complete source. This book covers many of the exciting alternatives that now exist, allowing you to choose the options that will enhance your patients' vision.

PRESBYOPIA: A SURGICAL TEXTBOOK

Amar Agarwal, MS, FRCS, FRCOphth

448 pp., Hard Cover, 2002, ISBN 1-55642-577-5, Order #65775, $110.00

This dynamic book not only presents the concepts necessary to understand presbyopia, but also offers the surgical possibilities for treating the condition. It covers the scleral, corneal, and lenticular modifications to treat presbyopia, dissects each technique, and explains how to manage complications of each technique. The most recent treatments, cataract or clear lens surgery, as well as the no-anesthesia procedure, are discussed in full detail. It is the ideal resource for ophthalmologists who currently perform presbyopic treatment as well as those who desire to move into it.

THE LITTLE EYE BOOK: A PUPIL'S GUIDE TO UNDERSTANDING OPHTHALMOLOGY

Janice K. Ledford, COMT and Roberto Pineda, MD

160 pp., Soft Cover, 2002, ISBN 1-55642-560-0, Order #65600, $14.95

The Little Eye Book: A Pupil's Guide to Understanding Ophthalmology is an easy-to-understand introduction to the field of eye care. This book is written with the non-physician in mind, so you won't be bogged down with heavy details, yet every basic fact that you need is right here. With photographs as well as drawings and helpful tables and charts, this conversational-style text packs a big punch. Perfect for anyone who works in the eye care industry or with patients, but isn't an ophthalmologist.

Contact us at

SLACK Incorporated, Professional Book Division
6900 Grove Road, Thorofare, NJ 08086
1-800-257-8290/1-856-848-1000, Fax: 1-856-853-5991
E-Mail: orders@slackinc.com or www.slackbooks.com

ORDER FORM

QUANTITY	TITLE	ORDER #	PRICE
	Customized Corneal Ablation	64884	$215.00
	The Little Eye Book	65600	$14.95
	Presbyopia: A Surgical Textbook	65775	$110.00
	Subtotal		$
	Applicable state and local tax will be added to your purchase		$
	Handling		$4.50
	Total		$

Name: _____

Address: _____

City: _____ State: _____ Zip: _____

Phone: _____ Fax: _____

Email: _____

• Check enclosed (Payable to SLACK Incorporated)_____

• Charge my: _____ _____ _____

Account #: _____

Exp. date: _____ Signature: _____

NOTE: *Prices are subject to change without notice.*
Shipping charges will apply.
Shipping and handling charges are Non-Returnable.

CODE: 328